The International Library of Bioethics

Founding Editors

David N. Weisstub
Thomasine Kimbrough Kushner

Volume 95

Series Editor

Dennis R. Cooley, North Dakota State University, History, Philosophy, & Religious Studies, Fargo, ND, USA

Advisory Editor

David N. Weisstub, Faculty of Medicine, University of Montreal, Montréal, QC, Canada

Editorial Board

Terry Carney, Faculty of Law Building, University of Sydney, Sydney, Australia

Marcus Düwell, Philosophy Faculty of Humanities, Universiteit Utrecht, Utrecht, Utrecht, The Netherlands

Søren Holm, Centre for Social Ethics and Policy, The University of Manchester, Manchester, UK

Gerrit Kimsma, Radboud UMC, Nijmegen, Gelderland, The Netherlands

Daniel P. Sulmasy, Edmund D. Pellegrino Center for Clinical, Washington, DC, USA

David Augustin Hodge, National Center for Bioethics, Tuskegee University, Tuskegee Institute, AL, USA

Nora L. Jones, Center for Urban Bioethics, Temple University, Philadelphia, USA

The *International Library of Bioethics* – formerly known as the International Library of Ethics, Law and the New Medicine comprises volumes with an international and interdisciplinary focus on foundational and applied issues in bioethics. With this renewal of a successful series we aim to meet the challenge of our time: how to direct biotechnology to human and other living things' ends, how to deal with changed values in the areas of religion, society, and culture, and how to formulate a new way of thinking, a new bioethics.

The *International Library of Bioethics* focuses on the role of bioethics against the background of increasing globalization and interdependency of the world's cultures and governments, with mutual influencing occurring throughout the world in all fields. The series will continue to focus on perennial issues of aging, mental health, preventive medicine, medical research issues, end of life, biolaw, and other areas of bioethics, whilst expanding into other current and future topics.

We welcome book proposals representing the broad interest of this series' interdisciplinary and international focus. We especially encourage proposals addressing aspects of changes in biological and medical research and clinical health care, health policy, medical and biotechnology, and other applied ethical areas involving living things, with an emphasis on those interventions and alterations that force us to re-examine foundational issues.

More information about this series at https://link.springer.com/bookseries/16538

Michael Boylan
Editor

Ethical Public Health Policy Within Pandemics

Theory and Practice in Ethical Pandemic Administration

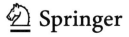

Editor
Michael Boylan
Department of Philosophy
Marymount University
Arlington, VA, USA

ISSN 2662-9186 ISSN 2662-9194 (electronic)
The International Library of Bioethics
ISBN 978-3-030-99691-8 ISBN 978-3-030-99692-5 (eBook)
https://doi.org/10.1007/978-3-030-99692-5

© The Editor(s) (if applicable) and The Author(s), under exclusive license to Springer Nature Switzerland AG 2022, corrected publication 2022
This work is subject to copyright. All rights are solely and exclusively licensed by the Publisher, whether the whole or part of the material is concerned, specifically the rights of translation, reprinting, reuse of illustrations, recitation, broadcasting, reproduction on microfilms or in any other physical way, and transmission or information storage and retrieval, electronic adaptation, computer software, or by similar or dissimilar methodology now known or hereafter developed.
The use of general descriptive names, registered names, trademarks, service marks, etc. in this publication does not imply, even in the absence of a specific statement, that such names are exempt from the relevant protective laws and regulations and therefore free for general use.
The publisher, the authors, and the editors are safe to assume that the advice and information in this book are believed to be true and accurate at the date of publication. Neither the publisher nor the authors or the editors give a warranty, expressed or implied, with respect to the material contained herein or for any errors or omissions that may have been made. The publisher remains neutral with regard to jurisdictional claims in published maps and institutional affiliations.

This Springer imprint is published by the registered company Springer Nature Switzerland AG
The registered company address is: Gewerbestrasse 11, 6330 Cham, Switzerland

*Dedicated to All the Public Health Workers
and
All Medical Personnel
Who have risked their lives
During the COVID-19 Pandemic,
So that others might live*

Preface

This book began as a response to the COVID-19 pandemic in its early stages in March, 2020. At the current time in the summer of 2022, it seems as if the SARS Corona Virus-2 and its variants will be around for a long time. Vaccination seems to be a key to controlling the virus, but getting vaccination rates to 70% and above seems to be difficult to achieve for most countries. This is because (A) poorer countries do not have access to the vaccines or because (B) within wealthier countries there are those who equate vaccination as giving up their individual rights to make their own choices (individualism). This stands in contrast to the community perspective of public health. These factions are at odds with each other and threaten the implementation of effective response to the disease.

Therefore A & B are obstacles in controlling the spread of the disease and limiting the deaths caused therein. This is curious, since with other diseases, vaccination is not so problematic. People regularly agree to and have access to inoculations against childhood diseases, and those for adults—like shingles, tetanus, pneumonia, TB, et al. What makes this disease outbreak different? Time will tell, perhaps. What we do know is that within pandemics certain ethical protocols are necessary to lessen the inequality in civic responses nationally and internationally. This volume seeks to explore some of the more important policy issues that will be necessary to enable an effective and ethically justifiable response to pandemics now and in the future. We hope that these essays spark public debate on these questions so that we might formulate the best possible responses to pandemic public policy going forward.

Arlington, USA   Michael Boylan

Contents

Part I Theoretical Background

1 **Introduction** 3
   Michael Boylan

2 **The Context and Foundations of Ethical Public Health Policy** 13
   Michael Boylan

3 **The Common Good and Individual Rights in Pandemic Times: The Case of Sweden's COVID-19 Strategy** 43
   Per Bauhn

4 **Formal Epistemology Meets a Coronavirus: Rational Decision and the Response to Covid-19** 63
   Sahotra Sarkar

5 **Reevaluating Value in Public Health Policy: Values as Iterative Rational Inquiry** 81
   Peter Tagore Tan

6 **Pandemics and Race** 95
   Takunda Matose and Paul C. Taylor

Part II Public Policy and Administration

7 **Is There a Duty to Treat in a Pandemic?** 119
   Wanda Teays

8 **Principlist Pandemics: On Fraud Ethical Guidelines, and the Importance of Procedural Transparency** 131
   Jonathan Lewis and Udo Schuklenk

9 **Public Tasks During Contagious Disease Pandemics: A Rights-Based Perspective** 149
   Klaus Steigleder and Johannes Graf Keyserlingk

10	**Allocating and Prioritizing Health Care in Times of Scarcity and Abundance** .... Rita Manning	167
11	**Addressing Pandemic Disparities: Equity and Neutral Conceptions of Justice** .... Debra A. DeBruin	195
12	**COVID-19 in Skilled Nursing Homes and Other Long-Term Care Facilities (LTCFs): Could Stronger Public-Health Measures Have Made a Difference?** .... Rosemarie Tong	219
13	**The UN System, COVID-19 Responses, and Building Back Better: Toward an Inclusive, Accessible and Sustainable World** .... Akiko Ito	237

Correction to: Ethical Public Health Policy Within Pandemics C1
Michael Boylan

Index 245

Contributors

Per Bauhn Linnaeus University, Kalmar, Sweden

Michael Boylan Department of Philosophy, Marymount University, Arlington, VA, USA

Debra A. DeBruin Center for Bioethics, University of Minnesota, Minneapolis, MN, USA

Akiko Ito New York, NY, USA

Johannes Graf Keyserlingk Ruhr-Universität Bochum, Bochum, Germany

Jonathan Lewis Centre for Social Ethics and Policy, University of Manchester, Manchester, UK

Rita Manning San Jose State University, San Jose, CA, USA

Takunda Matose Edmond J. Safra Center for Ethics, Harvard University, Cambridge, MA, USA

Sahotra Sarkar University of Texas, Austin, TX, USA

Udo Schuklenk Department of Philosophy, Queen's University, Kingston, ON, Canada

Klaus Steigleder Ruhr-Universität Bochum, Bochum, Germany

Peter Tagore Tan Department of Philosophy, Mount Saint Mary's University, Los Angeles, CA, USA

Paul C. Taylor Department of Philosophy, Vanderbilt University, Nashville, TN, USA

Wanda Teays Mount Saint Mary's University, Los Angeles, CA, USA

Rosemarie Tong Department of Philosophy and Healthcare Ethics, Center for Professional and Applied Ethics, Charlotte, USA

Part I
Theoretical Background

Chapter 1
Introduction

Michael Boylan

Abstract This Introduction sets out the broad context of the book through the Theoretical Background section and the Public Policy and Administration section. The focus of the book is the theory and practice of public health policy during infectious pandemics. Our shared experience with the COVID-19 pandemic shows how important this is. It is hoped that this book will stimulate conversations on these topics.

Keywords Public Health Policy · Pandemics · Ethics · Social and Political Philosophy

I have structured this project in the following way: First, I have divided this book into two parts: (1) The Theoretical Background and (2) Public Policy and Administration (the application of the theoretical background). This bifurcation of theory and practice has been my organizing principle in all my books on practical, applied ethics over the years.

In this introduction, I will give the reader a glimpse at the relation between the two large sections of the book as well as the justification of topics chosen. Let us begin with the theoretical section. My Introduction essay addresses this in two ways: (a) first, I set out the long-removed and short-removed history of pandemics and how public policy has reacted. Many of these policy responses are neither effective or ethical. This first part of the essay is meant to set out some of the social and political factors that went into the reaction to these public health emergencies. (b) Second, I set out a groundwork for public health ethics. This framework owes much to my earlier writings in both ethical theory and public health ethics.[1] Because of space considerations, I can only set out the highlights of the ethical theory and how it grounds public health ethics.

In Chapter 3, Per Bauhn sets his model concerning "public health responses" upon the theoretical distinction between seeing the Covid-19 threat through two lenses: (a) a utility-based approach versus (b) a rights-based approach. Now at this point

---

M. Boylan (✉)
Department of Philosophy, Marymount University, Arlington, VA, USA
e-mail: Michael.Boylan@marymount.edu

© The Author(s), under exclusive license to Springer Nature Switzerland AG 2022
M. Boylan (ed.), *Ethical Public Health Policy Within Pandemics*, The International Library of Bioethics 95, https://doi.org/10.1007/978-3-030-99692-5_13

in the essay, many readers might connect the utility-based approach with vaccine mandates, lockdowns, masking, et al. against the rights-based approach that would support the anti-vaxers and their ilk. However, Bauhn, by making reference to James Griffin and then especially to Alan Gewirth, shows that the most important criterion is "needfulness for action" which Gewirth supports via the Principle of Generic Consistency. Bauhn examines the various worldviews of the two sides and shows how they actually *flip* from what was initially expected in setting out his two poles. When the Swedish agency in charge of public health policy thought they were moving towards a position that emphasized both—with a lean towards "rights-based," they were actually moving towards "utility-based" because the fundamental aspect of Gewirth's primary concern in the supportive state toward providing a framework by which all prospective purposive agents (PPAs) might realize their ability to act, *requires* scientifically-based public health restrictions so that the "rights-based" approach requires legislation that might include vaccination and mask mandates. Politicians who want to pander to those who want to ignore the legitimate rights-claims to freedom to act and the goods that will allow that (with the end of maintaining or acquiring well-being), are *really* utility-*based*. And Sweden, as a case study, failed to make the correct theoretical assessment that underlies these public policies, and, as such, had higher mortality outcomes than other Scandinavian countries that required more public health mandates.

In Chapter 4, Sahotra Sarkar uses the methodology of philosophical epistemology to sort out the claims of the various stakeholders that follow from their held values. Starting at the beginning in China, Sarkar documents how fundamental ignorance of biology and epidemiology color the responses of various segments among the peoples of the world. There is a paucity of data that should have been easier to ramp-up, since we saw this virus-type earlier in the 2002–2003 SARS outbreak. But what is really operational in this political milieu are the underlying values of the stakeholders in each community. One dimension is the relative social worth of "citizen health" versus "citizen economic well-being." Obviously, the former would suggest *group sacrifice* while the latter would prioritize keeping the economic engine running even if it meant the death of the underpaid workers who are so essential to the operation of the economy.

Now science can estimate what the effects of certain sorts of public health measures might have on a given population, via the reproduction number R_o number. What science does is descriptively set out the probability of various policy initiatives in keeping the reproduction number as low as possible. But it does *not* show how these should be brought forth in rational decision theory. This is because decision theory needs to have parameters that will first describe what is to be ultimately valued and how possible trade-offs are to be assessed.

Sarkar then puts forth formal models of analysis that seek to clarify the best ways to assess the up-sides and down-sides of possible policy avenues. These multi-criteria analysis models become more complicated as they seek to account for permutations of different sorts of utility criteria. In the end, it is the creation of value hierarchies that will allow for the establishment of rationally-based public health policies.

In Chapter 5 Peter Tan explores the role of values in public policy formation. Giorgio Agamben suggested that governments might use a biological threat as a pretext to take an over- amount of control over people's lives: a form of totalitarianism. This conundrum is based upon a misunderstanding of how values should play a role in policy formation. Tan sets up two ways to understand value: (a) a fixed realm—such as Agamben's value of autonomy, and (b) a developing process that is constantly being worked and developed/refined. Tan believes that the latter is the truer and more useful for creating public policy.

To this end, Tan creates a model that relies upon Charles Peirce's pragmatic analysis of human inquiry formation, along with Jürgen Habermas's concept of performative contradiction in public discourse. This two-part process will reveal where values begin and how they are justified.

Step one is that public health policy must be the product of an iterative process that engages the language of values that can be publicly discussed. Step two is to free the public health policy from any performative practical contradictions. When the stated policy does not match what is happening on the ground, corrections must be implemented.

Lastly, the planning and roll-out of the public health policy must be transparent and structured to engage in public feedback that is taken seriously.

The structure of value is patterned after the structure of human inquiry that is continuously being created and revised. These values are intertwined with reason and can be assessed for their rational content which will allow one to evaluate their central role in the development of public health policy.

Chapter 6 is the last essay in the theory section of the book. Matose and Taylor discuss how pandemics can act as both a racialized and racializing phenomenon. This is because first, race is brought in to the *explanans* of the public health pandemic *explanandum*. And second, that this sort of *argumentum ex ignoratia* can lead to unequal public health outcomes. Finally, racist inputs can lead to higher death rates among those targeted.

The first point means that race must be taken seriously when planning and assessing a public health response to a medical pandemic. The authors put forth a consensus race theory that supplants classical race theories that have been responsible for the rise of racial oppression. Consensus race theory is a critical, revisionary alternative to the classical race theories that have done so much to shape the modern world. In consensus race theory a critical structure is created in the realms of politics, economics, sociological dynamics, et al. to ascertain how patterns of advantage and disadvantage are created that are not functionally based upon achieving work-based outcomes. The fundamental statistical inconsistencies call for causal factors that would account for these.

The second point is illustrated via the example of distribution of smallpox vaccines after Jenner's discovery. In the public health policy concerning distribution of these vaccines, the so-called "worth" of potential victims (based upon race) unethically entered into the public health planning of its distribution. Such calculations affect the statistical outcomes of victims. These unethical biases made their way through so-called scientific circles as eugenics caught the imagination of these "luminaries."

The third point glances historically at how various plagues always seemed to hit minority populations the hardest. From the plague to cholera epidemics, it was the racialized groups whose mortality percentages were the highest.

These are very important dynamics that are often left out of the theoretical perspective on how we should conceptualize ethical public health policy.

Chapter 7 begins the *application* section of the book. Here the essays focus upon particular practical/ethical problems raised by how we should apply and administer the theorical considerations that went into properly constructing a public health policy.

Wanda Teays begins this section with an inquiry on the extent of the moral and professional duty to provide medical treatment by doctors, nurses, and staff. Do physicians, nurses, and other healthcare workers have a duty to treat during a pandemic? Is working in a pandemic different from the ethical/professional duty during other medical contexts?

Teays cites the American Medical Association's 2020 statement that these are not ordinary times—implying that we need to do some examination on how this change might affect moral/professional duty.

Teays cites several cases from Monkey Pox to Ebola. Many caregivers became sick, and some died. Knowing this risk, is it incumbent upon the medical community provide care? Is there a maximum acceptable risk? Certainly, the responsibility to treat during a mass casualty incident is different from the responsibility to treat during an infectious disease. In the former case we are talking about working overtime while in the latter case we may be talking about working for the last time.

Sometimes decisions about acceptable risk have to be made during a short time interval. Patients present themselves at hospitals requesting care. It is certainly difficult for individuals trained to give that care to turn patients away, but it is probably better to consider these dynamics before patients show up at the emergency department.

Teays then examines professional responsibility from the perspective of oaths and codes. "Do no harm" is not environmentally specific. How far does promoting beneficence go? Most of these oaths and codes are meant to apply to circumstances in which the healthcare worker's life is not in jeopardy. Paraphrasing Judith Thomson, if we cannot be good Samaritans, perhaps we could become decent Samaritans. But what this means in clinical settings is left unclear by most codes of professional standards concerning risk to the health and life of physicians.

Teays then examines the arguments in favor of there being a duty to treat in pandemic times and the arguments against such a duty before coming up with her own position.

In Chapter 8, Jonathan Lewis and Udo Schuklenk examine principalism as a strategy for ethical action-guidance in pandemics. Using David DeGrazia's definition, principalism is: (1) Any ethical theory that emphasized principles, (2) Features more than one basic principle, (3) Leaves some of its principles unranked relative to each other. Lewis and Schuklenk then bring forward Beauchamp and Childress as an example of a bioethical principalist approach: respect for autonomy, beneficence, non-maleficence, and justice constitute an example of a principalist approach.

1 Introduction 7

Then Lewis and Schuklenk summarize some of the debate that has arisen on this principalist approach since it was put forward in the 1970s. The result of this discussion suggests seeking out: (a) coherence between the principles, (b) restrictions on the origins and operation of the necessary reflective equilibrium, and (c) formation of considered judgments under justifiable epistemic conditions. Otherwise, the principalist approach is actually an exercise in ethical intuitionism of the individual making the judgment.

Concerning pandemics, one model put forth by Canada's Public Health Ethics Framework, suggests a five-step process that is meant to give better action-guiding structure across various policy making venues: 1. Identify the issue and gather the relevant facts, 2. Identify and analyze ethical considerations and prioritize the values and principles upheld, 3. Identify and access options in light of values and principles, 4. Select the best course of action, and 5. Evaluate. However, some of the same problems that haunted biomedical ethical principalism find themselves appearing here, as well.

What the authors put forward is a model in which public transparency of the justifications for specific pandemic guidelines are discussed by diverse panels that develop procedures for consistent, explicit criteria for interventions that are based upon epistemically justifiable alternatives for action.

In Chapter 9, Klaus Steigleder and Johannes Graf Keyserlingk put forth a rights-based approach that is consistent with that put forward by Per Bauhn in Chapter 3. Steigleder and Keyserlingk start out by positing the state as the proximate political entity that is responsible for providing the conditions for freedom and well-being to its citizens.[2] All people have the *right* for these conditions and since rights and duties are correlative, the society at large (in a proximate way) and the world (in a remote way) have the duty to provide these conditions to those within their boundaries.

This is not a libertarian conception that advocates "egg carton communities"[3] but the notion of the supportive state and the community of rights set out by Alan Gewirth. As such, the duty bearers must also exhibit concern for those who do not possess those goods of agency necessary to allow the agent to pursue freedom and well-being (one component, of which, is health). The policy question is how to make this happen in the most efficient and equitable fashion for all groups and individuals within the state (or extended political units in the region or globally).

The "costs" and "benefits" and their relative calculus may be different in various societies that have more or less a community sensibility already existing withing their traditions. This can create two perspectives: from within (internal) and from without (external). These two perspectives vary among cultural traditions such that the creation of public policies within pandemic conditions must reflect these differences in the way they deliver the basic goods of agency to people within their countries (first) and then to others. The first-order metaethical duty[4] is the same, while the execution of it will vary according to societal resources. However, the wealthier nations bear a general duty to be prepared, as much as is possible, for public health emergencies (such as pandemics) and to assist other nations in preventative measures since these are the most effective.

In Chapter 10, Rita Manning begins her essay by reviewing the early stages of the COVID-19 pandemic by noting how shortages of essential hospital equipment (such as ventilators) and supplies required an allocation formula. Unfortunately, this occurred regionally and locally such that there were conflicts between strategies—and some were so poorly thought out that needless deaths were the result. Clearly, allocation of medical goods and services is a crucial problem in pandemics.

In section one of her paper Manning considers basic concepts of allocation and distributive justice. Key terms, such as "rationing," "triage," and "prioritization" are brought forth and discussed. The contexts of care (micro and macro) along with the structure of the healthcare system (private and mixed systems of healthcare delivery) are also key. Further, is the status of certain goods as "entitlements" and being essential for continuance of life along with the temporal conditions such as being in a crisis. Finally, vulnerable populations are examined.

In section two of her paper Manning considers features of essential goods that must be allocated fairly. The agencies that control this in the U.S. vary—with states at the vanguard and the Federal government using specialized public health agencies (like the Center for Disease Control) to offer advice on policy considerations.

In section three Manning discusses who is responsible for allocating these goods and how such responsibility is authorized. The models she brings forward for analysis are: consequence-based (Utilitarianism), virtue ethics (AMA Code of Ethics), and principled-based (examples from Rawls, Kant, and, from a different perspective, libertarianism)—also existing structural documents like the Universal Declaration on Human Rights can play a role.

Finally, in section four Manning sets out how principles of justice can be used to drive a principled allocation with special attention to the Crisis Standards of Care that apply directly to the current pandemic.

Debra DeBruin begins Chapter 11 citing the tremendous toll that the COVID-19 pandemic has had upon the nations of the world. This has raised issues of distributive justice particularly among Black individuals, Indigenous individuals, and People of Color: BIPOC populations.

First of all, as she points out in Table 11.1, the number of infections, hospitalizations, and deaths vary according to race and ethnicity. The toll, that these exact, is also unequal. This claim is born out in Table 11.2 which focusses upon hospitalization rates per 100,000 in various age and race/ethnicity groupings compared to Whites. These facts show that there is clearly health disparity in BIPOC populations.

In Table 11.3, this disparity is shown to carry through to mortality (the worst possible outcome). BIPOC population mortality is many times higher than White populations. This exacerbates a trend in pre-pandemic mortality rates so that some of this disparity may be due to unequal access to healthcare in general which gets worse when a health emergency (such as a pandemic) comes to the fore. Thus, part of the inequity of care within the United States is the fact that our healthcare system has structural flaws that are biased against BIPOC populations.

Because these routine, profound disparities are built into the healthcare system, it is no surprise that they become even more evident when extra pressure is exerted upon the system during a pandemic.

1 Introduction 9

Some of these disparate outcomes can be addressed in a way that does recognize BIPOC populations, as such (like living and work arrangements—the so-called *neutral approach*). But any comprehensive approach must address BIPOC populations directly (*beyond neutrality*).

DeBruin then sets out a middle ground approach which combines neutral and beyond-neutral approaches taking what works best in each. By working both sides of the spectrum, it is possible that healthcare may be improved for BIPOC populations both within the pandemic and afterwards.

In Chapter 12 Rosemarie Tong explores how COVID-19 affected nursing homes and other long-term care facilities (LTCFs). She begins by recounting her experience in 2007 as co-chair of the North Carolina's Department of Public Health Task Force on Ethics and Pandemic Influenza Planning. The purpose of the task force was to set out ethical guidelines in advance of a pandemic. The task force had a diverse membership. They principally examined: (1) Healthcare workers' responsibility to provide care during a pandemic, (2) The responsibility of workers in critical industries to continue at their jobs, (3) Balancing the rights of individuals with the duty to protect the public, and 4. Prioritization of limited resources during pandemics. However, what they failed to see was that residents of long-term care facilities (LTCFs) and other congregate living situations, such as prisons and homeless shelters, would be disproportionately affected by an infectious disease outbreak.

The medical needs of those 75+ years of age is a growing, vulnerable population and is predicted to constitute 23% of the U.S. population by 2060. Taken with the fact that there have been a number of pandemic outbreaks in the past century or so, and the need to create public health policies to protect especially vulnerable populations, it becomes a necessary task for us to attend to as soon as possible.

Concerning the responsibility to provide care during a pandemic Tong refers to a 2003 survey that found 80% of physicians willing to continue care during a pandemic outbreak, but that number drops to 55% when the care might threaten their own health and to 40% who were willing to risk their lives to do so. The North Carolina task force recommended giving healthcare workers who were endangering themselves, priority in resources for their own care and prevention.

Among those in critical industries (from caregivers in nursing homes to supermarket workers) many take such risks for low pay and long hours. Because the NC Ethics Task Force was focused upon hospitals, these individuals were not singled out, but probably should be a part of a comprehensive public health policy during pandemics.

The rights of individuals and the duty to protect the general populace have been a point of some conflict during the COVID-19 pandemic, but the NC Ethics Task force argued that the duty to the general population supervened individual displeasure at being inconvenienced during the maintenance of public health measures designed to protect the community.

Finally, is the issue of allocation of resources during the pandemic. The NC Ethics Task force set out that priority should be given to: (a) the functioning of society; (b) reducing the spread of the disease; (c) protecting those who have the most years to live; (d) every group has an equal claim for healthcare resources; (e) protecting those who have the most stages of life still ahead of them (quality of life).

Having clear guidelines for public health policy during pandemics helps ensure that the number of hospitalizations and deaths will be as low as possible.

In the last chapter of the book Ikiko Ito brings an international perspective to the problem. Ito, who works at the United Nations in a leadership capacity, is in a good position to comment on the international response to the pandemic. Though the pandemic has touched virtually every country in the world, it has not affected all citizens in those societies equally. Those who daily face discrimination—such as women and girls with physical disabilities, those who have invisible or psychological disabilities, migrants, refugees, and racial and other minorities—face a higher impact (hospitalization and fatality) than others in that society. The U.N. and various nations who have extra resources have tried to address these issues of justice and fairness, though the need is very great.

The U.N.'s Inter-Agency Support Group on the Convention on the Rights of Persons with Disabilities (IASG-CRPD) and the UN Partnership on the Rights of Persons with Disabilities (UNPRPD) have instigated international dialogue along these lines to create policy guidelines and muster assistance among member states. These also include data assessments and good practices that have worked elsewhere. For example, making COVID-19 testing more available to those who are wheelchair-bound can be a life-saver to many.

Making health information readily available as the pandemic progresses is also of critical importance. But many public health measures that have been in place, such as lockdowns and social distancing, can have a higher negative impact on those with disabilities. It is important that this sub-population not be left behind. So, by continuing to focus on this sub-population is essential in order to give them the equal right of an expectation for health and safety—especially during a pandemic that is so virulent. The WHO has listed special guidelines to help toward protecting disabled individuals around the world. The problems are enormous and the patterns for response through community outreach, etc. continue to grow. It is important for international organizations be at the forefront for these efforts.

Notes

1. My principal works in ethical theory are: Boylan (2004a, 2011, 2015, 2021). My principal works in public health ethics are: Boylan (2004b, 2008)—a second edition of this book is due out in 2023. For critical examination of my theoretical ethical position see: Gordon (2008), *Journal of Applied Ethics and Philosophy* (September, 2016) special theme issue on my theory of natural human rights. Discussion of my treatment of Immigration from my book, *Morality and Global Justice: Justifications and Applications* in a Theme Issue: *Journal of Applied Ethics and Philosophy* "Author Meets the Critics: Michael Boylan's Morality and Global Justice" *Journal of Applied Ethics and Philosophy* 4 (2012): 34-45. "Michael Boylan" by Robert Paul Churchill in Chatterjee's (2012).

2. For an example of the structure of such a state see the depiction of the "supportive state" in Gewirth (1978: 318–320); and the "community of rights" in Gewirth (1996: 59–60).
3. The term "egg carton communities" is one that I coined in Boylan (2004a: 115–116). These are communities in which individuals see themselves as totally separated from others with no duties or obligations to others: just like eggs in an egg carton that are set out so they don't touch and break!
4. First order metaethical duties are those that govern the creation of normative theories of distributive justice. For Alan Gewirth it is the *Principle of Generic Consistency*, see Gewirth (1978: 135) and Michael Boylan's *Personal Worldview Imperative* Boylan (2004a: chapter two).

Bibliography

Boylan, Michael. 2004a. *A Just Society*. New York and London: Rowman & Littlefield.
Boylan, Michael. 2004b. *Public Health Policy and Ethics*. Cham, Switzerland: Springer.
Boylan, Michael. 2015. *Natural Human Rights: A Theory*. Cambridge: Cambridge University Press.
Boylan, Michael. 2008. *International Public Health Policy and Ethics*. Cham Switz.: Springer.
Boylan, Michael. 2011. *Morality and Global Justice: Justifications and Applications*. Boulder, CO: Westview (rpt. Routledge 2020).
Boylan, Michael. 2021. *Basic Ethics*, 3rd ed. London and New York: Routledge.
Chatterjee, Deen, ed. 2012. *Encyclopedia of Global Justice*. Heidelberg, DE: Springer.
Gewirth, Alan. 1978. *Reason and Morality*. Chicago: University of Chicago Press.
Gewirth, Alan. 1996. *The Community of Rights*. Chicago: University of Chicago Press.
Gordon, John-Stewart., ed. 2008. *Morality and Justice: Reading Boylan's 'A Just Society.'* New York and London: Lexington.

Chapter 2
The Context and Foundations of Ethical Public Health Policy

Michael Boylan

Abstract This essay begins by examining a few historical examples of pandemics in the context of a schema of common categories of comparison. It then uses this historical framework to give context to the developing COVID-19 pandemic. The second part of the essay examines the moral basis of public health and uses these frameworks to suggest several key policy strategies that should be adopted in the face of this or any future infectious pandemic.

Keywords Antonine Plague · Spanish Flu pandemic · HIV/AIDS pandemic · Ebola pandemic · SARS and MERS pandemic · COVID-19 pandemic · Ethical Grounds for Public Health Policy

2.1 Prologue

This essay begins in the middle of things. This is how one often finds herself when there is an infectious disease, public health crisis. At the beginning are various symptoms presenting among a population or populations. Are the symptoms connected causally? Is a bacterium, virus, or a fungal protist acting as the causal agent? Is this causal agent also spread among people by other people—community spread? Who is most susceptible? Are sub-groups of a population (*demos*) more at risk for some particular reason (*en-demos*) or is it moving in the direction of the entire population (*epi-demos*). Perhaps it's spreading wildly everywhere (*pan-demos*)?[1]

Since this essay is being written in the middle of a pandemic caused by the pathogen SARS-CoV-2 that causes the spread of the disease COVID-19, whose biological mechanics are still being studied, there is much about the facts of the virus and the effects of the disease that are still unknown.[2] This means that this essay (and other essays in this book) cannot view the COVID-19 pandemic as a finished case, but as one in-progress. However, by combining a few, select examples of pandemics from history, we may be able to discern certain commonalities that

M. Boylan (✉)
Department of Philosophy, Marymount University, Arlington, VA, USA
e-mail: Michael.Boylan@marymount.edu

might be useful in assessing pathogenic development along with appropriate, ethical public health responses.

In this regard, I will briefly touch upon the Ancient Greek World before skipping to the 1918 Spanish Flu pandemic; the HIV/AIDS pandemic circa 1980, onwards; Ebola circa 1989, onwards; SARS circa 2003/MERS 2012 onwards; and COVID-19 current.[3]

In the second part of this essay, an ethical framework is set out that is intended to be a guide for public health policy, in general and in particular to pandemics—such as the current COVID-19 pandemic.

2.2 Introduction

We start our select history with the Hippocratic writer of *The Sacred Disease* (epilepsy), "I am about to discuss the disease called "sacred" (*hieres*). It is not, in my opinion, any more divine or more sacred than other diseases, but has a natural cause (*phusin prophasin*)."[4] *Disease,* especially multiple instances of symptoms within a small sample space of people is atypical. Most ancient Greek texts that have come down to us are clinical: one-to-one in orientation. One slight exception to this is the Hippocratic physician (probably Cnidian, a physician from the island of Cnidos)[5] who wrote *Epidemics III* (*Epedemion gamma*) that sets out symptoms, a crisis, and the result—most often death.[6] The book is meant to be a clinical handbook for the attending physician to assist in diagnosis. It is assumed that the attending physician would treat the symptoms that present according to the contraries: hot, cold, wet, and dry.[7] As these are pre-humor theory texts, there was little that the physician thought he could do except try and balance too much *hot* with *cold* (and vice versa) and too much *wet* with *dry* (and vice versa).[8]

What we should bring away from these two texts is: (1) That disease (from the earliest times) has by physicians largely been seen to be caused by physical causes and not divine causes[9]; and (2) That in the search for these physical causes of disease, the physician needs to rely upon empirical evidence to assess what disease is presenting and therefore lay the groundwork for treatment and prognosis based upon what other patients have.

In the ancient world probably the most devasting event we have record of is the Antonine Plague (circa 165–180 C.E.). What makes this event so vivid is the fact that one of the greatest of ancient physicians, Galen, was at the center of it.[10] Though Galen does not give consistent, systematic description of symptoms, scholars have thought that it is probably an early form of small pox (though a minority suggest an early form of measles). We do know that it was described by Galen to be a big plague (*megalas loimos*) which creates an extreme common disease event (*epidemon*). Fatalities are hard to quantify but some estimates suggest as many as 5 million Europeans or one-third of various recorded populations. At one time as many as 2,000 Romans per day were dying.

Some side notes from Rebecca Flemming which deserve attention are: (1) It seemed important to those in Rome and Italy to blame the disease on a foreign entity—in this case from the far east (China via Persia); (2) There seemed to be a recognized connection between infected armies spreading disease as they entered towns (though there is no macro civil response to this fact); (3) That marginalized peoples (especially those enslaved)—who become victims, don't much matter to mainstream society—in fact (for some), the infestation of cattle is thought to be a greater problem. (4) Galen continues in the midst of a wide-spread outbreak to continue treating one patient at a time while those in political power ignore and do not solicit any generalized civil reaction (public health).

Some of these responses from two thousand years ago resonate with contemporary reactions to pandemics—especially the one we are experiencing at the writing of this essay (COVID-19). The most salient, is the lack of a public health response to a killer plague (*megalas loimas*) which is widespread (*epidemon*).

2.2.1 How Do We Assess Infectious Diseases?

Before moving to our starting point in the modern era, the 1918 Spanish Influenza, it is useful to set out a few key factors that will be common to all the pandemics that we will examine (as a means for structuring the setting for ethical evaluation of public health responses).

A. First, there is *communicability*. This is measured by the means of transmission and how easy it is to avoid it. For example, measles is very communicable and the transmission is airborne. We all have to breathe to stay alive so this makes measles especially difficult to control. Another source is contact with a person with the disease (either directly or via a third entity (like a solid surface such as a door knob) that was in contact with that person). Rhinovirus transmits like this. Then there is a bite from an outside agent, e.g., an insect—such as a mosquito (malaria and yellow fever transmit like this). Then there is contact with the bodily fluids of an infected individual, HIV/AIDS and Hepatitis transmit like this. Finally, there is contact with contaminated water or food; cholera transmits like this. The agents of transmission are generally bacteria, viruses, and/or fungi (or other protists)—ringworm and athlete's foot transmit via fungi while malaria transmit via protists.

B. Second, is the *probability and degree of Human harm*. The probability of substantial human harm refers to the symptoms and how long lasting and harmful they are to an individual who undergoes no treatment. For example, rhinovirus has a high probability of causing symptoms of a stuffy nose, sore throat, and a headache, but most people can rid themselves of the virus within 5–14 days with no permanent effects. Other diseases have either lower or higher probability thresholds of possible infection and greater or lesser degrees of human harm. When assessing human harm, sometimes the infectious agent causes the harm directly to the body attacking a bodily system, like respiration—such as influenza. Other infectious agents stimulate auto-immune reactions (causing the body to attack itself—e.g., lupus, celiac disease, Sjögren's syndrome, et al.).

Finally, if one were to take the anthropocentric standpoint,[11] infections of other animals and/or plants can have deleterious effects upon humans that can cause disease by cross-over (such as HIV from monkeys and Marburg virus disease from bats). Other practical effects of plant pandemic can be the loss of valuable [to humans] products—such as trees and the Dutch Elm pandemic in North America. The Irish Potato Famine of 1845-1849 did not *directly* kill people but took away a primary dietary source of nutrition that led *a fortiori* to human mortality.

C. Third are the *civil reactions*. These follow three sorts of response: (1) Prophylactic (via isolation or quarantine of infected populations; inoculation against the pathogen (somewhat after the initial outbreak as this takes time for discovery and human testing); (2) Effective Treatment (also a time intensive approach that seeks to control/minimize the disease or to rid the body of the pathogen; (3) Finally, when all else fails, there is herd immunity response that kicks in when 70–85% of the population (the survivors) have effective antibodies to combat the disease lowering the *Reproduction Number*: R_x (where x approaches 0). This may be called the evolutionary answer (though it may come at a high human cost of lost lives and human suffering).[12]

2.3 Part One

2.3.1 *A Brief View from Select Pandemics*

Using the assessment criteria above, let's take a brief look at some of the more recent pandemics that express themselves through one or more of the categories to have caused excessive human harm and the public health responses to the same.

Spanish Flu: 1918–1919: The so-called "Spanish Flu" actually showed its first symptoms in the United States at a military base in Kansas, March 11, 1918.[13] It then went to Europe—probably through troop movements during the last phases of World War I. Very soon, thereafter, the King of Spain, Alfonso XIII, contracted the disease (though some say he got scarlet fever instead). He recovered. After that, the disease was pinned upon Spain—who, in turn, pinned it upon France. However, the first case was in the United States! Why is it so important to *nationalize* the blame for a virus that carries no passport?[14]

According to David Killingray, though the British Empire had dealt with epidemics before through yellow fever, sleeping sickness, small pox, cholera, and the bubonic plague, they were unprepared for effective public health responses to this strain of flu.[15] The infection rate was much higher (up to 40% of the world's population) and there was more consequential human harm (21–50 million dead).[16]

Most at risk were the young and healthy (so that World War I soldiers fit into this category).

In the case of this pandemic, the first wave was not too far from normal in infection rates and human harm causing civil reactions to be rather restrained. It was the second wave of the viral infection that occurred in the autumn hitting Asia (especially in India and then moving east). Again, Killingray believes that part of the cause of this was the British shipping industry that carried the flu from Europe to India and to Hong Kong.

The communicability of the disease was very high—especially for particular subpopulations. *The British Medical Journal*[17] estimates that incidence rates among native populations around the world was as high as 80% in some locales. In general, white populations in the Commonwealth Nations and the United States was as high as 60%. Among the military, the British Navy was around 30% and the British Army around 20%. (Interestingly enough, those military who had been exposed to poisonous gas during the war had their incidence rate drop to 4.7%). This can be compared to similar "in season" flu populations today that have up to an 8.3% incidence rate.

From the same source, the probability of human harm (in this case fatality) was greater than 2.5% overall for those who became sick with this strain of the flu. This can be compared to 0.1% for flu outbreaks in general populations today.

Further, the human harm continues beyond mere fatalities. In one study that focused upon the U.S. population 22+ years after the outbreak, the aftermath among the offspring of pregnant women who were affected exhibited: (1) Reduced educational attainment; (2) Increased physical disabilities; (3) Lower modal incomes throughout life; and (4) Decreased socio-economic status (due to #1–#3).[18]

Concerning civic, public health responses, though there were sporadic efforts that varied city-by-city, no effective, comprehensive public health measures were undertaken even though there had been prior influenza epidemics in 1889–1890. Some examples of what *was* done in the United States includes first New York City where the sick were (in many cases) quarantined from the healthy. Public health "runners" went about the city taking notes on which areas of the city seemed to be worse. The city's board of education engaged in health education about hygiene and what symptoms to note about sickness (and what course of action to take). New laws concerning public hygiene (such as anti-spitting laws) were enforced.[19] Then, as infections and deaths mounted, schools were closed.[20] African Americans were given systematic, inferior treatment due to attitudes concerning biological inferiority and general racism. They were put into segregated, sub-standard hospitals without state-of-the-art equipment. Because of this, their mortality rates exceeded their percent of the population.[21]

In San Antonio, Texas (a major city in that era) the public health response was three-fold: ban children from schools, quarantine the sick, and prohibit large public gatherings. This was moderately effective.[22]

In Pittsburgh, Pennsylvania (a manufacturing city at the time one-third the size of Philadelphia), there were inconsistent standards. This was caused by a political tug of war between the governor and the mayor. Once people showed signs of clear sickness, they were home quarantined. But this wasn't adequate as Pittsburgh soon had the worst rate of infection and fatality. The general population was sicker than normal before the flu, due to the manufacturing plants and the smoke they produced. Public gatherings were permitted including publicly sponsored concerts. Housing was crowded among the low-paid mill workers. The public sanitation system was sub-par with open sewers that had excrement floating about. Once again, African American populations were hit the worst. This public health response was a terrible failure.[23]

HIV: 1981 onwards: The second pandemic that I wish to gloss is the HIV/AIDS pandemic. According to United States' Center for Disease Control, from 1981 to 2006, 22 million people died of AIDS (500,000 in the United States). In 2005 2.8 million died from AIDS worldwide and 4.1 million were newly infected.[24] As of 2019 the total number of deaths due to HIV/AIDS worldwide is 32.7 million (with 690,000 in 2019 alone).[25] This is one measure of the quantity of human harm that has to be seen in the context of the diminished life-style of those on HIV antiretrovirals.[26]

On the issue of communicability, data from Canada gives some important details.[27] Anal sex-receiving semen has an infection rate of 1.4% (or 1–71 episodes); anal sex-giving semen has an infection rate of 0.11% (or 1–750 episodes). Vaginal sex-receiving semen has an infection rate of 0.08% (or 1–1,250 episodes), vaginal sex-giving semen has an infection rate of 0.04% (or 1–2,500 episodes). There are no statistics in this report on oral sex. Therefore, on this side of the pandemic analysis, communicability is lower than the 1918 Influenza pandemic. There is also an easy prophylactic device, the condom, which can reduce risk even further.

On the side of human harm, there is the mortality rate for those who contract HIV and develop AIDS. At its height in the 1980s (pre-treatment), those who contracted HIV in the United States were studied by the University of California, San Francisco Medical Center. In this study those who retained HIV and then developed AIDS died at up to a 50% rate.[28] This is a very high mortality rate for a pandemic. Now that antiretroviral treatment is available in much of the world, this mortality rate has dropped precipitously. In 2019 there were an estimated 38 million with HIV/AIDS (36.2 million adults and 1.8 million children). 1.8% of these infected individuals died.[29]

Treatment today via pre-exposure prophylaxis (PREP) and via post-exposure prophylaxis (PEP) can greatly lessen the transmission of HIV among people who are HIV negative. For those who are HIV positive, there are medications (antiretroviral therapy, ART) that can lower the levels of HIV so that the risk of transmission to others via sex is greatly diminished.[30]

The story of civic public health responses to the HIV/AIDS pandemic varied by country. One of the major problems facing public health officials was that in most countries in the world there are strong social taboos concerning sex outside of marriage and (at this time especially) concerning gay sex. These taboos created problems for public health officials to effectively instigate a public health response.

Donald P. Francis did a retrospective of the first 30 years of the HIV/AIDS public health reactions in the United States (and some of these problems listed resonate with some other countries).[31] The United States lacked an early understanding of epidemiology of infectious disease at the political levels. Because of this ignorance, a rapid public health response (critically necessary for all epidemics and pandemics) was lacking. People got side tracked into focusing on issues of sex, homosexuality, and intravenous drug users as a moral issue. Some religious zealots even proclaimed that this plague was a penalty from God for those "sins" of the victims (another version of *blame the victims*).[32] This re-invigorated the ancient quarrel between science and religion. The result was a public policy paralysis as politicians did not want to anger their base by letting a scientific medical question be addressed by public health scientists.

The U.S.A. CDC (Center for Disease Control) showed early on that there was a problem that needed immediate intervention, but the U. S. President, Ronald Reagan, did not understand the role of a President in a public health crisis. The refusal to listen to public health experts made the problem worse than it had to be and increased the number of lives lost. There was even a reticence for some time at recommending condoms for those engage in sex in high risk groups. This was because of the "religious right" who did not want to seem like they were encouraging sex—except among married people in their churches who might expand those churches and their money and power.

The tale of the tape here is a very bad start, and a gradual change over time that has largely put the pandemic into a controlled—yet still present and virulent—mode. There is continued hope for the future (40 years later) going forward.

Ebola: 1976, 2014, 2019: The next pandemic that we will briefly examine in this chapter are the various Ebola outbreaks that began in in the Democratic Republic of the Congo in 1976 in a village near the Ebola River. Since then, they have spread to Uganda, Gabon, Guinea, Liberia, Sierra Leone and Nigeria. The original transmission was between animals (bats and non-human primates to humans). The original mode of transmission is thought to have been the eating of infected bats and non-human primates. There is no data on how many exposures in this mode will cause human infection, however; the disease between humans is *highly* contagious—so we might be able to extrapolate here, as well. The principal outbreak to date was 2014–2016, which is touched upon below. As of 2019 another outbreak has begun in the Democratic Republic of the Congo and is still in its early phases.

The human-to-human transmission occurs from contact with bodily fluids: sweat, blood, urine, feces and then having that contact enter the blood stream via open cuts, contact with eyes, ears, nose, and mouth. Contact with corpses of infected individuals is also significant. This can cause problems due to social customs on funerals and "showing respect to the deceased" by touching or kissing the corpse. Overall, the infection rate per 100,000 in West Africa was 100 => 300 per 100,000.[33] Even healthcare workers (in Sierra Leone), who take significant caution in treating patients, were infected in the 2014 epidemic period at 5.4%. This shows how contagious the disease is.[34] The disease is not thought to be transmitted via airborne, aerosol contact.

Sexual contact with an infected person is contagious when giving or receiving semen (slightly higher risk). Those who are exposed in these ways have a high rate of infection (sometimes > 90%).[35] When this is paired with mortality rates that are generally 60%-70%, but can approach 90% in some circumstances, the Ebola Virus

Disease (EVD) is very dangerous among infectious diseases.[36] Once infected there are three stages of the disease. A. (after 2–21 days) fever, headache, myalgia; B. (just after stage one) gastro phase: diarrhea, vomiting, abdominal pains; C. (just after stage two) collapse of neurological functions and massive internal bleeding. These three phases generally take 1–3 weeks + after first symptoms. Death generally occurs quickly—generally before a month is finished. After the second week, the recovery rate increases significantly (up to 75%).[37]

The only real treatment is fluid and electrolyte replacement—low effective rate.

The combination of high communicability with high rate of mortality that proceeds rapidly, makes Ebola a formidable disease. In the time-span of April to October in 2014 in the countries of Senegal, Mali, Nigeria, Guinea, Sierra Leone, and Libera, there were 17, 145 cases and 6,070 deaths (35% mortality rate).[38]

The civil, public health reaction to the disease has varied. In Canada (and by extension the United States) the African pandemic was presented sometimes as an issue of national security and at other times as one of public health.[39]

Within Africa, the center of the various outbreaks, some popular beliefs have gotten in the way of effective public health measures. These beliefs include: (a) God will protect me against EVD; (b) traditional healers will be more effective than modern doctors; (c) people can become infected via airborne transmission; (d) it is a Western bioterrorism experiment against African nations.[40]

Because there is little continuity between countries for a coordinated public health response, there is no standard position on: (1) The compassionate use of experimental drugs for treatment along with new, untried vaccines; (2) There needs to be more money allocated towards infection control; and (3) There needs to be a long-term commitment toward creating a international public health infrastructure for the future.[41]

At the writing of this essay the Ebola pandemic has started again (where it first began) in the Democratic Republic of Congo, 2019. The public health measures just set out have limited the number of cases involved and have contained the death rate: As of 23 July 2020—250,000 exposure contact tracings; 200,000 tests administered; 3,481 cases reported resulting in 2,299 deaths (66%), a decrease from the 2014 outbreak.[42]

This latest flare-up shows that proper public health responses can curb the numbers of cases as well as the mortality. Sometimes there are those who will not trust modern science, but these outliers must be overcome for the health of the larger community. Since outbreaks are likely for the future, this should be a measure of support for those who seek to be resolved to use tried and true techniques for reigning in a virulent pandemic.

SARS: 2003/ MERS: 2012: Severe Acute Respiratory Syndrome (SARS) caused by the SARS corona virus was first detected by the World Health Organization (WHO) in February 2003.[43] It was spread, as most corona viruses, by airborne saliva aerosol. The infection rate indoors is around 3%. The incubation period is 2–7 days but that can expand to 10 days.[44] On March 12, 2003 the WHO issued a health alert describing a new unrecognizable flulike disease that was infecting healthcare workers. By August there were 8,422 cases and 916 deaths (11%) from 29 countries—far higher than the flu 0.1% in 2019 in the U.S.[45] This turned out to be a rehearsal for subsequent outbreaks of H5N1 and H1N1. This offered an opportunity for public health agencies around the world to prepare themselves. Some did (particularly in east Asia) and most did not.[46]

In the time where the pandemic was just beginning (February 2003), a 64-year-old physician was treating a patient with atypical pneumonia in his home in Guangzhou, China. The physician developed symptoms of a respiratory complaint but felt well enough to travel to Hong Kong to go sightseeing with his brother-in-law. Little did he know that he was in the early stages of "severe acute respiratory syndrome." He became a spreader. The resulting pandemic caused WHO to issue new public health guidelines that helped ameliorate the later H1N1 and H5N1 outbreaks.[47]

Various other developments of similar viruses originated in Saudi Arabia, MERS (also a corona virus). Initially, the infection began among camel workers. With many of the same symptoms as SARS, the initial infection rate was about the same (though males were slightly higher), but the mortality rate was higher, 65% versus 10% for SARS.[48]

The public health reaction to these two outbreaks has been varied. There have been no concerted international efforts because unless bodies pile up in very high amounts, it can be difficult to garner general response among nations.[49] One way to measure how well the nations of the world took these pandemics as a wake-up call to create policies and institutional capabilities, is to see which nations in the world have done comparatively better in yet one more novel corona virus outbreak.

COVID-19: At the initial writing of this essay in October, 2020 we are at another link in the chain of novel corona viruses that we have just touched on. SARS-CoV-2 causes COVID-19. Like the other corona viruses SARS-CoV-2 attacks the respiratory system, but may also affect other organs as well. The communicability so-far with the virus is 2.4% in the U.S.A. with a mortality rate among the infected group of 2.8%. World statistics for comparison are not as accurate for a variety of reasons.[50] As noted above, the infection rates and mortality rates of those infected is more than double the flu in the United States. Because it is so early on in the pandemic, it is not useful to note total mortality because this is subject to change. But within the first 9 months total deaths in the U.S.A. are around 208,000 and worldwide around 995,000.[51]

One critical factor in trying to create a strategy for treatment and for a vaccine is to discover just how SARS-CoV-2 reacts within human hosts. William A. Haseltine, who worked extensively on the HIV treatments, set out viruses into two group: (a) those that are "hit and run" like polio—if you can survive it, there is long-term acquired immunity so that you won't get it again; and (b) that are "catch and keep it" like HIV or the common herpes zoster that begins as chicken pox and lives in the spine and may later cause shingles.[52] This is an important facet of understanding SARS-CoV-2, and is, at the writing of this essay, unknown.

What can be commented on is the initial public health reaction to SARS-CoV-2.

The countries that are doing best at the initial stages of the COVID-19 crisis are those that took the SARS and MER pandemics seriously. Countries such as Japan,

South Korea, and Germany come to the fore.[53] Also, some countries in Africa have also learned and are better prepared.[54]

Concerning general public health responses in this early phase, it is remarkable that there has been a lack of international cooperation to a global pandemic.[55] Part of this may be attributed to then President of the United States, Donald Trump, who was intent on pursuing an isolationist foreign policy. As in other pandemics, there is also an unproductive "name-calling" blaming the virus upon China: "the Chinese virus." This has exacerbated prejudice on those of Asian descent within the United States and harmed these individuals unfairly.[56]

One last problem (that was also mentioned above in other public health infectious disease pandemics) is the dissemination of accurate information to the populations of the world's countries. One set of misinformation concerns the nature of the disease and how it should be confronted. Another is wild facts about some international nefarious agent who may be instigating this outbreak for national defense purposes.[57]

2.3.2 Conclusion of Part One

In this brief, select history of the pandemics over the past century, there are certain facts that stand out. First, it is important that governments in the countries affected recognize that this is a medical emergency that should be handled by health care professionals: doctors, nurses, and epidemiologists. Second, bringing in local traditions and religious leaders who connect it to supernatural dynamics are not helpful (as was said by the Hippocratic writer of *The Sacred Disease* many centuries ago). Still, this continues to happen. Third, using the crisis to demonize other countries (as an "indirect attack") or social groups within a country (such as LBGTQ individuals during the HIV/AIDS pandemic—that is still ongoing) is counterproductive to the task of keeping everyone safe and getting on the other side of the pandemic.

Unfortunately, many political leaders around the world think only of how impotent they are and have no vision of getting around denial and moving forward to actively confront the public health crisis through ethically and scientifically based policies that are laser-focused on the real problem of ridding ourselves of the public menace at hand.

2.4 Part Two

2.4.1 Grounding Public Health Ethics

In the last section of this essay, I will set out an outline of the ethical responsibility within public health ethics—particularly regarding pandemics.[58]

There are at least two sorts of imperatives to maintain public health[59]: (a) prudential, and (b) moral. In the former case an agent advocates policy supporting public health because it makes the environment in which the agent lives more desirable for the agent, himself. In this case (for example), one would like to rid his area of cholera because if cholera is allowed to spread, then the agent, himself, might catch cholera. In such situations the agent is thinking only of his own advantage. This has two discernable effects: (1) public health is merely an extension of particular agents' own personal needs, and (2) [as a result of #1] public health policies will only be supported when there is a political mandate to do so based upon coalitions of people advocating their shared self-interest.

Should public health be merely a line-item in the intercourse of self-interested policy maneuvering or should it be governed by some other sort of principle? Part Two will discuss this first alternative and demonstrate its shortcomings. Then it will propose a different ground of public health policy based upon a worldview model and fundamental human rights.

2.4.2 *Prudential Grounds for Public Health*

The prudential model is based upon a principle of selfish egoism and extended egoism (the political expression of selfish egoism). Continuing with the cholera example, agents are only after their own self-interest. Thus, these agents will support a policy if and only if they believe that policy will directly benefit them. In the cholera example, someone living outside a city might only support a public health effort for sanitation if he believed the danger of contracting cholera was getting dangerously close to infecting him or his family. The risk must be immanent. There must be a clear and present danger of his being harmed. This sort of agent is willing to support only those projects that directly benefit him. From the agent's point of view, this is the most efficient allocation of resources. ("Efficient" here means not spending public money on other people apart from the agent. Thus, the adage, *if the program doesn't help me, it's a wasteful program.*)

Others will support policies that they see are in their "enlightened self-interest." These might include preventative measures that may (indirectly) help others whether or not there is an imminent threat or a clear and present danger to themselves. These individuals are acting from self-interest but have *a longer view of things*. They see prevention as the most efficient allocation of resources because reacting in the midst of a crisis is notoriously expensive. These individuals would point to the adage, *an ounce of prevention is worth a pound of cure*. In this way the "enlightened self-interest" version of egoism sees public health measures as some sort of insurance policy that will efficiently address potential problems. ("Efficiency" here means using fewer public dollars to address an issue that may have an impact upon the agent, himself. Though there is some waste involved because [i] the problem might not arise and [ii] the solution may help many others apart from the agent—still, the cost savings from acting early offsets this other sense of waste.)

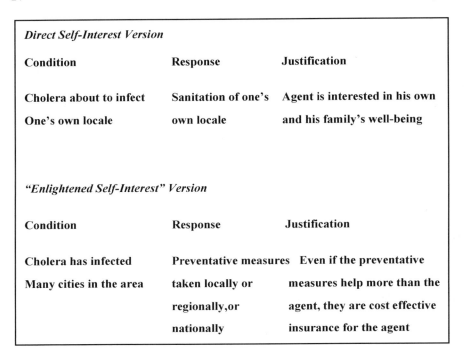

Fig. 2.1 The direct and "enlightened self-interest" versions of prudential justification of public health policies via extended egoism

These two strategies can be summarized in the Fig. 2.1.

Though these two sorts of prudential justification share the category of extended egoism, they otherwise are quite distinct. In the direct form, the agent views "efficiency" solely in terms of how it benefits himself. In other words, all money spent upon others is "wasteful." This is because only the agent, himself, counts. If a public program does not benefit him directly—right now—it is wasteful.

To some (including the author) this view of policy wastefulness is problematic. The reason I would give for this is that it violates the Personal Worldview Imperative: "All people must develop a single comprehensive and internally coherent worldview that is good and that we strive to act out in our daily lives."[60] Direct egoists are forced to adopt an inconsistent position of creating a worldview in which *they* count for more than *others*. But on what grounds is this assertion put forth? Merely that the agent sees and values her own claims for goods above all others. But what is the basis of this valuation? Simply that the agent is self-absorbed to the extent that she dismisses other people's claims as being of lesser weight *because* they are not the agent's own claims. But why this an inequality in claim valuation? The basis is centered in the original assessment by the agent that she is more important than other agents merely because she says so. However, if other agents make the same claim, then a contradiction develops immediately. (Logical contradictions within individual worldviews violate the Personal Worldview Imperative.)

In Fig. 2.1, the "enlightened self-interest" version of prudential justification via extended egoism, the agent understands that it may be more fiscally efficient to create programs that treat problems before they arise (preventative). This is done because it spends less of the public's money and will cause the agent to have lower taxes, etc. This sort of agent views such policies as insurance effectively meted in an efficient social manner. Efficiency here has to do with lower net social costs *but only for the sake of the agent himself*. There is no altruism involved nor connection with the general good. Because the "enlightened" egoist (along with the direct egoist) asymmetrically values his rights claims above others, and because this is an inconsistent position, he is also subject to the same negative evaluation (as per the Personal Worldview Imperative).

Some would assert that the addition of "extended" to egoism is significant. This is because it is thought that if one accepts a policy that extends beyond the self to include others, then it automatically becomes moral. The inclination to this position is most often brought forth by utilitarians.[61] However, this assessment is incorrect. In the case of direct egoists, the only reason that they support extended versions of their vision is to protect themselves. This is a far cry from signing on to the position that one endorses the happiness/pleasure of the group. Endorsing the happiness/pleasure of the group as primary, *means* that the individual has renounced the vision that the individual's own happiness is primary (an essential maxim to direct egoists). And yet, it is easy to see why some utilitarians might like to make this claim. This is because nineteenth century utilitarianism was "sold" on the scientific principle of selfish egoism (to which most in the audience would agree) and then this was extended to the group. The extension to the group constituted the "moral turn" and made a prudential theory into a moral theory. However, this move has been called into question by no less than the prominent utilitarian, Henry Sidgwick, himself.

> I do not mean that if we gave up the hope of attaining a practical solution of this fundamental contradiction [between egoistic and general hedonism] … it would be reasonable for us to abandon morality altogether; but it would seem necessary to abandon the idea of rationalizing it completely. We should doubtless still, not only from self-interest, but through sympathy and sentiments protective of social well-being, imparted by education and sustained by communication with other men, feel a desire for the general observance of rules conducive to general happiness …. But in the rarer cases of a recognized conflict between self-interest and duty, practical reason, being divided against itself, would cease to be a motive on either side; the conflict would have to be decided by the comparative preponderance of one or the other of two groups of non-rational impulses.[62]

When put up against it, there is no compelling rational reason why the direct egoist should accept the claims of the general happiness as primary and action guiding. This is because the very foundation of the direct egoist is that he is committed to his own self-advancement above all else. To single one's self out asymmetrically over all others is generally not the worldview of one willing to share and to be cooperative.[63] It is the worldview of the free rider, exploiter, or *kraterist* dedicated to the laws of *feng*.[64] Thus, it seems to this writer that there is no way that the direct egoist might be construed as anything other than a prudential agent bargaining about preferment that he feels is his due.

"Enlightened egoists" fare no better. The fact that they will permit extended policies that do not directly benefit them is *not* a sign of cooperation but rather is indicative of their understanding of what constitutes "efficiency." The enlightened egoist, just like the direct egoist, is only concerned about herself. However, the manner of *effecting her self-interest* is different. The tactics of attaining personal advantage are set in terms of a strategy that spends less total money. But why should the enlightened egoist care about the least amount of social money being spent? Shouldn't she be as the direct egoist and consider efficiency solely in terms of money spent upon herself? No. This is because the more generalized efficiency calculation is based upon a premise that if social funds are used effectively, then either taxes (upon the agent) will be lower or there is more social money left over to spend upon efficient programs to benefit herself. In either case, the enlightened self-interest agent is in no way cooperative or interested in the general happiness, but only seeks a unique strategy of efficiency that differentiates herself from the direct egoist.

If it is true that both direct and enlightened egoists are logically inconsistent in their views (as per Fig. 2.2), and if logically inconsistent views are rejected by the Personal Worldview Imperative, then both of these positions should be rejected as foundations for Public Health.

2.4.3 *Moral Grounds for Public Health*

2.4.3.1 How Does Morality Relate to Public Health?

In part two of this essay, it has been argued that both the direct and enlightened egoists fall prey to logical inconsistency—even in their extended forms and so are not suitable justifications for public health policy. In its stead, this essay will suggest that moral grounds for public health are more certain because they give a clear and intersubjective foundation. In order to avoid the problems of egoism that lead to the contradictions, the moral theory chosen must be one that is deontologically or virtue-ethics derived. The reason for this is that of the classes of moral theories, the anti-realist theories devolve into egoism (individual or group) and the realistic moral theories that are subject to maximizing individual or group happiness amount to the same thing. Only deontologically-based or virtue-based theories can rely on an assessment of the right action, per se (in the case of deontologically-based theories) or the right action that a person of virtue (one possessing the fundamental virtues of wisdom, self-control, courage, and justice (including feminist theories of care)).[65]

To begin, it is essential to address the difficulty presented from the prudential worldview: the inconsistent claims of asymmetrical preference. These may be addressed directly in the following argument.

> 1. "I, Ms. Greed, value my claims for x, y, and z"(where x, y, and z, are goods of agency in short supply)—Fact
> 2. Others also value x, y, and z—Fact
> 3. The speaker's claims hold positive asymmetric weight over competing rights claims—Assertion (essential to selfish egoism)
> 4. Ms. Greed is a speaker--Fact
> 5. Ms. Greed's claims are more important than any other competing rights claims—1-4
> 6. Mr. Grasping is among the competing rights claimers—Fact
> 7. Mr. Grasping is a speaker--Fact
> 8. Mr. Grasping's claims are more important than any other competing rights claims (including Ms. Greed's)—3, 6, 7
> 9. There can be only one agent whose claims are more important than any other competing rights claims—Fact
>
> ———————
>
> 10. The formula espoused in premise #3 is logically inconsistent—5, 8, 9

Fig. 2.2 The logical inconsistency within the egoist's worldview

The Argument for the Moral Status of Basic Goods

1. Before anything else, all people desire to act—Fact
2. Whatever all people desire before anything else is natural to that species—Fact
3. Desiring to act is natural to *homo sapiens*—1,2
4. People value what is natural to them—Assertion
5. What people value they wish to protect—Assertion
6. All people wish to protect their ability to act beyond all else—1,3,4,5
7. The strongest interpersonal "oughts" are expressed via our highest value systems: religion, morality, and aesthetics—Assertion
8. All people must agree, upon pain of logical contradiction, that what is natural and desirable to them individually is natural and desirable to everyone collectively and individually—Assertion
9. Everyone must seek personal protection for her own ability to act via religion, morality, and/or aesthetics—6.7

10. Everyone upon pain of logical contradiction must admit that all other humans will seek personal protection of their ability to act via religion, morality, and/or aesthetics—8,9
11. All people must agree, upon pain of logical contradiction, that since the attribution of the basic goods of agency are predicated generally, that it is inconsistent to assert idiosyncratic preferences–Fact
12. Goods that are claimed through generic predication apply equally to each agent and everyone has a stake in their protection—10,11
13. Rights and duties are correlative—Assertion

14. Everyone has at least a moral right to the basic goods of agency and others in the society have a duty to provide those goods to all—12, 13

For the purposes of this essay, premise #11 is perhaps the most controversial. This is because it declares that when predication occurs generally, then all instantiations share (via logical heritability) in that general characterization. Thus, if Mary is a human and if humans are rational animals, then Mary's claim to being human is true in virtue of "rationality" (or rationality and the ability to care)[66] being heritable from the generic attribution. Mary is rational not because she is Mary, but because she is human. Thus, for Mary or any other agent to assert idiosyncratic preference (the basis of asymmetric claims) is for Mary to make a logical mistake. When making reference to generically predicated properties, it is a logical mistake to declare that they arise from some disposition of the individual agent, herself. Instead, the agent (upon pain of logical contradiction) must admit that generic features of action are predicated and apply generally. Because of this, humans (with respect to these generically predicated properties) are interchangeable (with respect to rights claims to essential goods of agency). Each counts the same.

But what are these goods that may be predicated of all people in virtue of being human? This is a difficult question, but one version of these goods is as follows:

The Table of Embeddedness

BASIC GOODS—Level One: *Most Deeply Embedded*[67] (That which is absolutely necessary for Human Action): Food, Clean Water, Clothing, Shelter, Protection from Unwarranted bodily harm (including basic healthcare).

Level Two: *Deeply Embedded* (That which is necessary for effective basic action within any given society),

- Literacy in the language of the country.
- Basic mathematical skills.
- Other fundamental skills necessary to be an effective agent in that country, e.g., in the United States some computer literacy is necessary.
- Some familiarity with the culture and history of the country in which one lives.
- The assurance that those you interact with are not lying to promote their own interests.

- The assurance that those you interact with will recognize your human dignity (as per above) and not exploit you as a means only.
- Basic human liberties such as those listed in the U.S. Bill of Rights and the United Nations Universal Declaration of Human Rights.

SECONDARY GOODS—Level One: *Life Enhancing,* Medium to High-Medium Embeddedness,

- Basic Societal Respect.
- Equal Opportunity to Compete for the Prudential Goods of Society.
- Ability to pursue a life plan according to the Personal Worldview Imperative.
- Ability to participate equally as an agent in the Shared Community Worldview Imperative.[68]

Level Two: *Useful,* Medium to low Medium Embeddedness,

- Ability to utilize one's real and portable property in the manner she chooses.
- Ability to gain from and exploit the consequences of one's labor regardless of starting point.
- Ability to pursue goods that are generally owned by most citizens, e.g., in the United States today a telephone, television, and automobile would fit into this class.

Level Three: *Luxurious,* Low Embeddedness,

- Ability to pursue goods that are pleasant even though they are far removed from action and from the expectations of most citizens within a given country, e.g., in the United States today a European Vacation would fit into this class.
- Ability to exert one's will so that she might extract a disproportionate share of society's resources for her own use.

What this Table of Embeddedness does is to suggest what goods are comparatively more embedded to action. If the desire to act is the most primary human desire, then the Table of Embeddedness provides a hierarchical ranking of those goods in order of necessity. It thus becomes a document defining *triage* in public health crises.

It would seem that the recognition of the fundamental character of action (seen generically) is what is meant by morality—that I describe as the science of right and wrong in human action.[69] Under this guise, what generally supports the possibility of human action (and its effective action) must be a primary principle of morality. If this is true, then under a social interpretation of distributive justice, a country must allocate the basic goods (level-one) for all citizens before all else (subject to the caveat of 'ought implies can').[70]

With respect to infectious disease pandemics, 'Public Health' as a good of agency would fall under Basic Goods, level-one (protection from unwarranted bodily harm, including basic healthcare). Because pandemics also have economic consequences, it is also possible that other goods of agency would also be involved.[71] Public health is therefore broadly concerned with supplying the goods necessary for human action and eliminating impediments to the same.[72]

Because even a narrow event (such as a pandemic) may have an impact more broadly, a few general observations on public health, per se, are in order. Such a definition can be interpreted from two angles: (a) a collection of healthy humans, and (b) the maintenance of a healthy society—seen from the perspective of the macro group. From the perspective of (a) it is better to be broader in our scope and include the first three levels of goods because without these people cannot be effective actors in society. If purposive action is most essential to our nature as humans living in a social world, then removing those impediments will provide opportunity for all to exercise their autonomy subject merely to reasonable social constraints (such as those described in the Personal Worldview Imperative). Thus, from the perspective of (a) what is being advocated is a set of policies that will empower as many people as possible to be able to act as they wish in society (subject to reasonable social constraints). Public health is about supporting the individual health of each person (understood as allowing her those goods requisite for effective action).

In sense (b) the concern is with creating a *society* that (seen as a sociological unit) is healthy. Such a society would be one in which no segment of the society is being left out. Thus, if one viewed his society and found an identifiable social group (with robust boundaries) that was being excluded from full and equal participation in the society, then that *society* would be unhealthy. To create a healthy social unit, the application of distributive justice along the lines of the Table of Embeddedness would be an important step toward bringing back society's health. Thus, under interpretation (b) public health is about making sure that the first three levels of the goods of agency are given to all at some appropriate functional level.[73] In this way the state as a social unit may become healthy.

The duties entailed by both the (a) and (b) approaches, begin with level-one basic goods, those goods that biologically are requisite for human action. From the public health perspective, the lack of these, severely limits an agent's ability to act. Without adequate food and clean water, children are more likely to become mentally retarded. Adults are likely to develop other diseases and mental illness. Without adequate clothing and shelter people can die. Without proper sanitation for the same, individuals are subject to added external and internal disorders that will severely affect their ability to act. Finally, without reasonable freedom from bodily harm, the agent's attention is turned toward the attacking entity with the result that free deliberation is severely limited. This bodily harm can come in the form of: sickness, accident, crime, war, and domestic abuse (among others). Thus, since all agents have a claim to possess (at least) level-one basic goods, the first responsibility of public health is to provide these (as much as possible)[74] to all agents living within the society. Under this interpretation of public health, homelessness, poverty, disease, common accidents (like carpal tunnel syndrome), crime, civilian war casualties, domestic abuse (among others)[75] are all issues of public health (in both senses). Since this essay focusses upon ethical policy within infectious pandemics, it is here that policy-makers must concentrate.

2.4.4 Ethical Grounds for Pandemic Public Health

Using the principles set out in the previous section along with the brief glosses on selected pandemics in part one, a few observations can be made concerning the ethical direction that ought to be taken when countries and the world faces pandemics. Taken together, the most important tenets might be summarized as in Fig. 2.3.

1. Starting from the beginning, Fig. 2.3 sets out that it is essential that there not be categories of preferred population groups when allocating resources to fight a pandemic. This would require a healthcare system that was equally available for all. In order to effect this, the country would have to have either universal healthcare or special emergency healthcare to cover those infected. This requirement is a tall order for most poor countries of the world, but it doesn't stop there: The United States of America (one of the richest countries in the world) does not have either universal healthcare or any formal plans for those suffering from COVID-19 (at the writing of this essay).
2. When deciding how to allocate goods, Fig. 2.3 contends that the standard should be an assessment of the goods at stake. People's lives (Basic good, Level-one) would get priority over less embedded goods. A couple of examples include: (a) education delivery in the manner that many would want (Basic Good Level-two), i.e., in-person teaching in schools (as opposed to online teaching which might better protect Basic Good Level-one goods for all involved). If in-person (aka face-to-face) constitutes a significant risk to students, professors (teachers), or the families or community at large, then the safer public health option wins on the basis of The Table of Embeddedness. Again, policies that limit Basic Goods Level-two liberties such as required mask wearing, quarantines, or the closure of certain businesses like restaurants and bars that have close human contact (a loss of a Basic Good Level-two good of agency to protect a Basic Good Level-one good of agency), then the safer public health option wins on the

---

1. The lives and basic human rights of all individuals should be considered equal as per the Argument for the Moral Status for Basic Goods

2. Public Policy should follow the priorities of The Table of Embeddedness.

3. Epidemiologists and scientists should be given control of the process

4. Global and not merely individual national responses

5. Not a time for finger-pointing nationalism

6. Not a time for political exploitation

7. Not a time for using the pandemic as an excuse to further marginalize minorities

---

Fig. 2.3 Essential guidelines for pandemic public health

basis of the Table of Embeddedness. Secondary goods restrictions are similarly affected.

These restrictions also affect social protests needed to protect justice within the community: participants should observe mask wearing and social distancing. This is done on principle to protect the community's health (which for each individual in the community constitutes a Basic Good Level-one). Obviously, other material good acquisition and luxury good acquisition would give way to needs of fighting the pandemic to save lives and fundamental health—even if these policies cause disruption in the leisure-travel industry.

In the United States, such a response by Congress has not always been to allocate goods in this way. Personal Protective Equipment (PPE), ventilators, construction upgrades for containing contagion, and hospital support was sometimes overridden by economic support to large companies. Thus, such policies as putting Secondary Goods Levels two and three above Basic Goods, Level-one are immoral.[76] The ethical strategy is to follow the Table of Embeddedness when making tough choices of spending limited funds.

3. Figure 2.3 asserts that it would seem to be prudentially sound to let people trained for a particular problem solve those sorts of problems when they arise. Socrates used to ask who you would turn to when you needed your shoe to be repaired: obviously a cobbler. The same holds true for a public health crisis. Epidemiologists, physicians, scientists trained in virology and pharmacology, et al. should be put to the fore in creating public policy to help contain the pandemic. Politicians and others with self-interest who are not so-trained, should step aside and let the experts dictate the next step. This becomes *ethical* because there is an ethical duty to be knowledgeable about the world and let science and logic supervene over belief and self-interest.[77]

4. Working together in a multinational approach is better than one nation working exclusively by itself. This is because of expanded resources in cooperative approaches and the advantages of more intelligent scientists seeing the problem from different angles. By sharing this information, it is an advantage to all. Let's call this maxim *the principle of diverse community deliberation*. At the writing of this essay (October, 2020), the United States has decided to take a solitary position (sometimes referred to as "America First") and has withdrawn from the World Health Organization.[78] Since this works against the principle of diverse community deliberation, it violates #3 in not aspiring to the most knowledgeable scientific solution, and as such is unethical.

5. Finger-pointing nationalism has been around from our examples beginning with the ancient Greeks to the Spanish Flu to the COVID-19 pandemic. There is no scientific benefit in this exercise. It is merely a political exercise for the benefit of various civil leaders who do not wish to lose power over the outbreak of the pandemic. #3 and #4 above show how anything that moves us away from a scientific solution to a medical problem is unethical. *A fortiori* the same holds here, as well.

6. In times of crisis, there is always a longing for *order* and *the way things were before*. These are two conditions that lend themselves to political despots (and

aspiring despots). For the ethical standpoint, this creates a conflict of interests: (a) the interests of the people versus (b) the interest of the despot. The moral theory outlined above is crystal clear about what *ought* to be the case, but history has shown us that "ought" and "is" do not always coincide. It is up to the World Community to try and keep such *strongman* tactics in check for the good of all the people on earth.

7. Whenever times get bad, it is the least advantaged of society who are put into a position of absorbing the most pain. The least advantaged have the least amount of political power and leverage so they are, in practice, the bullseye for passing on the pain of the moment. This, violates #1 and #2 above (which are ethical principles) so that this kind of response is ethically prohibited. Even though this is unfortunately the case, in the COVID-19 crisis in the United States, poor African Americans and Latinx and Indigenous populations outnumber the general population in infection and death rates.[79]

2.4.5 Conclusion for Part Two

Part Two has sought to engage the moral versus the prudential grounds of public health and then briefly to apply these guidelines to pandemics, in general as set out in Part One. There are many potential pitfalls in setting out public health policy. But having the right orientation will create a situation in which—even if mistakes are made, that the overall direction is requisite over gamesmanship and *kraterism* of prudential grounding.

The way to this general strategy is to view ethics as an essential part of the grounds of public health. The prudential grounds for policy will lead to a skewed outcome that will not achieve the avowed goal for all living in the country (and around the word). In the case of the collection of healthy individuals (interpretation-a) this means that money and influence will provide the goods of public health only to the wealthy (whether they deserve their wealth or not). This violates the moral dictum of viewing each person without idiosyncratic preference (the argument for the moral status of basic goods, premise #11).

In the case of the healthy unit, efficiency (as measured by various social science statistics) becomes a crucial player. However, if it is the *supreme arbitrator*, then the result will be a plutocracy in which only the wealthy will have the essential basic goods of agency.

Efficiency is important, but it must give way to moral equity as a distribution formula by which society might provide as many of the basic goods of agency to all. Only this sort of policy-orientation will create something approaching *balance* in the society. And since health is balance,[80] it is only this sort of strategy that will create a healthy society (interpretation-b).

No matter how you understand public health, it is only by moral means that the enterprise, itself, makes sense. Idiosyncratic preference (that stands behind the prudential approach) is itself irrational. If rationality is (at least) a necessary condition to authentic human action,[81] then if we pursue prudential concerns over moral imperatives (when the two are in conflict) and when those *moral* imperatives are rationally more primary, then following the prudential path of idiosyncratic preference will result in our social/political degradation. We will become co-conspirators in devolution of society itself.

Our individual and collective futures lie in not allowing this to happen.

Notes

1. *Demos*, is from Ancient Greek referring to people, in the sense of a common group. "*En*" refers to something within—thus the modern English "endemic" taken medically would refer to a particular subgroup. "*Epi*" when used with the accusative means "on, to, against"; with the genitive means "on the surface of, in the direction toward, in the time of"; with the dative means "on, depending on." Obviously, the primary sense here is the genitive sense "of the common people" and being an early indicator of connection in time and place. "*Pan*" means "all" (in the sense of the universal quantifier in logic). This exercise in etymology may be useful for precise expression of meaning.
2. For some good, basic background on corona viruses (of which SARS-CoV-2 is a member) see: https://www.youtube.com/watch?v=8_bOhZd6ieM (accessed August 14, 2020) and https://raw.githubusercontent.com/milo-lab/SARS-CoV-2/master/versions/SARS-CoV-2_BTN.pdf (accessed August 14, 2020).
3. This is obviously not meant to be a comprehensive list, but rather illustrative of key, recent pandemics and how they presented and the public health responses that resulted. In the last portion of this essay, some thoughts on ethical foundations for public health are put forth as a standard by which these selective cases can be judged.
4. Hippocrates (1923b).
5. For a discussion of the methodological differences of the Cnidean medical writers in the Ancient Greek world with other contemporary writers see Boylan (1983, 14–18).
6. Hippocrates (1923a).
7. One quick way to connect to the Galenic categorization of symptoms comes from Sigerist (1961). There are four categories of symptoms: Choleric (full of *thumos* and *epithumos* spiritedness, desire, and drive—even to the extreme [due to an excess of yellow bile, connected with the root *fire* and exhibited most often in the summer]); Melancholic (sad and depressed—even to the extreme [due to an excess of black bile, connected with the root *earth* and exhibited most often in the autumn]); Phlegmatic (sluggish [a lack of *thumos*] –even to the extreme (due to an excess of phlegm, connected with the root *water* and exhibited most often in the winter); and Sanguine (socially oriented, talkative, calm (even in the midst of circumstances that should make one concerned (due to an excess of blood connected with the root, *air* and exhibited most often in

the spring))). The point of Galenic medicine is to create balance. If one is too much of one of the four humors, then try to balance it with a counter-active, e.g., if one is phlegmatic, then offer him/her citrus fruit which will counter the phlegm and create a stimulus of yellow bile that will make the patient more active again.
8. For a comprehensive account of this in the context of ancient medicine, see: Nutton (2013). For an examination of the theory behind the medicine at the time see: Boylan (2015, ch. 2).
9. There are various exceptions to this as set out by Boylan (2015, 3–17).
10. Three very good accounts of Galen and his role in the Antonine Plague are: Flemming (2019, 219–244), Boudon-Millot et al. (2010), Gourevitch (2013, 77–127 [esp. 72–75 on small pox]), and Duncan-Jones (1996). For reference to an extensive bibliography on this subject see: Lo Cascio (2012) and Elliott (2016).
11. Of course, one need not adopt the anthropocentric standpoint and opt for the biocentric ethical standpoint, instead. For a brief gloss of the arguments behind these two positions see: Boylan (2021a, ch. 4).
12. For some discussion on how to think about herd immunity see: Thompson (2019), Cunningham (2017), and de Cellês et al. (2016).
13. For a discussion of the historical spread of the disease—especially in the British Empire—see: Killingray (2003).
14. This behavior exists today as (at the initial writing of this essay) President Trump on multiple occasions blames Covid-19 on China: https://abcnews.go.com/Politics/chinas-ambassador-us-slams-trump-covid-19-blame/story?id=72187153 (accessed August 25, 2020). Cf. Ranger and Sacks (1992).
15. Killingray, *loc. cit.*
16. The standard figures of the Spanish Flu pandemic were 21–24 million, but work done by Johnson and Mueller (2002), put the figure rather higher—to at least 50 million.
17. Jefferson and Ferroni, (2009).
18. Almond (2006).
19. Aimone (2010).
20. Stern et al. (2010).
21. Gamble (2010).
22. Martinez-Catsam (2013).
23. Higgins (2010).
24. The United States Center for Disease Control report as of 2006: https://www.cdc.gov/mmwr/preview/mmwrhtml/mm5531a1.htm (accessed August 29, 2020).
25. Source is the United Nations: https://www.unaids.org/en/resources/fact-sheet (accessed August 29, 2020).
26. https://www.hiv.gov/hiv-basics/staying-in-hiv-care/other-related-health-issues/other-health-issues-of-special-concern-for-people-living-with-hiv (accessed August 29, 2020).

27. https://www.catie.ca/en/pif/summer-2012/putting-number-it-risk-exposure-hiv.
28. http://hivinsite.ucsf.edu/InSite?page=kb-01-03#S1.4X (accessed August 31, 2020).
29. https://www.hiv.gov/hiv-basics/overview/data-and-trends/global-statistics (accessed August 31, 2020).
30. https://www.hiv.gov/hiv-basics/hiv-prevention/reducing-sexual-risk/preventing-sexual-transmission-of-hiv (accessed September 1, 2020).
31. Francis (2012). For a brief scan of international reaction see: Iqbal and Zorn (2010), Rodney et al. (2010), Enoch and Piot (2017), Eba (2016), Mondal and Shitan (2015).
32. Jonsen and Stryker (1993).
33. Incident Management System: Ebola Epidemiology Team on Morbidity (2014).
34. Kilmarx et al. (2014).
35. Durojaye and Mirugi-Mukundj (2015).
36. Beeching et al. (2014). This is a comprehensive, clinically-oriented article.
37. Ibid.
38. Kana et al. (2016).
39. Humphries et al. (2017).
40. Kpanake et al. (2016).
41. Gericke (2015).
42. https://www.who.int/emergencies/diseases/ebola/drc-2019 (World Health Organization, accessed September 21, 2020).
43. https://www.who.int/health-topics/severe-acute-respiratory-syndrome#tab=tab_1 (accessed September 24, 2020).
44. Ibid.
45. https://www.cdc.gov/flu/about/burden/2018-2019.html (accessed September 24, 2020).
46. Koh and Sing (2010).
47. Nuttall and Dye (2013).
48. Zhou et al. (2014) and Dyer (2013).
49. This point is made by: Rollet (2014) and Arie (2014).
50. https://www.cdc.gov/coronavirus/2019-ncov/hcp/faq.html (accessed October 2, 2020). The world rates which are far less in the infection rate but around the same for the death rates of those infected need to be tempered by the fact that infection numbers are not readily available in all parts of the world because of lack of infrastructure and because sometimes there are political pressures to under-report infection numbers. Though the gross fatalities in the U.S.A. and the world have risen significantly, the CDC is now emphasizing vaccination rates in order to cut the rate of transmission. 99.5% of the deaths recently in the U.S. (summer, 2021) have been among the unvaccinated: https://www.bing.com/search?FORM=AFSCVH&PC=AFSC&q=cdc+coronavirus+update (accessed July 17, 2021).

51. Ibid. Of course, the U.S. deaths are now (July, 2021) over 600,000 and world deaths over 4,000,000.
52. Haseltine (2020), cf. Haseltine and Wong-Staal (1988).
53. For a comparative list see: https://time.com/5851633/best-global-responses-covid-19/ (Accessed 4 October, 2020). For some background on the Asian nations see: Staniec (2020).
54. Somse and Eba (2020).
55. Sachs (2020a, b).
56. https://www.washingtonpost.com/nation/2020/03/20/coronavirus-trump-chinese-virus/ (accessed October 1, 2020).
57. For some examples see: Fuentes (2020) and Jackson and Lieber (2020).
58. For an expanded exposition of my position see: Boylan (2004b).
59. It should be noted from the outset that the purview of this essay is public health within some given society. This is not to imply that I do not believe that there are international responsibilities involved in maintaining public health, but merely that the sovereignty structure of the world at present makes this sort of discussion more readily applicable. I do believe that ultimately these responsibilities should extend internationally. The appropriate agencies to administer these programs need to have greater authority than the present U.N. programs or those of the World Health Organization or the World Bank. (The WHO's actions in regard to the recent SARS outbreak is a case in point.) At this moment in history, it seems that the only way to execute duties is first through one's sovereign state and then remotely via these fledgling international bodies.
60. Boylan (2014b, ch. 6).
61. This has been a much discussed position in utilitarian thinking from the beginning. For a sample of the development of this notion see: (I) Historical Sources: Austin (1885), Bentham (1789), Hutcheson (1775), Mill (1863), Paley (1785), and Sidgwick (1907). (II) Contemporary Sources: Baier (1989), Bailey (1997), Johnson (1991), Korsgaard (1983), Lyons(1965, 1994), Schneewind (1977), Slote (1985), Smart and Williams (1973), Regan (1980), Thomson (1992).
62. Sidgwick (1907, 508).
63. Of course, some like Donald Regan will demur. This is because he (and others like him) puts forth an ethos of cooperation under which utilitariansim might flourish. See: Regan (1980).
64. *Kraterism*, is a term I use to denote those who believe that their use of power legitimates its exercise just in case it is successful. "Might makes right" is one version of this. *Feng* is a term I use after the Anglo-Saxon verb, 'fengon' that means "to snatch or take—generally with force". The connotation is that it is a decisive and aggressive taking—rather like a "commandeering." The word is prominent in *Beowulf* as an important element of the competitive worldview of the contending parties. For a further discussion of this see: Boylan (2004a, 151–153).
65. For an overview of these theories as they address problems in the world see: Boylan (2021b). Note, that in this book I place feminist ethics within the parameters of virtue ethics.

66. The interpretation of "completeness" in the personal worldview imperative entails care as an outcome of empathy + sympathy. See Boylan (2004a, chapter 2).
67. 'Embedded' in this context means the relative fundamental nature of the good for action. A more deeply embedded good is one that is more primary to action.
68. "Each agent must strive to create a common body of knowledge that supports the creation of a shared community worldview (that is complete, coherent, and Good) through which social institutions and their resulting policies might flourish within the constraints of the essential core of commonly held values (ethics, aesthetics and religion)," from Boylan and Brown (2002, 16), cf. Michael Boylan (2004a, b, chapter 5).
69. This has been my key contention in Boylan (2004a, 2010, 2014a). In the first and last of these references I examine other possible grounds, cf. Boylan (2021).
70. Boylan (2001, 19–20, 103), and Boylan and Brown (2002, 24).
71. This sense of "health" goes beyond being free from accident and disease. Health is not merely the lacking of something bad, but the possession of something good (the goods of agency). This implies a sense of health as a balance. Such a notion is holistic and in keeping with the Personal Worldview Imperative. Some current work that take up issues involved in this position includes: Steinberg (2000), Stux et al. (2001), Gairett (1994), and Weil (1988).
72. Some would say that such a definition seems to exclude environmental concerns. Such a general stance has been taken by Cranor (2001) and Ellis and Ravita (1997). However, I would demur to such attacks by citing my essay in which I use the above framework to defend environmental protection, see: Boylan (2001).
73. What I mean by an "appropriate" functional level here is really rather simple. If Jamal needs 2,000 cal a day in order to function well, then any reasonable delivery of these calories according to our latest ideas of nutrition would be functionally appropriate. Jamal need not have the very best organically grown tomatoes, but he does deserve nutritious, wholesome food that will meet his dietary needs.
74. The caveat "as much as possible" here refers again to the "ought implies can" dictum. If there is no cure for AIDS or breast cancer, one cannot provide the agent relief from its devastations. However, this does not mean that one should be resigned to this reality. Rather, the society should devote resources to cure these diseases and work cooperatively with other societies doing the same.
75. The "others" might include issues indirectly related to these—such as gun control is related to crime and to domestic violence—or other categories fitting into the slots of level-one goods.
76. For a gloss on this see: https://www.theguardian.com/us-news/2020/jun/09/us-congress-billions-coronavirus-aid-relief-package (accessed October 7, 2020); and https://www.ama-assn.org/delivering-care/health-equity/congress-digs-deep-fixing-health-inequities-exposed-covid-19 (accessed October 7, 2020).

77. I make the argument for this in Boylan (2021b, chapter 3).
78. https://www.bbc.com/news/world-us-canada-53327906 (accessed October 7, 2020).
79. https://www.nytimes.com/2020/04/08/nyregion/coronavirus-race-deaths.html (accessed October 7, 2020).
80. For an argument on this claim see: Boylan (2014a).
81. I should note here that I do NOT believe that rationality, alone, is both necessary and sufficient. The Personal Worldview Imperative sets out various understandings of the term "good." These include ethics, religion, and aesthetics (among others). The components in these various axiological criteria will certainly involve more that merely rationality. However, in the spirit of Plato's *Meno*, I would contend that all these other criteria are tethered by rationality. This means they inform and influence the scientific determination of the right and wrong in human action.

Bibliography

Aimone, Francesco. 2010. The 1918 Influenza Epidemic in New York City: A Review of Public Health Response. *Public Health Reports* 125 (Supplement 3): 71–79.

Almond, Douglas. 2006. Is the 1918 Influenza Pandemic Over? Long-Term Effects of in Utero Influenza Exposure in the Post-1940 U.S. Population. *Journal of Political Economy* 114 (4): 672–712.

Arie, Sophie. 2014. Would Today's International Agreements Prevent Another Outbreak Like SARS?". *British Medical Journal* 348: 1–3.

Austin, John. 1885. *The Province of Jurisprudence Determined*, ed. Robert Campbell, 5th ed., 2 vols. London: John Murray.

Baier, Annette. 1989. Doing Without Moral Theory? In *Anti-theory in Ethics and Moral Conservatism*, ed. Stanley G. Clarke and Evan Simpson. Albany, NY: State University Press of New York.

Bailey, James Wood. 1997. *Utilitarianism, Institutions, and Justice*. New York: Oxford University Press.

Beeching, Nicholas J., Manuel Fenech, and Catherine F. Houlihan. 2014. Ebola Virus Disease—Clinical Review. *British Medical Journal* 349: 1–15.

Bentham, Jeremy. 1789. *An Introduction to the Principles of Morals and Legislation*. Oxford: Oxford University Press.

Boudon-Millot, Véronique, Jacques Jouanna, and A. Pietrobelli, ed., trans., comment. 2010. *Galion: Ne pas se chagriner*. Paris: Les Belles Lettres.

Boylan, Michael. 1983. *Method and Practice in Aristotle's Biology*. Lanham, MD and Oxford: UPA/Rowman & Littlefield.

Boylan, Michael. 2001. Worldview and the Value-Duty Link to Environmental Ethics. In *Environmental Ethics*, ed. Michael Boylan. Upper Saddle River, NJ: Prentice Hall.

Boylan, Michael. 2004a. *A Just Society*. New York and Oxford: Rowman & Littlefield.

Boylan, Michael. 2004b. The Moral Imperative to Maintain Public Health. In *Public Health Policy and Ethics*, ed. Michael Boylan, xvii–xxxiv. Dordrecht: Springer.

Boylan, Michael. 2010. *Morality and Global Justice*. Boulder, CO: Westview.

Boylan, Michael. 2014a. Health as Self-Fulfillment. In *Medical Ethics*, ed. Michael Boylan, 2nd ed., 58–64. Malden, MA and Oxford: Wiley-Blackwell.

Boylan, Michael. 2014b. *Natural Human Rights: A Theory*. Cambridge: Cambridge University Press.
Boylan, Michael. 2015. *The Origins of Ancient Greek Medicine—Blood: A Philosophical Study*. New York and London: Routledge.
Boylan, Michael, ed. 2021a. *Environmental Ethics*, 3rd ed. Malden, MA and Oxford: Wiley-Blackwell.
Boylan, Michael. 2021b. *Basic Ethics*, 3rd ed. New York and London: Routledge.
Boylan, Michael, and Kevin Brown. 2002. *Genetic Engineering*. Upper Saddle River, NJ: Prentice Hall.
Cascio, Elio Lo, ed. 2012. *L' impatto dela "peste Antonina"*. Bari: Edipuglia.
Cranor, Carl F. 2001. Learning from the Law to Address Uncertainty in the Precautionary Principle. *Science and Engineering Ethics* 7 (3): 313–326.
Cunningham, Aimee. 2017. Zika Epidemic Ebbs but Threat Remains. *Science News* 192 (8): 12.
de Cellês, Matthieu Domenech, Felicia M.G. Magpantay, et al. 2016. The Pertussis Enigma: Reconciling Epidemiology, Immunology, and Evolution. *Proceedings: Biological Sciences* 283 (1822): 1–10.
Duncan-Jones, R. 1996. The Impact of the Antonine Plague. *JRA* 9: 108–136.
Durojaye, Ebenezer T., and Gladys Mirugi-Mukundj. 2015. The Ebola Virus and Human Rights Concerns in Africa. *African Journal of Reproductive Health* 312 (3): 48–55.
Dyer, Owen. 2013. MERS Will Spread While Natural Host Is Unknown. *British Medical Journal* 346 (7914): 6.
Eba, Patrick Michael. 2016. Towards Smarter HIV Laws, Considerations for Improving HIV-Specific Legislation in Sub-Saharan Africa. *Reproductive Health Matters* 24 (47): 178–184.
Elliott, Collin P. 2016. The Antonine Plague, Climate Change, and Local Violence in Roman Egypt. *Past and Present* 231: 3–31.
Ellis, Ralph, and Tracienne Ravita. 1997. Scientific Uncertainties, Environmental Policy, and Political Theory. *Philosophical Forum* 28 (3): 209–231.
Enoch, James, and Peter Piot. 2017. Homan Rights in the Fourth Decade of HIV/AIDS Response an Inspiring Legacy and Urgent Imperative. *Health and Human Rights* 19 (2): 117–122.
Flemming, Rebecca. 2019. Galen and the Plague. In *Galen's Treatise Περὶ Ἀλυπίας (De indolentia) in Context: A Tale of Resilence* Leiden: Brill. https://doi.org/10.1163/j.ctvrxk2wj.12. Accessed August 15, 2020.
Francis, Donald P. 2012. Commentary: Deadly AIDS Policy Failure by the Highest Levels of the U.S. Government: A Personal Look Back 30 Years Later for Lessons to Respond Better to Future Epidemics. *Journal of Public Health Policy* 33 (3): 290–300.
Fuentes, Gabriel A. 2020. Federal Detention and 'Wild Facts' During the COVID-19 Pandemic. *The Journal of Criminal Law and Criminology* 110 (3): 441–476.
Gairett, Laurie. 1994. *The Coming Plague: Newly Emerging Diseases in a World Out of Balance*. NY: Farrer, Straus, & Giroux.
Gamble, Vanessa Northington. 2010. 'There Wasn't a Lot of Concern in Those Days' African Americans, Public Health, and the 1918 Influenza Epidemic. *Public Health Reports* 125 (Supplement 3): 114–122.
Gericke, Christian A. 2015. Ebola and Ethics: Autopsy of a Failure. *British Medical Journal* 350: 1–2.
Gourevitch, D. 2013. *Limos kai Loimos: A Study of the Galenic Plague*. Paris: Éditions de Bocard.
Haseltine, William A. 2020. What We Learned from AIDS: Lessons From Another Pandemic for Fighting COVID-19. *Scientific American* 323 (October, 4): 37–41.
Haseltine, William A., and Flossie Wong-Staal. 1988. The Molecular Biology of the AIDS VIRUS. *Scientific American* 259 (October, 4): 52–63.
Higgins, James. 2010. 'With Every Accompaniment of Ravage and Agony:' Pittsburgh and The Influenza Epidemic of 1918–1919. *The Pennsylvania Magazine of History and Biography* 134 (3): 263–286.
Hippocrates. 1923a. Epidemics III. In *Hippocrates I*, tr. W.H.S. Jones. Cambridge, MA: Loeb.

Hippocrates. 1923b. The Sacred Disease. In *Hippocrates II*, tr. W.H.S. Jones. Cambridge, MA: Loeb.
Humphries, Brittany, Martha Radke, and Sophie Lavzier. 2017. Comparing 'Insider' and 'Outsider' News Coverage of the 2014 Ebola Outbreak. *Canadian Journal of Public Health* 108 (4): 1–15.
Hutcheson, Francis. 1775. *A System of Moral Philosophy*, 2 vols. London: Privately Published by His Son Francis.
Incident Management System: Ebola Epidemiology Team on Morbidity. 2014. Update: Ebola Virus Disease Epidemic—West Africa 2014. *Morbidity and Mortality Weekly Report* 63 (50): 1199–1201.
Iqbal, Zaryab, and Christopher Zorn. 2010. Violent Conflict and the Spread of HIV/AIDS in Africa. *The Journal of Politics* 72 (1): 149–162.
Jackson, Michael, and Paul Lieber. 2020. Countering Disinformation; Are We Our Own Worst Enemy? *The Cyber Defense Review* 5 (2): 45–56.
Jefferson, Tom, and Eliana Ferroni. 2009. "The Spanish Flu Through BMJ's Eyes. *British Medical Journal* 399 (7735): 1397–1399.
Johnson, Conrad D. 1991. *Moral Legislation: A Legal-Political Model for Indirect Consequentialist Reasoning*. Cambridge: Cambridge University Press.
Johnson, Niall P.A.S.., and Jeurgen Mueller. 2002. Updating the Accounts: Global Mortality of the 1918–1919 'Spanish' Influenza Pandemic. *Bulletin of the History of Medicine* 76 (1): 105–115.
Jonsen, A.R., and J. Stryker, eds. 1993. *National Research Council on Monitoring the Social Impact on the AIDS Epidemic*. Washington, DC: National Academic Press. https://www.ncbi.nlm.nih.gov/books/NBK234566/. Accessed September 3, 2020.
Kana, Musa Abubukar, Olufunmilayo Y. Elegba, et al. 2016. Ebola Viewed Through a Lens of African Epidemiology. *Journal of Epidemiology and Community Health* 70 (1): 6–8.
Killingray, David. 2003. A New 'Imperial Disease': The Influenza Pandemic of 1918–1919 and Its Impact on the British Empire. *Caribbean Quarterly* 49 (4): 30–49.
Kilmarx, Peter, Kevin Clarke, et al. 2014. Ebola Virus Disease in Healthcare Workers in Sierra Leone, 2014. *Morbidity and Mortality Weekly Report* 63 (49): 1168–1171.
Koh, David and J. Sing. 2010. Lessons from the Past: Perspectives on Severe Acute Respiratory Syndrome. *Asia Pacific Journal of Public Health* 23 (3): 132–136
Korsgaard, Christine. 1983. Two Distinctions in Goodness. *Philosophical Review* 88 (2, April): 169–195.
Kpanake, Lonzozou, Komlantsè Gossou, et al. 2016. Misconceptions About Ebola Virus Disease Among Lay People in Guinea: Lessons for Community Education. *Journal of Public Health Policy* 37 (2): 100–172.
Lyons, David. 1965. *Forms and Limits of Utilitarianism*. Oxford: Clarendon Press.
Lyons, David. 1994. *Rights, Welfare, and Mill's Moral Theory*. Oxford: Oxford University Press.
Martinez-Catsam, Ana Luisa. 2013. Desolate Streets: The Spanish Influenza in San Antonio. *The Southwestern Historical Quarterly* 116 (3): 286–303.
Mill, John Stuart. 1863. *Utilitarianism*. London: Parker, Son & Bourn, 1863, rpt. 1979, Hackett Publishers.
Mondal, Md., Nazrul Islam, and Mahendran Shitan. 2015. HIV/AIDS Epidemic in Malaysia: Trend Analysis from 1986–2011. *Southern African Journal of Demography* 16 (1): 36–56.
Nuttall, Isabelle, and Christopher Dye. 2013. The SARS Wake-Up Call. *Science* 339 (6125): 1287–1288.
Nutton, Vivian. 2013. *Ancient Medicine*, 2nd ed. London and New York: Routledge.
Paley, William. 1785. *The Principles of Moral and Political Philosophy*. London: R. Faulder.
Ranger, Terence, and Paul Sacks, eds. 1992. *Epidemics and Ideas: Essays on the Historical Perceptions of Pestilence*. Cambridge: Cambridge University Press.
Regan, Donald. 1980. *Utilitarianism and Co-operation*. Oxford: Clarendon Press.
Rodney, Patrica, Yassa Ndjakani, et al. 2010. Addressing the Impact of HIV/AIDS on Women and Children in Sub-Saharan Africa: PEPFAR, The U.S. Strategy. *Africa Today* 57 (1): 64–76.

Rollet, Vincent. 2014. Framing SARS and H5N1 as an Issue of National Security in Taiwa: Process, Motivations, and Consequences. *Extrême-Orient, Extrê-Occident* 37: 141–170.

Sachs, Jeffrey D. 2020a. Perspective COVID-19 and Multilateralism. *Consilience* 22: 1–5.

Sachs, Jeffrey D. 2020b. COVID-19 and Multilateralism. *Horizons*, 30–34.

Schneewind, J.B. 1977. *Sidgwick's Ethics and Victorian Moral Philosophy.* Oxford: Oxford University Press.

Sidgwick, Henry. 1907. *The Methods of Ethics,* 7th ed. London: Macmillan.

Sigerist, Henry. 1961. *A History of Medicine.* Oxford: Oxford University Press.

Slote, Michael. 1985. *Common Sense Morality and Consequentialism.* London: Routledge.

Smart, J.J.C., and Bernard Williams. 1973. *Utilitarianism: For and Against.* Cambridge: Cambridge University Press.

Somse, Piere, and Patrick M. Eba. 2020. Lessons from HIV to Guide COVID-19 Responses in the Central African Republic. *Health and Human Rights* 22 (1): 371–374.

Staniec, Cyrus. 2020. Cruising into a Global Pandemic (Early Lessons from the Indian Ocean). *Phalanx* 53 (2): 46–49.

Steinberg, Esther M. 2000. *The Balance Within: The Science Connecting Health and Emotions.* NY: W. H. Freeman.

Stern, Alexandra Minna, et al. 2010. School Closures. *Public Health Reports* 125 (Supplement 3): 63–70.

Stux, Gabriel, et al. (eds.). 2001. *Clinical Acupunture: Scientific Basis.* Berlin: Springer.

Thompson, Helen. 2019. This Number [the R_x] Helps Explain Why Measles Is so Contagious. *Science News* 195 (10): 32.

Thomson, Judith Jarvis. 1992. On Some Ways in Which a Thing Can Be Good. *Social Philosophy and Policy* 9 (2): 96–117.

Weil, Andrew. 1988. *Health and Healing.* Boston: Houghton Mifflin.

Zhou, Zie, Hin Chu, Cum Li, et al. 2014. Active Replication of Middle East Respiratory Syndrome Coronavirus and Aberrant Induction of Inflamatory Cytokines and Chemokines in Human Macrophages: Implications for Pathogenesis. *Journal of Infectious Diseases* 209 (9): 1331–1342.

Chapter 3
The Common Good and Individual Rights in Pandemic Times: The Case of Sweden's COVID-19 Strategy

Per Bauhn

Abstract In this chapter I intend to problematize the relationship between conceptions of the common good and individual rights in pandemic strategies, using the Swedish COVID-19 pandemic strategy as an example. The common good can be understood as either utility-based or rights-based. A utility-based conception of the common good aims at maximizing good consequences for society as a whole, while a rights-based conception of the common good aims at protecting important individual rights. It would perhaps be natural to assume that a utility-based conception of the common good would justify a pandemic strategy that is restrictive of individual rights, such as freedom of assembly and freedom of movement, for the sake of securing collective goods such as public health. Likewise, it would perhaps be natural to assume that a rights-based conception of the common good would justify a more permissive pandemic strategy, emphasizing individuals' right to freedom as a central aspect of the common good that the strategy should protect. However, as the case of Sweden suggests, a pandemic strategy might be utility-based and permissive at one and the same time. Moreover, its very permissiveness makes the strategy morally problematic from a rights-based perspective, as it allows the pandemic to spread and threaten the basic well-being of a large number of people.

Keywords Common good · Utility · Rights · COVID-19 · Sweden

3.1 Sweden's Pandemic Strategy

With a number of deaths from COVID-19 "putting it among Europe's worst-hit countries",[1] Sweden's strategy to fight the pandemic has received global attention. The strategy has been characterized by a lack of formal restrictions, such as lockdowns and curfews, and a reliance on recommendations issued by the Swedish Public Health Agency (PHA). Sweden has been heralded as "pioneering an approach of relying on voluntary compliance while most other countries promulgated

P. Bauhn (✉)
Linnaeus University, Kalmar, Sweden
e-mail: per.bauhn@lnu.se

legally enforced measures to assure compliance".[2] While many European countries, including Sweden's neighbours Denmark, Norway, and Finland, closed restaurants, bars, shopping centres, hairdressers, nightclubs, and gyms, prohibiting people from coming together in groups numbering more than ten individuals, Sweden allowed facilities to remain open and only prohibited public events involving more than 500 (later 50) people. Private parties, however, could go on without any interference from the police and people were allowed to come together for drinks after work in bars and restaurants as before the pandemic.

(As the pandemic resurged during late autumn and winter 2020–2021, a COVID-19 Act was introduced on January 10, 2021, banning public as well as private events and gatherings of more than eight people in clubs and "other places that can be rented".[3] The Act also made it mandatory for gyms, sport centres, and public baths to calculate the maximum number of simultaneous visitors with each visitor having 10 square metres at her disposal. However, the Act did not ban people from coming together in larger numbers in private homes, nor did it introduce curfews, bans on travels, or any other similar emergency regulations).

As the number of deaths in COVID-19 increased to exceed by far the death toll of all its Nordic neighbours taken together, the Swedish strategy has come to be hotly debated and questioned. (In mid-January 2021, while Denmark had 32.31 deaths per 100,000 inhabitants, Norway 10.22, Finland 11.45, and Iceland 8.20, Sweden had 106.03 deaths per 100,000 inhabitants.[4]) In January 2021 the medical journal *The Lancet* published an article by Mariam Claeson, former director of the Global Financing Facility (GFF) for Every Woman Every Child at the World Bank, and Stefan Hanson, an infectious disease physician, in which they criticized the Swedish pandemic strategy. They pointed out that at the time of their writing, in late December 2020, the Swedish COVID-19 deaths per 1 million population was 4.5 to ten times higher than the corresponding numbers for neighbouring Nordic countries, and continued:

> This difference between Nordic countries cannot be explained merely by variations in national cultures, histories, population sizes and densities, immigration patterns, the routes by which the virus was first introduced, or how cases and deaths are reported. Instead, the answers to this enigma are to be found in the Swedish national COVID-19 strategy, the assumptions on which it is based, and in the governance of the health system that has enabled the strategy to continue without major course corrections. From the onset of the COVID-19 pandemic, the Public Health Agency ... embarked on a de-facto herd immunity approach, allowing community transmission to occur relatively unchecked.[5]

Summing up the first eight months of the pandemic, Jonas Ludvigsson, an epidemiologist and senior pediatrician with a more sympathetic view of the Swedish strategy, notes that "Sweden's response was less invasive than many other countries, with no general lockdown. It focused on mitigation: slowing, but not stopping, the pandemic. Physical distancing was recommended in public spaces, but mandatory in bars, restaurants and at events. Visits to nursing facilities were banned. Kindergartens and schools for children up to 16 stayed open, but closed for older children for three months. There were no enforced quarantines for infected households or geographical regions, and face masks were not recommended outside health care."[6]

The Swedish pandemic strategy has been described as one of "nudging" rather than ordering or decreeing. Instead of closing borders and enforcing testing of returning winter holiday travellers in February and March 2020, the reaction of the Swedish government was remarkably passive: "For instance, direct flights from Iran and northern Italy were admitted even after the corona outbreak in these locales had become known to Swedish authorities. Passengers arriving from those stations were not screened when disembarking the flights, let alone quarantined."[7] Critics have pointed to this "nudging strategy" as an important reason for the rapid spread of the coronavirus in Sweden in the spring of 2020: "Early decisions had to be mandatory ones. To wait for public opinion to realize the stakes and mobilize itself voluntarily was futile."[8]

Certainly, the PHA issued recommendations about working from home whenever possible, about not making unnecessary travels on public transport and not meeting with people outside one's immediate family, about keeping distance, washing hands, and sneezing into one's elbow. But these were recommendations, not bans or prohibitions, and certainly not anything like the state of emergency introduced in Finland in the spring of 2020, during which borders were shut down and travel to and from the Uusimaa region (containing the capital Helsinki) was prohibited. Moreover, unlike the case in many other countries, the Swedish recommendations did not involve wearing face masks until January 2021, and then only on public transport and only in rush hours, with no penalties attached to non-compliance.

From the above accounts, it might appear as if the Swedish pandemic strategy was guided by a rights-based conception of the common good, prioritizing the individual right to freedom over the goal of preventing the spread of the coronavirus. However, I will argue that the Swedish strategy instead was driven by a utility-based conception of the common good and that it had a higher tolerance for the loss of human lives than would have been consistent with a rights-based conception of the common good.

3.2 Moral Conflicts in Pandemic Times: The Common Good vs. Individual Rights

Conflicts between public health and individual liberties are certainly not unique to pandemic times. We can here think of how advocates of an unrestrained market often have tried to prevent political interferences motivated by environmental or public health concerns. Here is Michael Walzer with one example: "Even something so simple, for example, as the provision of uncontaminated milk to large urban populations requires extensive public control; and control is a political achievement, the result (in the United States) of bitter struggles, over many years, in one city after another. When the farmers or the middlemen of the dairy industry defended free enterprise, they were certainly acting rationally in their own interests. The same thing can be said of other entrepreneurs who defend themselves against the constraints of inspection, regulation, and enforcement. Public activities of these sorts may be of the highest value to the rest of us; they are not of the highest value to all of us."[9]

John Rawls famously argued that "liberty can be restricted only for the sake of liberty itself".[10] However, he also maintained the value of protecting the common good: "Government is assumed to aim at the common good, that is, at maintaining conditions and achieving objectives that are similarly to everyone's advantage."[11] Given the reasonable assumption that it is to every citizen's advantage to avoid being the victim of a pandemic disease, and given that the pandemic itself may pose a threat to people's freedom (as they cannot move around freely without endangering their own health), it could be argued that the conflict between individual rights to various freedoms and pandemic restrictions might be more apparent than real. Still, even if pandemic restrictions may protect citizens' long-term freedom, they certainly restrict their short-term freedom.

In this context, we should also recognize that there are certain freedoms the suppression of which cannot be justified by the need to fight the COVID-19 pandemic – such as the freedoms of information and expression. The suppression of these freedoms actually played an important part in the outbreak of the pandemic, as the Chinese authorities initially were more concerned to stop the spread of information about the new coronavirus than they were to stop the spread of the virus itself.[12]

Now, the classical defence of individual rights to freedom has always come with the proviso that these rights do not protect actions that may unjustifiably harm others. Immanuel Kant argued that the kind of society best suited to enable human beings to develop all their natural capacities is one "which has not only the greatest freedom ... but also the most precise specification and preservation of the limits of this freedom in order that it can co-exist with the freedom of others".[13] According to John Stuart Mill, "the only purpose for which power can be rightfully exercised over any member of a civilized community, against his will, is to prevent harm to others".[14] Mill's argument has a bearing on the justification of pandemic restrictions on the right to freedom:

> Why think that the rights we enjoy in normal times don't apply in the pandemic? Simply because in normal times, exercising these rights does not harm others (or does so only minimally or unpredictably), whereas in a pandemic, leaving your house, going to work, meeting other people, etc., has a much higher chance of significantly harming others. And if many of us do these things, then it is certain that many people will be greatly harmed as a result.[15]

So, what we are looking for here is a kind of compromise between individual rights and the common good that Isaiah Berlin once formulated as "the maximum degree of non-interference compatible with the minimum demands of social life".[16] Such a goal is also reflected in the "Ethical Guidelines in Pandemic Influenza", adopted by the US Centers for Disease Control and Prevention, stating that a government should apply "the least restrictive practices that will allow the common good to be protected".[17] However, in order for us to make any use of such a principle, we need to know how to understand the concept of the common good.

According to one encyclopedia discussion of the concept, the common good of a political community "requires personal sacrifices only when these are indispensable to the maintenance of an organized community", adding that such sacrifices might be required not only in times of war: "Floods and pestilence supply equally compelling occasions for common efforts".[18] To fight a "pestilence" like COVID-19 will certainly require common efforts, but different conceptions of the common good may justify different kinds of personal sacrifices. I will here explore two different ways of conceptualizing the common good, one utility-based and the other rights-based, and with the help of these two conceptions I intend to clarify the aims and moral problems of the Swedish pandemic strategy.

3.3 A Utility-Based Conception of the Common Good

A utility-based conception of the common good defines this good as the greatest possible quantity of happiness, well-being, or satisfied preferences of some community. Utility-based conceptions of the common good have little use for the idea of individual rights. The common good of a community, according to Jeremy Bentham, the nineteenth century originator of utilitarianism, is simply "the sum of the interests of the several members who compose it", and "interest" is here to be understood in terms of happiness: "An action then may be said to be conformable to the principle of utility, or, for shortness sake, to utility (meaning with respect to the community at large), when the tendency it has to augment the happiness of the community is greater than any it has to diminish it."[19] Hence, utility is equivalent to the common good and "[t]he business of government is to promote the happiness of the society".[20]

Contemporary utilitarians tend to prefer to frame their discussion of the common good in terms of *preferences* rather than in terms of happiness. As rational persons, aware of the possibility that our present preferences may change in the future, R. M. Hare suggests that we embrace the goal that "the satisfaction of our now-for-now and then-for-then preferences should be maximized".[21] Accordingly, the contents of the common good – the maximal satisfaction of the preferences of a given community – will depend on the actual preferences of the members of that community. As Hare points out, "what ... principles of substantive justice are the best for a particular society to adopt will vary according to the circumstances of that society. These will include the propensities of its members; the fact that they are quite happy about social inequalities and would be made unhappy by the disturbance of them may make it best for them to have principles of justice which accord weight to them, until such time as social attitudes change."[22] Accordingly, the value of institutionalizing personal and political liberties in some particular community will depend on contingent empirical beliefs about such liberties promoting the goal of maximizing satisfied preferences within that community: "If these were shown to be false, then the same philosophical views about the nature of the moral argument involved might make me advocate slavery and tyranny."[23]

A utility-based conception of the common good, however, rests on two controversial assumptions. First of all, there is the assumption that it is possible to aggregate the happiness of individuals into a collective happiness. But does this collective happiness capture the moral quality of a community? Is a society with a large population, each member of which enjoys very little happiness, to be preferred over a society with a much smaller population, each member of which enjoys a lot of happiness, simply because the first society (due to its having so many members) has a higher total sum of happiness? (This is the so called *repugnant conclusion*—that a utilitarian whose only aim is to maximize the total sum of happiness is committed to prefer a society where everyone is in fact quite miserable.[24])

Second, utilitarianism assumes that we can aim to maximize happiness (or preference satisfaction) for a collective of individuals in much the same way as an individual person can aim to maximize happiness within her own life. At the personal level, we may well accept some sacrifices here and now (for instance, in terms of hard work) for the sake of increased well-being (for instance, in terms of having more money or higher social status) later on. However, if we try to maximize happiness for a *collective* of individuals in the same way as we try to maximize happiness for ourselves, we are likely to run into moral problems. The idea of maximizing collective happiness builds on the illusion that the sacrifices experienced by some individuals and the happiness enjoyed by some other individuals can be brought together in a net happiness experienced by the collectivity. However, as there is no collective being capable of enjoying that net happiness—there is "no *social entity* with a good that undergoes some sacrifice for its own good"[25]—what we do is simply to make some individuals unhappy and some other individuals happy, and that is all. But to inflict sacrifices on some people for the sake of making some other people happy is morally problematic, to say the least. It not only offends against the moral principle, associated with Immanuel Kant, that human beings should never be treated as merely means,[26] but also comes disturbingly close to Aristotle's description of slaves as human tools.[27]

When it comes to formulating a pandemic strategy from the point of view of a utility-based conception of the common good, the expected total consequences of various interventions will decide whether these interventions should be undertaken in the first place. Lives saved is just one factor among many others to be considered, and it is not necessarily the most important one.[28] According to philosophers sympathetic to utilitarianism, "utilitarianism does not necessarily seek to save most lives, but would aim to achieve the most well-being overall, including elements of both length of life and quality of life".[29] Now, people who get sick and die of course suffer a loss of well-being, but so do all those people who would be confined to their homes or lose their jobs as a result of curfews and lockdowns initiated to prevent a pandemic from spreading. The utility-based conception of the common good will be especially sensitive to the impact any pandemic strategy will have on societal institutions, such as hospitals and schools, due to their importance for the overall and long-term well-being of the population as a whole. For the same reason, what impact a strategy has on the economic strength and productivity of the political community is highly relevant according to a utility-based conception of the common good.

3.4 A Rights-Based Conception of the Common Good

A rights-based conception of the common good defines this good as the fulfilment of the moral rights of each and every member of some community. Arguing from the opposite end of utilitarianism, Robert Nozick famously defended an idea of moral rights that would go far to curtail any collectivist version of the common good. According to Nozick, such an idea of the common good would erase morally important boundaries between individuals, making each and every one of them a resource to be used for the benefit of the others:

> Each person has a claim to the activities and the products of other persons, independently of whether the other persons enter into particular relationships that give rise to these claims, and independently of whether they voluntarily take these claims upon themselves, in charity or in exchange for something. ... This process whereby they take this decision from you makes them a *part-owner* of you; it gives them a property right in you.[30]

Now, while Nozick manages to point out serious weaknesses in the utilitarian position, he is himself notoriously vague when it comes to delivering a positive argument for rights. Except for the peremptory declaration that "[i]ndividuals have rights, and there are things no person or group may do to them (without violating their rights)",[31] he does not provide his readers with any justification of the rights that play such an important role in his reasoning. Nozick's argument is based on intuitions, just as utilitarianism.

However, it is possible both to provide individual rights with a stronger foundation than mere intuitions and to formulate a conception of the common good that is consistent with and supportive of such rights. According to a theory of human rights developed by the Chicago philosopher Alan Gewirth, all human agents, simply by being agents, must claim rights to the necessary conditions of successful agency. By definition, agents want to achieve the ends for which they act—the point of any action is to achieve some goal that motivates the action in the first place. Of course, different agents have different ends. Some want to climb mountains, others are content to cultivate their garden. But common to all agents are certain conditions without which they either could not act at all or act only with limited chances of success. Hence, since every agent views the realization of the end of her action as something good, all agents must view as *necessary goods* the conditions without which successful agency in general would not be possible. (Here it can be noted that the philosopher and economist Amartya Sen's discussion of well-being in terms of people's "opportunity to achieve outcomes that they value and have reason to value"[32] has a similar focus on the needs of human agency; likewise, the philosopher James Griffin has related human rights to "normative agency" and the conditions required for "being able to make something good of our lives".[33])

Gewirth specifies the necessary conditions of successful agency as *freedom* and *well-being*. Freedom involves the ability to control one's behaviour in accordance with one's own unforced and informed choice, while well-being involves general physical and psychological conditions of agency (basic well-being), as well as the ability to maintain one's capacity for agency (nonsubtractive well-being) and the ability to expand that capacity (additive well-being). Basic well-being includes being alive and healthy, enjoying physical integrity and mental equilibrium; nonsubtractive well-being includes not being exposed to theft, slander, fraud, and similar attacks on one's capacity for successful agency; additive well-being, finally, includes having access to education, opportunities for earning an income, as well as possessing self-esteem and virtues such as prudence, temperance, and courage that work to strengthen one's capacity for successful agency.

That freedom and well-being are necessary goods means that no agent can logically accept to be deprived of them, since that would be inconsistent with the very identity of being an agent—that is, someone who wants to realize the ends of her actions. Hence, every agent must claim *rights* to the necessary conditions of successful agency. In Gewirth's words, "the agent is saying that because freedom and well-being are necessary goods for him, other persons strictly ought at least to refrain from interfering with his having them. And this is equivalent to saying that he has a right to them, because the agent holds that other persons owe him this strict duty of at least noninterference".[34]

So far this rights-claim is not moral but prudential, emanating from the agent's self-interest, that is, from her interest in not having the necessary conditions of her own successful agency interfered with. However, since the sufficient reason for the agent's rights-claim is that she is an agent (or, at least, a prospective agent), she must accept the generalization that *all* agents have rights to freedom and well-being: "This generalization is a direct application of the principle of universalizability; and if the agent denies the generalization, then … he contradicts himself. For on the one hand in holding, as he logically must, that he has the rights of freedom and well-being because he is a prospective purposive agent, he accepts that being a prospective purposive agent is a sufficient condition of having these rights; but if he denies the generalization, then he holds that being a prospective purposive agent is not a sufficient condition of having these rights."[35] Accordingly, every agent must rationally accept that all agents have rights to freedom and well-being; that is, every agent must rationally accept that there are *human rights* to freedom and well-being.

Now the rights of all agents to freedom and well-being will also play an important part in a rationally justified conception of the common good. Given that freedom and well-being are necessary goods for all agents, the common good of any political community must include the actual possession of these goods by each and every one of its members.

In pandemic times, a Gewirthian rights-based conception of the common good would not only justify but make mandatory governmental interventions of various kinds to protect citizens' right to basic well-being. These interventions may include restrictions on citizens' freedom of movement and assembly when this is necessary to prevent the spread of a potentially lethal illness. But an important part of the justification of restrictions on individual liberties imposed by governments in times of a pandemic comes from the fact that individual agents already have a moral duty not to expose each other to harmful actions, that is, actions that violate the right to basic well-being. And not only do agents have a duty not to harm each other, but, according to Gewirth, the right to basic well-being implies that agents also have a mutual duty to rescue each other from basic harm when they can do so at "no comparable cost" to themselves.[36]

Governments imposing pandemic restrictions on their citizens can then be viewed as making them fulfil this duty: "[C]onsidering the grave harms that even a single individual can cause through spreading an infectious disease, and that can in some cases be prevented through quarantine and isolation, enduring the constraints involved in quarantine and isolation might, *depending on the circumstances*, represent a moral obligation that is justified by a duty of easy rescue. The relevant question is if and when the cost to individuals is small enough."[37]

Likewise, business owners and companies would have a duty to do what they can to protect their employees and customers from being infected, even if this would have a negative impact on their profit margin. Such a duty to protect would include actions such as providing employees with opportunities for working from home and, when this is not an option, to take steps to make the workplace as safe as possible, providing employees with facemasks and disinfectants, and enabling them to practice social distancing by redesigning the workplace and spacing the use of common areas such as lifts and dining rooms.[38]

As the above explanation suggests, a Gewirthian rights-based conception of the common good acknowledges that some rights can only be accomodated at the cost of overriding some other rights. Life and health are protected at the cost of foregoing economic gain and limiting social interaction and freedom. However, this is because some rights are more important than others. Gewirth outlines a *criterion of degrees of needfulness for action* that enables his theory to handle conflicts of rights without having to invoke any kind of utilitarian considerations. According to this criterion, "[w]hen two rights are in conflict with one another, that right takes precedence whose object is more needed for action".[39] Hence, in case of a conflict, the right to basic well-being takes priority over the rights to nonsubtractive and additive well-being. The criterion of degrees of needfulness for action explains this priority by pointing to the fact that basic well-being is more important to agency than nonsubtractive and additive well-being, in the sense that without basic well-being we will not be able to act at all or only to a generally reduced extent, while lack of nonsubtractive and additive well-being will only affect our capacity to perform particular actions but otherwise leave our general capacity for agency unaffected. Hence, in case one has to choose between stopping one's car and rescue a gravely injured person or being in time for a meeting that will secure a profitable employment for oneself, one has to give priority to the basic well-being of the injured person over one's own additive well-being.

The criterion of degrees of needfulness for action would justify a pandemic strategy that limits the rights to freedom of movement and assembly for the sake of preventing deaths and other losses of basic well-being; it would also justify lockdowns that deprive business owners and their employees of income for the sake of preventing deaths and serious cases of illness. However, it would not justify a pandemic strategy that itself would cause people to suffer a loss of basic well-being, such as a lockdown that makes it impossible for people to feed themselves. It is also important to note that the ranking of rights suggested by the criterion of degrees of needfulness for action does not mean that a Gewirthian rights-based conception of the common good would be insensitive to the losses involved when less important rights are overridden. That certain rights can be overridden does not change the fact that they are still rights and that we should do what we can to minimize the negative effects of not being able to uphold them:

> If schools are closed, leaving low-income children without school breakfasts and lunch, authorities should arrange for children and families to receive food at home. Paid sick leave should be afforded to people temporarily out of work due to quarantines, isolation, business closures, or lack of childcare. People with disabilities and their caregivers should receive funding to ensure that their needs are met and to cover extra costs, such as for home delivery of food and other necessities.[40]

People forced to stay at home in a lockdown society might develop depressive and other psychiatric illnesses or suffer from domestic violence; hence, governments have a moral responsibility to care for these people and to find ways of relieving them of their distress. This responsibility applies to the COVID-19 pandemic, as "the evidence from national stay-at-home orders suggests that isolation, mental illness, domestic abuse, the burdens of care-giving, and hunger have been on the rise".[41]

Hence, from the point of view of a rights-based conception of the common good, if a government shuts down businesses or orders its citizens to isolate themselves for the sake of preventing a pandemic from spreading, it is also morally obligated to try to compensate them for this invasion of their rights. However, in this context it is also important to ensure that compensations to the business sector have a human rights focus rather than a focus on just keeping the economy going. Relief and support should be designed to help vulnerable individual citizens and employees rather than redistributing tax-payers' money to corporations that have chosen to register in tax havens or continue to pay out dividends to its shareholders while at the same time demanding that the state look after their employees.[42]

3.5 Understanding the Swedish COVID-19 Strategy and Its Conception of the Common Good

The Swedish pandemic strategy, including its view of how to protect the common good, was not formulated by the Swedish government, but by its "expert authority", that is, the Public Health Agency (PHA). Accordingly, "the core executive, i.e. the Prime Minister and other Cabinet ministers and their staff, would not be operationally involved in the crisis management".[43] At the outbreak of the pandemic the government chose to take a back seat to the PHA, satisfying itself with repeating the recommendations issued by that agency.

This was also how the PHA perceived the situation. "We are the ones holding the baton", Johan Carlson, the Director-General of the PHA, confidently told reporters in March, 2020, comparing himself and the PHA to the conductor of an orchestra.[44] It has been argued that one reason why the Swedish response to the pandemic was so relaxed was that the PHA was left in an unopposed position to control the contents of the strategy: "Crucially, ... there was never sufficient pressure on the agency from any quarter to effect change during the initial phase of the pandemic, even as the agency's strategy appeared to be going wrong in late spring 2020. This ... was due to the organisational insulation from political influence that the agency had already acquired".[45]

Now, to understand the conception of the common good implicit in the Swedish COVID-19 strategy, one needs to clarify its underlying normative beliefs. These beliefs are not always stated explicitly, but are sometimes implied in, for instance, risk assessments. A risk is conventionally defined as "the chance of an undesirable outcome".[46] Accordingly, the risk of a possible outcome will depend in part on how undesirable it is, and the undesirability will in turn reflect the normative beliefs of the people making the risk assessment—in this case, beliefs that certain outcomes *should* or *must* be avoided.

According to Johan Carlson, the Director-General of the Swedish PHA, the focus of the Swedish pandemic strategy has been "to avoid overresponding" and, more specifically, "to avoid a forced lock down, penalties etc.".[47] When the Swedish Civil Contingencies Agency in early February 2020 asked other governmental agencies and authorities to describe their analysis of the coronavirus pandemic, the PHA replied that its aim was "to calm authorities so that they do not overreact" and to "handle the public" with regard to people who are "worried or spread untrue information"; the focus was on preventing "wrongful scenarios" emanating from "ignorant authorities, regions, or political decisions".[48] From the outset, then, the Swedish strategy was just as much concerned with possible harmful effects of attempts to contain the pandemic as with the harmful effects to be expected from the pandemic itself. This suggests a utility-based rather than a rights-based conception of the common good, focusing on consequences for the society in general rather than on the rights of individual citizens not to be infected.

When the PHA has defended its strategy, it has focused on structural and institutional achievements rather than on the impact on human lives. In October 2020, Anders Tegnell, the state epidemiologist, claimed that the Swedish pandemic strategy during spring had been "reasonably successful", since "the Swedish healthcare was never overwhelmed".[49] At the time, close to 6,000 persons had already died from COVID-19, and Sweden had among the highest rates of COVID-19 deaths per million people in the world.[50]

Of course, it could be argued that protecting health-care institutions is valuable because they in turn protect the well-being of human individuals, and that hence there is no conflict between protecting health-care institutions and protecting the lives of individual human beings. However, there is still a difference between having as one's immediate goal to protect human lives, and having as one's immediate goal to protect health-care institutions while having the protection of individual human lives as only a secondary or indirect goal, allowing many people to die in the process. Moreover, if the goal was to protect health-care institutions from being overwhelmed, why not then aim for a more restrictive strategy that would limit the number of people who got infected with the coronavirus in the first place? If the spread of the coronavirus had been prevented early in the spring of 2020 by restrictions similar to those that proved effective in the other Nordic countries, it is reasonable to assume that Sweden could have managed *both* to save more lives *and* to lessen the burden on its health-care sector. Presumably, the architects of the Swedish strategy believed that the overall societal costs of lockdowns, travel bans, stay-at-home orders, and similar invasive methods would be too high—that is, these restrictions would be inconsistent with a utility-based conception of the common good.

The Swedish strategy had as one of its goal to "flatten the curve", rather than stopping the virus from spreading: "[W]e aim to flatten the curve, slowing down the spread as much as possible—otherwise the health-care system and society are at risk of collapse", the Swedish state epidemiologist Anders Tegnell explained in an interview with the journal *Nature*.[51] Here, once again, the primary focus is on protecting institutions, not individual human lives. This can be contrasted with the strategy implemented by, for instance, New Zealand. There the Prime Minister, Jacinda Ardern, early on decided to "adopt a more aggressive and ambitious approach than just 'flattening the curve', aiming to position New Zealand to achieve eradication of the virus within its borders".[52] In adopting this strategy, and in implementing a lockdown already late in March, 2020, Prime Minister Ardern noted the fact that New Zealand at the time had only 102 corona cases, but added "so did Italy once" and now that country faced a situation in which "hundreds of people are dying every day". If the spread of the virus were to be left unchecked, the Prime Minister concluded, "tens of thousands of New Zealanders will die".[53]

Another assumption of the PHA was that lockdowns and similar invasive kinds of restrictions would not work, simply because people would not obey them. Hence, the PHA argued that "the less onerous the restrictions on personal behaviour, the more sustainable they would be."[54] While this seems a reasonable enough assumption, it also implies that one is willing to accept a certain number of extra deaths for the sake of not inconveniencing the Swedish public too much. Here we should note a study, made by the US Department of Health and Human Services, claiming that "European countries that implemented more stringent mitigation policies earlier in their outbreak response ... might have saved several thousand lives relative to countries that implemented similar policies, but later."[55] Hence, refraining from introducing "stringent mitigation policies" in times of a pandemic can be expected to come with a price in human lives.

Certainly, the Swedish PHA did claim that its strategy to combat COVID-19 was intended to "minimise mortality and morbidity in the entire population and to minimise other negative consequences for individual persons and society".[56] But this very combination of goals allows for utilitarian trade-offs between saving lives and other goals. Minimizing "negative consequences for individual persons and society" implies that preventing COVID-19 deaths is not necessarily the top priority. A lockdown may save lives but also disrupt the national economy, create unemployment, and deprive people of their livelihood, which in turn also may have negative consequences for people's health. Depending on how much value a utilitarian assigns to a person's life (which in turn might depend on the person's age, productivity, and so on), she might come to the conclusion that the common good is better served by accepting a certain spread of the coronavirus than by introducing a lockdown.

Now, the Swedish PHA has never made any statement to the effect that it embraces a utility-based conception of the common good. However, perhaps the PHA does not need to be explicit about its moral assumptions as utilitarian ways of thinking are well entrenched in the history of the Swedish welfare state. For instance, it has been observed about Sweden that "[a]s an old no-nonsense eugenic social democracy, it can assume a health utilitarian line".[57] (The word "eugenic" in this quote refers, among other things, to a law recommending sterilization for eugenic reasons; the law, proposed by a Social Democratic government in 1934, was in force until 1976.)

It has been argued that the "strong emphasis on individual responsibility as a specific trait of the Swedish strategy is closely related [to] the postmodern emphasis on individuality and opposition to authority".[58] This conclusion does not seem to fit the facts of the case. First of all, as we have seen above, the Swedish strategy was not focused primarily on upholding the rights of individuals, but on protecting societal institutions and collective well-being. Second, those who criticized the strategy were quickly reminded that authorities were not to be opposed without repercussions. At one point it was considered almost tantamount to treason to suggest that the PHA's way of dealing with the pandemic might be mistaken. An epidemiologist who had criticized the PHA strategy was accused by her head of department for undermining the work of the PHA and for being "a danger to society".[59]

In a *Financial Times* interview in September 2020 Anders Tegnell, the state epidemiologist, dismissed lockdowns as "using a hammer to kill a fly".[60] This brings to mind Director-General Carlson's fear of "overresponding" to the pandemic. But it also suggests a preparedness to accept at least a certain spread of the coronavirus and thereby also a certain number of COVID-19 deaths for the sake of not having to bring in the "hammer".

Johan Giesecke, former state epidemiologist and consultant to the PHA, agreed: "[O]ur most important task is not to stop spread, which is all but futile, but to concentrate on giving the unfortunate victims optimal care".[61] Giesecke was also quoted arguing that the many deaths of old people that occurred in Sweden should be considered as a reasonable price to be paid for avoiding a lockdown: "People who will die a few months later are dying now. And that's taking months from their lives, so that's maybe not nice. But [compare] that to the effects of the lockdown."[62]

The implication here is that the deaths of people who would have died in a short time anyway is not such a great loss compared to the restrictions suffered by the rest of the community if there is a lockdown. This is the "Fair innings argument" – the idea that "the young have stronger claims to lifesaving interventions than older persons because they have had fewer opportunities to experience life. The false implication arising from this argument is that saving 1 year for a young person is valued more than saving 1 year of life for an older person."[63] Utilitarian thinking is here combined with ageist stereotypes, normalizing that old people die when they get sick and, consequently, also normalizing that less resources are spent on curing them compared to the resources spent on younger patients affected by the same disease.[64]

Such a way of thinking reduces a patient to her age cohort and ignores her individual life story and the values that come with it.

Utilitarians would agree with Giesecke's argument: "[T]reatment that saves people's lives for longer is to be preferred over treatments that save life for shorter periods. ... Because older people tend to die sooner than younger people, utilitarianism tends to favour saving the lives of the younger."[65] This way of thinking also affects how utilitarians perceive the value of lockdowns: "[I]f the pandemic largely affects patients with short life expectancy, the benefit of a lockdown (preventing deaths) would be smaller than a different illness that affected younger patients. ... [E]ven if lockdown were cost-effective, it would not be as cost-effective as different interventions that save babies or young people."[66]

Another line of argument that suggests a utility-based conception of the common good is the one about herd immunity. At one point, Anders Tegnell, the state epidemiologist, expressed his belief that "[e]ach country has to reach 'herd immunity' in one way or another, and we are going to reach it in a different way".[67] This statement is interesting, as the official position of the PHA has been that herd immunity is not part of the Swedish strategy, but only a possible result of it. The reason for this unwillingness to officially embrace herd immunity is, of course, that such a position would imply a willingness to let people get infected and die for the sake of achieving a collective immunity. In another interview, Tegnell added to the confusion about herd immunity by saying that "the main strategy was to have a slow transmission of COVID-19 so that the healthcare system could manage, but that herd immunity was 'not contradictory' with this", adding that "herd immunity was a 'great concept'."[68] Mail correspondence between Tegnell and his Finnish colleague Mika Salminen suggests that Tegnell in March 2020 also considered achieving herd immunity as a reason for keeping schools open during the pandemic.[69]

Although the PHA has been careful not to claim herd immunity as a goal of the Swedish strategy, both Tegnell and Giesecke have expressed themselves in a way that suggests that "post-infection immunity" would be a desirable consequence of the strategy. And here "the difference between a goal and a by-product might be considered largely semantic".[70]

3.6 Conclusions

In spite of its reluctance to interfere with individual rights to freedoms of movement and assembly, there are strong indications that the Swedish pandemic strategy emanated from a utility-based rather than a rights-based conception of the common good. If individual rights had indeed been at the centre of the PHA decisions, these decisions would have had as their focus to protect the right to basic well-being of all those people who got infected and later died from COVID-19. Then the loss of old people's lives would not have been considered as preferable to the costs of a lockdown—at least not as long as the lockdown itself did not produce outcomes in which people died or got seriously ill. Nor would it have been considered permissible to let people get infected and die as long as this did not overwhelm health-care institutions. Hence, even if the strategy avoided restrictions on individual rights to free movement and assembly, it can still be argued that it was lacking in respect of individual rights. Paradoxically as it may seem, its very unwillingness to limit various individual liberties made the Swedish pandemic strategy unprotective of Swedish citizens' right to basic well-being.

Notes

1. Savage (2020, 33).
2. Collins, Florin and Renn (2020).
3. Government Offices of Sweden, "COVID-19 Act allows stronger communicable disease control measures", at https://www.government.se/articles/2021/01/covid-19-act-allows-stronger-communicable-disease-control-measures/ [Accessed on January, 20, 2021].
4. Johns Hopkins Coronavirus Resource Center, "Cases and mortality by country", at https://coronavirus.jhu.edu/data/mortality [Accessed on January 21, 2021].
5. Claeson and Hanson (2021, 259).
6. Ludvigsson (2020, 2459).
7. Pierre (2020, 484).
8. Baldwin (2021, 287).
9. Walzer (1996, 81).
10. Rawls (1972, 244).
11. Rawls (1972, 233).
12. Spadaro (2020, 323).
13. Kant (1991, 45).
14. Mill (1998, 14).
15. Bramble (2020, 17).
16. Berlin (1997, 232).
17. Kinlaw, Barrett and Levine (2009, 187).
18. Braybrooke and Monahan (2001, 263).
19. Bentham (1948, 126–127).
20. Bentham (1948, 189).
21. Hare (1981, 105).
22. Hare (1981, 159).
23. Hare (1981, 167).
24. Parfit (1984, 387–388).
25. Nozick (1974, 32–33); emphasis in the original.
26. Kant (1964, 96; Ak. 429).
27. Aristotle (1981, 64–65 (1253b)).
28. Bellazzi and Boyneburgk (2020).
29. Savulescu, Persson and Wilkinson (2020, 626).
30. Nozick (1974, 172); emphasis in the original.
31. Nozick (1974, ix).

32. Sen (1999, 291).
33. Griffin (2008, 48).
34. Gewirth (1978, 79–80).
35. Gewirth (1978, 112).
36. Gewirth (1978, 218).
37. Giubilini et al. (2018, 185–186); emphasis in the original.
38. Tripathi (2020, 254).
39. Gewirth (1996, 45).
40. Gostin, Friedman and Wetter (2020, 10).
41. Anand et al. (2020, 294).
42. Bohoslavsky (2020).
43. Pierre (2020, 483).
44. Örstadius, Delin and Eriksson, "Så gick det till när regeringen gav taktpinnen till expertmyndigheten" [How the government handed over the baton to the expert authority], *Dagens Nyheter*, March 15, 2020, at https://www.dn.se/nyheter/sverige/sa-gick-det-till-nar-regeringen-gav-taktpinnen-till-expertmyndigheten/ [Accessed on January 16, 2020].
45. Andersson and Aylott (2020, 12).
46. Yoe (2012, 1).
47. Public Health Agency of Sweden, "The Swedish strategy about COVID-19", at https://www.folkhalsomyndigheten.se/the-public-health-agency-of-sweden/communicable-disease-control/covid-19/covid-19--the-swedish-strategy/ [Accessed on January 15, 2021].
48. Engström, "Folkhälsomyndigheten bromsade starten på krishanteringen av covid-19" [The Public Health Agency slowed down the start of the crisis management of COVID-19], at http://mengstrom.blogspot.com/2020/09/folkhalsomyndigheten-bromsade-starten.html [Accessed on March 17, 2021].
49. Eaton, "Trust is vital if you want to stop this disease", *New Statesman*, 23–29 October 2020, 16.
50. Our World in Data, "Cumulative confirmed COVID-19 deaths per million people", at https://ourworldindata.org/covid-deaths?country=~SWE#cumulative-confirmed-deaths-per-million-people [Accessed on February 28, 2021].
51. Paterlini, "'Closing borders is ridiculous': the epidemiologist behind Sweden's controversial coronavirus strategy", *Nature*, 21 April 2020, at https://www.nature.com/articles/d41586-020-01098-x [Accessed on 29 December, 2020].
52. Wilson (2020, 281).
53. Wilson (2020, 282).
54. Andersson and Aylott (2020, 3).
55. Fuller et al. (2021, 59).
56. The Public Health Agency of Sweden, "The Public Health Agency of Sweden's work with COVID-19", at https://www.folkhalsomyndigheten.se/the-public-health-agency-of-s.../covid-19/the-public-health-agency-of-swedens-work-with-covid-19/ [Accessed on December 29, 2020].
57. Häyry (2021, 48).
58. Lindström (2020, 4).

59. Vogel (2020, 161).
60. Milne, "Anders Tegnell and the Swedish Covid experiment", *Financial Times*, September 11, 2020, at https://www.ft.com/content/5cc92d45-fbdb-43b7-9c66-26501693a371 [Accessed on January 22, 2021].
61. Giesecke (2020, e98).
62. Bramble (2020, 11).
63. Jeffrey (2020, 497).
64. D'cruz and Banerjee (2020).
65. Savulescu et al. (2020, 623).
66. Savulescu et al. (2020, 623–624).
67. Paterlini, "Closing borders is ridiculous".
68. Irwin (2020, 5).
69. Emanuel Karlsten, "Så fick begreppet flockimmunitet fäste på myndigheten" ["How the concept of herd immunity gained a foothold in the [Public Health] Agency", *Expressen*, August 12, 2020, at https://www.expressen.se/nyheter/qs/interna-radslaget-om-flockimmunitet/ [Accessed on February 8, 2020].
70. Andersson and Aylott (2020, 5).

Bibliography

Anand, Paul, Bob Ferrer, Qin Gao, Ricardo Nogales, and Ellaine Unterhalter. 2020. COVID-19 as a Capability Crisis: Using the Capability Framework to Understand Policy Challenges. *Journal of Human Development and Capabilities* 21 (3): 293–299.
Andersson Staffan, and Nicholas Aylott. 2020. Sweden and Coronavirus: Unexceptional Exceptionalism. *Social Sciences* 9 (12): 1–19. Open access. DOI: https://doi.org/10.3390/socsci9120232.
Aristotle. 1981. *The Politics*. London: Penguin Books.
Baldwin, Peter. 2021. *Fighting the First Wave*. Cambridge: Cambridge University Press.
Bellazzi, Francesca, and Konrad v. Boyneburgk. 2020. COVID-19 Calls for Virtue Ethics. *Journal of Law and the Biosciences* 7 (1): 1–8. Advance online publication. Doi:https://doi.org/10.1093/jlb/lsaa056.
Bentham, Jeremy. 1948. An Introduction to the Principles of Morals and Legislation. In *A Fragment on Government and An Introduction to the Principles of Morals and Legislation*, ed. Wilfrid Harrison, 113–435. Oxford: Basil Blackwell.
Berlin, Isaiah. 1997. Two Concepts of Liberty. In *The Proper Study of Mankind*, ed. Henry Hardy and Roger Hausheer, 191–242. London: Chatto & Windus.
Bohoslavsky, Juan Pablo. 2020. COVID-19 Economy vs Human Rights: A Misleading Dichotomy. *Health and Human Rights Journal* 22 (1): 383–385.
Bramble, Ben. 2020. *Pandemic Ethics*. Sydney: Bartleby Books. Released in Open Access and available at https://philpapers.org/archive/BRAPE-7.pdf.
Braybrooke, David, and Arthur P. Monahan. 2001. Common Good. In *Encyclopedia of Ethics*, ed. Lawrence C. Becker and Charlotte B. Becker, 262–266. New York and London: Routledge.
Claeson, Mariam, and Stefan Hanson. 2021. COVID-19 and the Swedish enigma. *The Lancet* 397 (10271): 259–261.
Collins, Aengus, Marie-Valentine. Florin, and Ortwin Renn. 2020. COVID-19 Risk Governance: Drivers, Responses and Lessons to be Learned. *Journal of Risk Research* 23 (7–8): 1073–1082.

D'cruz, Migita, and Debanjan Banerjee. 2020. 'An Invisible Human Rights Crisis': The Marginalization of Older Adults During the COVID-19 Pandemic – An Advocacy View". *Psychiatry Research* 292: 1–9. Advance online publication. Doi: https://doi.org/10.1016/j.psychres.2020.113369.

Eaton, George. Trust is Vital if You Want to Stop this Disease. *New Statesman*, 23–29 October 2020: 16–17.

Engström, Mats. Folkhälsomyndigheten bromsade starten på krishanteringen av covid-19 [The Public Health Agency slowed down the start of the crisis management of COVID-19]. http://mengstrom.blogspot.com/2020/09/folkhalsomyndigheten-bromsade-starten.html [Accessed on March 17, 2021].

Fuller, James A., Avi Hakim, Kerton R. Victory et al. 2021. Mitigation Policies and COVID-19-Associated Mortality – 37 European Countries, January 23 – June 30, 2020. *Morbidity and Mortality Weekly Report* 70 (2): 58–62.

Gewirth, Alan. 1978. *Reason and Morality*. Chicago: The University of Chicago Press.

Gewirth, Alan. 1996. *The Community of Rights*. Chicago: The University of Chicago Press.

Giesecke, Johan. 2020. The Invisible Pandemic. *The Lancet*, 395 (10238), e98.

Gostin, Lawrence O., Eric A. Friedman, and Sarah A. Wetter. 2020. How to Navigate a Public Health Emergency Legally and Ethically. *Hastings Center Report* 50 (2): 8–12.

Government Offices of Sweden. COVID-19 Act Allows Stronger Communicable Disease Control Measures. https://www.government.se/articles/2021/01/covid-19-act-allows-stronger-communicable-disease-control-measures/ [Accessed on January 20, 2021].

Griffin, James. 2008. *On Human Rights*. Oxford: Oxford University Press.

Giubilini, Alberto, Thomas Douglas, Hannah Maslen, and Julian Savulescu. 2018. Quarantine, Isolation and the Duty of Easy Rescue in Public Health. *Developing World Bioethics* 18 (2): 182–189.

Hare, R.M. 1981. *Moral Thinking*. Oxford: Clarendon Press.

Häyry, Matti. 2021. The COVID-19 Pandemic: Healthcare Crisis Leadership as Ethics Communication. *Cambridge Quarterly of Healthcare Ethics* 30 (1): 42–50.

Irwin, Rachel Elisabeth. 2020. Misinformation and De-Contextualization: International Media Reporting on Sweden and COVID-19. *Globalization and Health* 16 (62): 1–12. Open access. Doi: https://doi.org/10.1186/s12992-020-00588-x.

Jeffrey, David Ian. 2020. Relational Ethical Approaches to the COVID-19 Pandemic. *Journal of Medical Ethics* 46 (8): 495–498.

Johns Hopkins Coronavirus Resource Center. Cases and mortality by country. https://coronavirus.jhu.edu/data/mortality [Accessed on January 21, 2021].

Kant, Immanuel. 1964. *Groundwork of the Metaphysic of Morals*. New York, NY: Harper & Row.

Kant, Immanuel. 1991. Idea for a Universal History with a Cosmopolitan Purpose. In *Political Writings*, ed. Hans Reiss, 41–53. Cambridge: Cambridge University Press.

Karlsten, Emanuel. Så fick begreppet flockimmunitet fäste på myndigheten ["How the Concept of Herd Immunity Gained a Foothold in the [Public Health] Agency". *Expressen*, August 12, 2020. https://www.expressen.se/nyheter/qs/interna-radslaget-om-flockimmunitet/ [Accessed on February 8, 2020].

Kinlaw, Kathy, Drue H. Barrett, and Robert J. Levine. 2009. Ethical Guidelines in Pandemic Influenza: Recommendations of the Ethics Subcommittee of the Advisory Committee of the Director, Centers for Disease Control and Prevention. *Disaster Medicine and Public Health Preparedness* 3 (S 2): 185–192.

Lindström, Martin. 2020. The COVID-19 Pandemic and the Swedish Strategy: Epidemiology and Postmodernism. *Social Science & Medicine – Population Health* 11: 1–5. Open access. Doi: https://doi.org/10.1016/j.ssmph.2020.100643.

Ludvigsson, Jonas. 2020. The First Eight Months of Sweden's COVID-19 Strategy and the Key Actions and Actors that were Involved. *Acta Paediatrica* 109 (12): 2459–2471.

Mill, John Stuart. 1998. *On Liberty*. In *On Liberty and Other Essays*, edited by John Gray, 1–128. Oxford: Oxford University Press.

Milne, Richard. Anders Tegnell and the Swedish Covid experiment. *Financial Times*, September 11, 2020. https://www.ft.com/content/5cc92d45-fbdb-43b7-9c66-26501693a371 [Accessed on January 22, 2021].

Nozick, Robert. 1974. *Anarchy, State, and Utopia*. Oxford: Basil Blackwell.

Kristoffer Örstadius, Mikael Delin, and Karin Eriksson. Så gick det till när regeringen gav taktpinnen till expertmyndigheten [How the Government Handed Over the Baton to the Expert Authority]. *Dagens Nyheter*, March 15, 2020. https://www.dn.se/nyheter/sverige/sa-gick-det-till-nar-regeringen-gav-taktpinnen-till-expertmyndigheten/ [Accessed on January 16, 2020.]

Our World in Data. Cumulative Confirmed COVID-19 Deaths per Million People. https://ourworldindata.org/covid-deaths?country=~SWE#cumulative-confirmed-deaths-per-million-people [Accessed on February 28, 2021].

Parfit, Derek. 1984. *Reasons and Persons*. Oxford: Clarendon Press.

Paterlini, Marta. 'Closing Borders is Ridiculous': The Epidemiologist Behind Sweden's Controversial Coronavirus Strategy. *Nature*, 21 April 2020. https://www.nature.com/articles/d41586-020-01098-x [Accessed on December 29, 2020].

Pierre, Jon. 2020. Nudges Against Pandemics: Sweden's COVID-19 Containment Strategy in Perspective. *Policy and Society* 39 (3): 478–493.

Public Health Agency of Sweden. The Public Health Agency of Sweden's Work with COVID-19. https://www.folkhalsomyndigheten.se/the-public-health-agency-of-s.../covid-19/the-public-health-agency-of-swedens-work-with-covid-19/ [Accessed on December 29, 2020].

Public Health Agency of Sweden. The Swedish Strategy about COVID-19. https://www.folkhalsomyndigheten.se/the-public-health-agency-of-sweden/communicable-disease-control/covid-19/covid-19--the-swedish-strategy/ [Accessed on January 15, 2021].

Rawls, John. 1972. *A Theory of Justice*. Oxford: Oxford University Press.

Savage, James. A Failed Strategy. *New Statesman*, 19–25 June 2020: 33.

Savulescu, Julian, Ingmar Persson, and Dominic Wilkinson. 2020. Utilitarianism and the Pandemic. *Bioethics* 34 (6): 620–632.

Sen, Amartya. 1999. *Development as Freedom*. Oxford: Oxford University Press.

Spadaro, Alessandra. 2020. COVID-19: Testing the Limits of Human Rights. *European Journal of Risk Regulation* 11 (2): 317–325.

Tripathi, Salil. 2020. Companies, COVID-19 and Respect for Human Rights. *Business and Human Rights Journal* 5 (2): 252–260.

Vogel, Gretchen. 2020. Sweden's Gamble. *Science* 370 (6513): 159–163.

Walzer, Michael. 1996. *Spheres of Justice*. Oxford: Blackwell.

Wilson, Suze. 2020. Pandemic Leadership: Lessons from New Zealand's Approach to COVID-19. *Leadership* 16 (3): 279–293.

Yoe, Charles. 2012. *Principles of Risk Analysis: Decision Making Under Uncertainty*. Boca Raton, FL: CRC Press.

Chapter 4
Formal Epistemology Meets a Coronavirus: Rational Decision and the Response to Covid-19

Sahotra Sarkar

Abstract Techniques from formal epistemology can be used to provide decision support during the formulation of societal policy responses to pandemics such as Covid-19. The complexity of these decisions arises from multiple sources including incompatible values of stakeholders. These differences in values result in conflicting objectives which can be studied using formal multicriteria decision analysis. An important component of multicriteria analysis is the construction of an objectives hierarchy (OH) to represent the conflicting values. This paper points out the benefits of constructing such a hierarchy through public deliberation. It shows all stakeholders where tradeoffs must be made between divergent values such as halting disease spread and unfettered economic activity.

Keywords Coronavirus · Covid-19 · Decision theory · Formal epistemology · Multicriteria analysis · Pandemic · SARS-CoV-19

4.1 Introduction

According to the official story of Covid-19, samples taken from the lungs of a pneumonia patient in Wuhan (China) on 30 December 2019 showed for the first time the presence of a previously unknown coronavirus (Horton 2020). The Chinese authorities reacted immediately, shut down the region completely and the rest of the country within three weeks. China promptly informed the world of the emergence of a new coronavirus disease. The rest of the world reacted in a disorganized *ad hoc* fashion. Though China was able to shut down the virus, a global pandemic erupted that is still not under control in much of the world.

However, given the lack of transparency on the part of Chinese authorities about what exactly transpired in Wuhan around that time, it is impossible to determine the extent to which the official story is true. It is known that local authorities acted severely against the first physician, the opthalmologist Li Wenliang, who tried to raise

S. Sarkar (✉)
University of Texas, Austin, TX, USA
e-mail: sakar@austin.utexas.edu

© The Author(s), under exclusive license to Springer Nature Switzerland AG 2022
M. Boylan (ed.), *Ethical Public Health Policy Within Pandemics*, The International Library of Bioethics 95, https://doi.org/10.1007/978-3-030-99692-5_3

an alarm about the possible emergence of a new coronavirus similar to the one that had caused the SARS (severe acute respiratory syndrome) outbreak in 2002–2003 (Green 2020).[1]

It is also true that, perhaps because they did not want a repetition of their perceived poor handling of the 2002–2003 SARS outbreak, the Chinese authorities in Beijing did immediately inform the World Health Organization (WHO) of the emergence of what came to be known as the SARS-CoV-2 virus (Horton 2020). They also isolated the virus and sequenced its (RNA) genome promptly and shared the results publicly on 12 January 2021. Meanwhile case counts exploded in Wuhan and China went into lockdown on 20 January.

At WHO, its director-general, Tedros Adhanom Ghebreyesus, convened the International Health Regulations (IHR) Emergency Committee to determine whether a declaration of a Public Health Emergency of International Concern (PHEIC), was warranted. Two criteria must be met for such a declaration: first, a disease outbreak must be "an extraordinary event which is determined to constitute a public health risk to other States through the international spread of disease" and, second, controlling the spread of the disease must "potentially require a coordinated international response" (WHO 2005). On 28 January 2020, after a month of discussion (some would say dithering), WHO finally declared a PHEIC thus setting into play legally binding rules "to prevent, protect against, control, and and provide a public health response to the international spread of disease" (Horton 2020, p. 5).

WHO eventually declared a Covid-19 pandemic on 17 March 2020. Part of the hesitation was due to there being no internal technical definition of "pandemic" within WHO. There was also a worry that the use of "pandemic" had previously been restricted to major global flu outbreaks and Covid-19 clearly presented a different and more dangerous situation than any flu outbreak. Also, for some WHO policymakers, declaring a pandemic was also a counsel of despair, suggesting that efforts should move away from containment to focus on mitigation. As Tedros put it: "Pandemic is not a word to use lightly or carelessly. It is a word that, if misused, can cause unreasonable fear, or unjustified acceptance that the fight is over, leading to unnecessary suffering and death" (WHO 2020). Tedros, therefore, went on to insist that WHO would not change course in spite of recognizing a pandemic, continuing to focus on prevention.

What followed next is well-known. There was no semblance of a coordinated global response. Baldwin (2021) has documented the extent to which responses varied from country to country; in the case of the United States the responses varied just as radically from state to state. According to Baldwin the presence of such variation belied the extent to which "the etiological understanding of Covid-19 was largely uniform across the globe" (p. 18). In a sense this is correct: there was no dispute that the causal agent of Covid-19 is the SARS-CoV-2 virus. Similarly it was beyond dispute that aerosolized virus constituted a major mode of disease transmission.

However, beyond this basic understanding, there was little consensus because of a profound ignorance about the basic biology of the virus and epidemiology of the disease. For instance, no one was sure how long the virus remained infectious on different surfaces or about the efficacy of different disinfectants applied to these surfaces. There was no agreement about the airborne transmissibility of the virus between individuals, that is, what constituted an adequate "social distance" to prevent transmission. No one knew the influence of temperature or humidity in the persistence of the virus. There was even less agreement about the performance of different materials as facial masks.

These disagreements were the result of a lack of data; not about interpretation of ambiguous data. The lack of data was surprising for two reasons: there is good reason to expect that some or the required information would have been collected during work on the SARS-CoV-1 virus that caused the 2002–2003 SARS outbreak. Moreover, experimentally, some of these data would not have been hard to collect so long as one had access to a biosecure laboratory. Measuring the permeability of a virus across a cloth membrane does not require overwhelming technological facility or experimental acuity.

Nevertheless, Baldwin is correct in his assessment that the differences in response to the pandemic on the part of different governing bodies cannot be explained by uncertainties and disagreements about scientific facts. Rather, he concludes, the differences arise from the differences in the political tools available, the extent to which governments could impose restrictions on the lives of citizens and the extent of compliance to these restrictions. These differences are no doubt important but, as this paper will argue that in the case of Covid-19 responses, as in many other contexts of public policy decisions, the policy differences reflect deeper normative disagreements. They fundamentally reflect values.

These normative differences are of two types: disagreements about what should be valued and to what extent (for instance, diseases control versus psychological or economic well-being), and disagreements about what constitutes acceptable risk. We will deploy techniques from formal epistemology to elucidate and structure these norms. We will consider only the first of these sets of normative disagreements in this paper leaving the latter for full attention for a different occasion. Section 2 will note the crucial but limited role of science in policy discussions in contexts such as the control of pandemics. Section 3 describes how formal epistemology frames the problem of making public policy decisions. Section 4 is a note on multicriteria analysis and its role in policy formulation in response to Covid-19. Section 5 organizes the values relevant to pandemic response decisions in an objective hierarchy. Section 6 consists of some final remarks.

4.2 The Role of Science

That science, in the form of established empirical facts and predictive models, has a role to play in pandemicrelated public health policy decisions should be obvious. However, one of the telling features of the ongoing Covid-19 pandemic has been science denial by populist politicians such as Bolsonaro of Brazil and Trump of the United States who have wilfully compounded cognitive incapacity with profound ignorance and arrogance. The result was a dramatic failure, measured by morbidity and mortality, to control the pandemic in these countries until mass vaccination changed the situation in the latter.

Nevertheless, it is important to establish the critical but delimited role for science *qua science* in such policy contexts. There are two aspects of the role of science that deserve explicit emphasis. Science does not determine policy. First, scientific facts should be accepted as providing a constraint on policy options: what, in the terminology of decision theory, we will call the set of feasible alternatives.

What the feasible alternatives are will depend on the fundamental and other objectives of the policy as explained below (in Sect. 5). However, once those objectives are set, science may show that some alternatives are not feasible. For instance, if herd immunity to Covid-19 is a community goal not subject to negotiation, and it requires resistance in 75% of the population, and the fraction of the population below 16 is 30%, a policy option of only vaccinating adults (older than 16) in the absence of significant exposure-induced immunity is not a feasible alternative even with a vaccine that is 100% effective. This is the situation faced in many parts of the United States today. Feasible alternatives must include vaccinating persons younger than 16 as, indeed, is the current recommendation from the Centers for Disease Control (CDC).

Science may also determine that some goals themselves are not feasible. Returning to the last example, suppose that the only vaccine available is the Chinese-developed Sinopharm vaccine with, at best, an efficacy rate of 79% (Baraniuk 2021). Now, suppose that herd immunity requires a resistance rate of 80% (which is a widely-accepted figure). Then a goal of achieving herd immunity is impossible: it is not a feasible alternative assuming, once again, that there is no exposure-induced immunity. (The reason is simple: assume everyone in the population is vaccinated with the Sinpharm vaccine. That means 79% of the population is resistant which is lower than the required 80%).

Even such a straightforward use of science is fraught with many assumptions which cannot be tested with high certainty: for instance, estimating the proportion of the population that has acquired immunity to Covid-19 through exposure is difficult to do with any reasonable level of accuracy. Moreover, the herd immunity (resistance) rate depends critically on a notoriously difficult-to-estimate parameter, the basic reproduction number (R_0), which is the number of individuals with whom an infected individual has infective contact. For Covid-19 it is estimated to lie between 2 and 4, not very high compared to other airborne infections such as measles ($12 \leq R_0 \leq 18$) but higher than that of typical flu ($1 \leq R_0 \leq 2$). R_0 values are heavily dependent on context. In the case, of the global measles outbreak of 2019, air travel significantly increase infective contact which also depended heavily on vaccine hesitancy (Sarkar et al. 2019; Gardner et al 2020). In practice, estimated R_0 values cannot even be directly tested.

A new type of uncertainty emerges when we move from these relatively straightforward scientific analyses to more complex situations such as predicting the future course of a pandemic. In the case of Covid-19 these predictions, as one would expect to be the case in all complex situations, have been based on scenario modeling, computational simulation of the future state of a system. The new source of uncertainty is that these simulations must incorporate human behavioral choices, what policies are enacted and the extent to which they are implemented. But these policies, and their acceptance, may themselves depend on the course of the pandemic and the policy options that have thus far been implemented. Individual choices alter the course that the pandemic would follow.

Scenario modeling must not only cope with the uncertainties thus introduced by individual behavior, but dependence on these behaviors make models well-nigh impossible to validate in the field. Future predictions must rely on antecedent assumptions about human behavioral choices. Unless these detailed assumptions are met in practice, a failure in prediction cannot be taken as definitive evidence of model failure. The details of the antecedent assumptions may include individual choices such as wearing masks, social distancing, and other isolation measures. It is hardly surprising that coarse-level predictions from Covid-19 scenario modeling have routinely not been successful (Ioannidis et al. 2020).

These uncertainties and lack of validation have left policy options for responding to Covid-19 radically underdetermined by established scientific results. Such a contingency has enabled policy makers to cherrypick policy options to suit their political predilections as they see fit. Stevens (2020) has documented how politicians in Britain have indulged in cherry-picking when it comes to setting pandemic policy. Baldwin (2021) has documented disagreements between scientific experts arising in part due to the impotence of the available science. However, according to him, when experts (including epidemiologists) make policy recommendations, they no longer play their role qua scientists; rather, Baldwin argues, they become politicians.

This brings us to the second important point to note about the relationship between science and pandemic policy: even independent of these uncertainties and other scientific difficulties, science does not determine what policy *should* be adopted because the latter involves normative strictures whereas the former does not. Claiming that policy options can just "follow the science" (Stevens 2020) falls afoul of the chasm between facts and values, that is, of the fact-value fallacy recognized by by Hume in the eighteenth century and since endorsed by most commentators within the philosophy community.

There are philosophers of various stripes who deny the fact-value fallacy including those who hold that there are moral facts to be found in nature. Moreover, any claim that science is value-free has been credibly challenged since the mid-twentieth century to such an extent that it has few strict adherents amongst philosophers of science today (Longino 1990). However, we do not have to rely on either the force of the fact-value fallacy or in the value-neutrality of science in order to defend a modest contextually delimited claim that, in situations such as that of determining appropriate pandemic response policy, scientific results do not have determinative policy implications by themselves.

All that our best science can lay out are the empirical consequences of policy choices and, even so, can do so with very little certainty in the case of Covid-19 because of the reasons that we have already seen. Put in another way, science can only provide conditional claims of the following sort: "If policy α is adopted in region ρ then the expected consequence is x." Science does not tell us whether we should find x desirable, acceptable, or beyond the pale. We will need normative analysis to decide whether we should implement α for ρ.

Some examples may help drive this important point home. For instance, if α is a policy that consists of avoiding shutdowns while implementing weaker isolation measures (as was practiced early on in the United Kingdom as well as in Sweden), then scientific analysis shows that SARS-CoV-2 exposure, morbidity and mortality would be higher *per capita* than for a policy α^0 that enforced a strict lockdown as had been adopted in China. However, the uncertainties are such that science cannot credibly predict the quantitative difference in these parameters between α and α^0. Science would also show that the economic cost of α would be lower than that of α^0 though, again, quantitative prediction of the extent of this difference would not be possible because of the uncertainties involved. Similarly science would presumably also show that the psychological cost of α, for instance, for young children would be lower than that of α^0.

What science does not determine is whether any community (country, province/state, municipality, etc.) should prefer α or α^0. This is where values must enter the story: what kind of life do we want to lead even in the presence of a pandemic. This not a scientific question. Nor is it an easy question: how do we balance, that is, find a tradeoff between Covid-19 morbidity and mortality on one hand and economic collapse and psychological distress on the other? What helps is a methodology from decision theory, multicriteria analysis (MCA) that forms part of formal epistemology. It allows us to structure our values, first, as individuals. However, if we do engage in this game as a public activity, with the aim of eventually elaborating a common value structure for all of us in a communal decision setting, MCA can facilitate rational group decisions in which there is transparency about how and why we choose between the feasible alternative policy options available to us.

4.3 Formal Epistemology and Decision Theory

Formal epistemology consists of the deployment of formal techniques for the analysis of epistemological problems. These formal techniques include, but are not limited to, those developed in mathematics, operations research, computer science, and logic. The term "formal epistemology" *seems* to have been invented only in the early 2000s when Branden Fitelson and I began organizing the annual Formal Epistemology Workshops (FEWs) but the discipline is of much older vintage and can be traced back at least as far as to the development of probability theory in the seventeenth century (Sarkar and Uebel 2015). Formal epistemology has both theoretical and practical components.

Theoretical problems within formal epistemology include statistical inference and model selection, both relevant to the Covid-19 response. Practical problems include making rational decisions and that is our current focus in this paper. That is the task of decision theory. What constitutes as rational is itself (expectedly) open to philosophical disagreement. Moreover, decision theory suffers from several well-known paradoxes when seemingly innocuous criteria of rationality lead to contradictions as in Arrow's impossibility theorem (Duddy and Piggins 2020). We will ignore these foundational problems to focus on the use of decision theory to clarify the structure of choices in pandemic response.

The most salient advantage of decision theory is that it forces explicitness about the factors that are incorporated in a decision. The first step is to specify the goal of a decision. Typically, in rational decision theory, the goal is implemented in form of a function to be optimized. As we will see below, this is where public discussions of policy response to Covid-19 seem to have been uniformly lacking in every place globally.

Baldwin's (2021) discussion suggests that politicians in all countries were optimizing (maximizing) the political acceptability of decisions. Thus it should come as no surprise that curtailment of individual freedom was considered acceptable in totalitarian regimes such as China but highly controversial in liberal democracies. Baldwin also suggests that epidemiologists, by the very nature of their profession, assumed that what should be optimized, in this case minimized, is the spread of disease. Alternatively, other medical personnel may perceive the goal to be optimized as the reduction of morbidity and mortality. Meanwhile, it is at least plausible that many opponents of isolation measures such as lockdowns and social distancing had as a goal the optimization of economic well-being. Those who also objected to masks may have psychological well-being in mind. Moreover, if a community's well-being in general is the goal, shouldn't that include psychological and economic well-being as well as freedom from disease?

In Sect. 5 we will consider how these goals can be identified and related to each other and usefully structured. Here, what deserves emphasis are four points. First, not only do these goals diverge, some of them are incompatible with each other. Optimizing for disease prevention through lockdowns is in conflict with optimizing for economic well-being: if people are restricted to their homes (for instance, through "shelter in place" orders in U.S. cities) economic activity is significantly restricted. Second, recognizing the divergence of goals helps explain the many political disagreements that emerged in discussions of appropriate policy responses to the pandemic. Returning to our earlier example, the divergence of the disease prevention and economic goals explains what is easily the most serious disagreement that emerged in communities across the world, typically at the national level.

Third, it is plausible that explicit discussion of these divergences between goals *may* have helped to mitigate if not entirely resolve some of these disagreements. (In Sect. 5 we will discuss how that may have been the case.) An explicit recognition of the incompatibility of goals brings with it the implication that, unless some sides in a dispute are to not to be accommodated at all, tradeoffs must be accepted between the goals. If this realization, in turn, leads to a willingness to compromise to some extent, as it should, that by itself enables making a rational decision in which all sides have a stake. Returning to the example we have been using, it was probably implicitly realized all along that those who advocated social isolation, lockdowns, etc., had different goals from those who demanded the opposite. It is possible that in some contexts that did not involve the degree of polarization seen in the United States and Brazil, recognizing tradeoffs would suffice to ease disagreements. This may happen even when the final policy adopted varies from case to case. For instance, faced with similar circumstances, Sweden chose to implement a more relaxed approach to virus control compared to the rest of the Scandinavian countries).

Fourth, and most importantly, we can have legitimate normative arguments about differences in goals. We can ask, what should be our goal? Is it really prevention of disease at all costs? Or is it general well-being with disease control only one component of that goal. Note that, once the decision is framed in this way, it becomes clear that the crucial issue for policy formulation is not scientific. The "follow the science" slogan, however emotive it may be, contributes nothing. Using formal decision analysis shows exactly why.

After the elaboration of goals, the next stage in a formal decision analysis is to establish the set of feasible alternatives, that is, the policy options that are on the table. The role of decision analysis is to help rank these feasible alternatives or at least identify the best of them. Each alternative is a policy option. Having to list all feasible ones explicitly forces us to incorporate the relevant operative constraints in our discussion.

For instance, are we really willing to tolerate community-wide morbidity as well as, say, mortality rates higher than 5% of the population? When such a question is explicitly posed, proponents of a policy of pursuing herd immunity through inaction may well come to admit that the policy is not feasible. This is what happened in the United Kingdom in March 2020 (Baldwin 2021, pp. 21–24). Until 23 March a newlyelected Conservative government followed a policy of avoiding lockdown measures and explicitly tolerated the rise of infections. The expectation was that recovered individuals would increase the proportion of the immune in the country and thus contribute towards achieving herd immunity.

However, a simulation analysis from Imperial College London that the number of deaths would exceed a quarter of a million and the health care system would be overwhelmed with the sick. (These predictions were no different from the what the government's own team had suggested much earlier.) Moreover, similar outcomes had induced lockdowns in other countries such as France and the U.K. government could no longer publicly avoid the question whether it was willing to tolerate this level of morbidity and mortality. It decided it was not and changed course to implement a lockdown. Going back to the issues discussed in Sect. 2, note that the role of science in this process was to make a prediction of the outcome from a policy option. Whether that option represents a feasible alternative was decided by values.

Similarly, we may ask whether we are willing to tolerate complete economic collapse leading to serious food shortages in order to minimize morbidity and mortality? If not, it may well be the case that total lockdown (with no ameliorative measures) over a long period of time is not a feasible alternative.

The value of formal decision analysis in contexts such as the Covid-19 pandemic lies primarily in the public deliberations it induced by explicit statement of goals and alternatives of a decision. This happens before *any* formal technique is brought to bear on the problem.[2] To reiterate the point being made in another way: recourse to formal decision analysis facilitates explicit public discussion of the values with the expectation that it would allow a community to bridge preferred policy differences.

4.4 A Note on Multi-Criteria Analysis (MCA)

Ultimately, this paper will argue that the deliberative use of formal decision analysis is the most important tool formal epistemology can contribute to situations such policy responses to a pandemic. Section 5 will expand on the only formal technique that will be needed for that purpose: the construction of an "Objectives Hierarchy" of values. However, to get to that stage will require many simplifying moves to make a complex decision tractable. This section will take up that task.

It is widely recognized that crises present complex decision problems (Cesta et al. 2014; Baldwin 2021). The simplest decisions are those in which individual agents make decisions with exactly one goal in mind, there is no uncertainty, and the decision chooses from a stable alternative set with unchanging information. The decisions required to formulate Covid-19 policy are the very opposite.

The first complication is that, in democratic societies, there are multiple stakeholders or agents whose preferences must somehow be accommodated into decisions even when some of them are ultimately given minimal value. There are many formal protocols for integrating group preferences; the most common method used in democratic societies through voting in its many guises (*e.g.*, ranked choice *vs.* singe mark voting). However, what matters here is not the number of individuals but the number of agents: a group of individuals can constitute a single agent when it comes to making decisions. For instance, when voters delegate policymaking authority to an elected body, that body then becomes a single decision-making agent. In principle, that is the situation in democratic societies.

However, in practice, democracies do not function quite that simply. The politicians who form the relevant elected bodies represent constituencies that can remove them from power in the next election. Political survival often requires establishing a perception of consensus between different interest groups or, at least, an accommodation of these differences. There is a rich literature within decision theory about the formation and operation of coalitions for this purpose (reviewed by Greenberg [1994]). However, it is unclear that these tools from decision theory are practically relevant in almost any situation. At least in the Covid-19 pandemic response, single agents (typically heads of governments such as governors in the United States) set policies claiming to reflect the consensus of experts. Typically, what these decisions reflected was the path of least resistance from stakeholders who were special interest groups.[3]

The two pertinent aspects of these decisions are, first, a single agent was ultimately responsible, and second, final decisions were the result of a deliberative process rather than the formal aggregation of different individuals' preferences. There are two implications. We can thus simplify our decision problem to be a single-agent decision where the decision maker is a deliberative body which acts as a whole. We can, therefore, orient the rest of our analysis towards producing a discussion that facilitates this deliberation.

Earlier sections of this paper emphasized the many uncertainties associated with Covid-19, in particular, uncertainties about the transmission of infection and course of the disease.[4] In a formal decision theory these uncertainties affect the relative ranking of the policy options that comprise the feasible alternative set. Typically, probabilities are used to model these uncertainties and take them into account.

In a fully quantitative analysis, each policy option has a *value* ascribed to it corresponding to the outcome of taking that action. For instance, let us suppose that a particular policy leads to 10 fewer infections than would otherwise have occurred. We could assign a value of 10 to it. Uncertainty is incorporated by ascribing a probability (between 0 and 1) to an outcome. In our example, suppose that the probability of 10 fewer infections is 0.8 (and 0 for all other values for the infection number). Then the *expected value* or *utility* of the policy is 8 rather than 10.[5]

It should be clear from the earlier discussion of this paper that, when it comes to the Covid-19 pandemics, ascription of definite probabilities to outcomes of policies would largely be a matter of guesswork. This means that any fully quantitative decision analysis would have to rely on ad hoc probability ascription of probabilities and no such analysis would be credible. One way to make progress in such a situation is to eschew quantification and attempt only to rank the feasible alternatives (Sarkar and Garson 2004). The trouble is that even rankings may be difficult to produce. We will acknowledge a residual problem here and return to it below.

There remain two other components of complexity. The first is the dynamic nature of the policy problem. We learn from policy failures and successes and this feedback changes how we rank different policy options or feasible alternatives. Moreover, as our experience of the pandemic increases new information and technologies emerge and even the feasible alternative set keeps on changing. The emergence of successful vaccines towards the end of 2020 was the most important game-changer. Whereas total lockdown was a viable policy response in May 2020, a year later it was not considered a feasible alternative even in countries such as Brazil and India which were experiencing massive increases in disease morbidity and mortality. Meanwhile, vaccination campaigns emerged as a viable (and highly desirable) feasible alternative. The changing nature of a problem to be solved means that policies must be *adaptive*, responding to the changes in problem characterization.

There are formal solutions of simple cases of adaptive decision problems based on a technique called dynamic programming (Bellman 1961). However, obtaining these solution is typically inordinately computationally expensive because the associated computational problems are intractable.[6] Rather, what is appropriate in most policy contexts, including the Covid-19 pandemic, is an adaptive approach that involves reiterating the decision process periodically to take into account the changes in problem structure. In practice this is what happens when policies are periodically reviewed, for instance, to change threat levels.

The final component of complexity remains: multiple incomplete values that are all perceived to be relevant to the goal of the decision. This brings us to multicriteria analysis (MCA). In MCA, each of these values is modeled as a criterion the satisfaction of which has to be optimized (maximized or minimized). There are a wide variety of MCA methods available. Some of these such as multiattribute value and utility theories (MAVT and MAUT) are consistent with standard economic theory. MAUT is a generalization of standard utility theory in which an alternative is evaluated according to multiple weighted criteria and these weighted scores are subsequently compounded (typically on a linear scale) to produce a final performance or utility measure. (When there is no uncertainty, we have MAVT instead of MAUT.)

Other methodologies, including the popular Analytic Hierarchy Process, are not compatible with standard economic theory and are, in that sense, arbitrary besides also being subject to well-known paradoxes.[7] MCA methods have been been systematically reviewed by Figuera et al. (2005) and Moffett and Sarkar (2007).

Many MCA techniques have already been deployed in the context of the Covid-19 pandemic. Mahato et al. (2020) have used the Analytic Hierarchy Process (AHP) to produce a Covid-19 risk map for India. Hussain et al. (2021) used the AHP to do a multicriteria impact assessment on an energy project due to Covid19 spread and associated safety parameters. Marti and Puertas (2021) used an outranking methodology, Technique for Order Preference by Similarity to the Ideal Solution (TOPSIS), to analyze the vulnerability of European countries with respect to health-related, social, and work-related criteria. Roselli et al. (2020) used MAUT to show how multiple criteria can be used to screen for Covid-19.

Finally, in an analysis that comes closest to the purpose of the present paper, Raboisson and Lhermie (2020) have emphasized the importance for MCA in devising Covid-19 response policy in the context of potentially ending the early lockdowns in mid-2020. They argue for the relevance of three criteria: economic activity, societal well-being, and disease containment. They explicitly recognize the problems posed by uncertainties and also point out that a dynamic response, one that was called adaptive earlier bin the present paper, would be necessary. However, they make no attempt to proceed with an analysis. We will now go beyond their analysis.

4.5 Objectives Hierarchies

In the context of complex environmental decisions, Moffett et al. (2006) pointed out that MAUT (which reduces to MAVT in the absence of uncertainty) is preferable to other MCA methodologies because, as a generalization of (single attribute or single criterion) utility theory, it is consistent with standard economic theory. Central to the use of these theories is an exploration of values relevant to a decision (Keeney 1992). These values are organized in a hierarchy that makes explicit how they are related to each other, which can subsume others and which are the most important. Sarkar (2018) argued that, because organizing these values require preference elicitation from a group of stakeholders in a public decision context, the resulting deliberative process can by itself produce a rational decision, and one that has sufficient purchase from all (or at least most) stakeholders to enable it to be politically implementable. Subsequent parts of the MCA methodology, which involve quantitative compounding of the performance of alternatives according to each criterion, would not even be necessary.

In the case of decisions on societal responses to Covid-19 such a strategy recommends itself for at least three reasons. First, given our general lack of experience with the new pandemic, assigning quantitative performance scores to different policies cannot be credibly accomplished. Consider a very simple example where the two policies to be evaluated (that is, two feasible alternatives) are social distancing requirements of either one or two meters and the relevant goal is to reduce morbidity and mortality. We do not know enough even to quantify the expected differences in morbidity and mortality due to these two policies.[8] Second, while we have been emphasizing the various uncertainties throughout this paper, there is also no credible method to quantify those uncertainties. The implication is that credible value or utility measures cannot be constructed. Third, though we have discussed a variety of values that are relevant to Covid-19 decisions, we have no reason to believe that our discussion so far has produced a complete or canonical list of values. But that is exactly what we wish to achieve through constructing an objectives hierarchy (OH).

In MAUT (and MAVT), an objectives hierarchy (OH) consists of a set of fundamental objectives with a tree of sub-objectives subsumed under each of them and with the lowest nodes (that is, the "leaves" of the tree) being associated with measurable attributes that have quantitative values. This means that at the bottom of the hierarchical tree are parameters which can be measured. The development of such a structure starts with the identification of fundamental objectives that are ends-in-themselves; that is, there is no further answer to the question, "Why is this objective important?" (Keeney 1992). Objectives lower in the hierarchy (sub-objectives) are important for what they contribute to the fundamental objectives. They are thus means-to-an-end.

Construction of the OH is driven by elicitation from stakeholders acting as a group through deliberation. The process involves the iterated use of variants of two questions: "What are the objectives of the decision?," and the one mentioned earlier, "Why is this objective important?" Answers to the first question provide the set of objectives for the OH, answers to the second establishes the structure of the hierarchy. The elicitation process stops at the top (of the hierarchy) when fundamental objectives are reached. It stops at the bottom when the lowest–level objectives that are identified can be associated with measurable attributes. Note that an objectives hierarchy is not canonical: more than one structure can accommodate stakeholder preferences equally adequately. In practice, informal discussion may allow a first pass at a putative objectives hierarchy, which can then be subject to iterated revision and discussion. We will encounter examples below of both the non-uniqueness of an OH and its iterated revision to accommodate preferences more faithfully.

Let us begin the process of eliciting an OH for policy responses to the Covid-19 pandemic. If we were policy-makers—or decision analysts providing support to them—we would be targeting stakeholders in public forums or dedicated focus groups or some other venue dedicated to the same purpose. There, a deliberative process of constructing an OH would begin.[9] Here we will be reconstructing plausible but imagined discussions and draw conclusions from them.

As Baldwin (2021) has pointed out, epidemiologist stakeholders will typically emphasize the objective of halting the spread of disease. We then ask: "Why is it important to stop the spread of disease?" If our stakeholder says that there is no further answer, stopping the spread of disease is a fundamental objective. Now, we would look at all other objectives the stakeholders offer. If they can all be organized in a hierarchy under this fundamental objective, then they are all sub-objectives and our OH has a unique fundamental objective. Such sub-objectives presumably would include goals such as preventing airborne transmission of the virus, preventing travel from regions with high infection rates, closure of public dining areas, various quarantine measures, and so on.

However, our stakeholders will include those who are not epidemiologists. Suppose one of them has the goal of preventing disease morbidity and mortality. This objective cannot be fully accommodated under the "Halt the spread of disease" fundamental objective. We must do more by treating those who are already infected. We ask: "Why is it important to minimize morbidity and mortality?" and begin constructing a new hierarchical structure. We would likely find multiple possibilities with equal plausibility. We could end up with at least these three plausible fundamental objectives: maximize population health (but, then, perhaps"Halt the spread of disease" should itself be one of its sub-objectives rather than a fundamental objective); maximize individual well-being (with a sub-objective of minimizing disease); or maximize population wellbeing.

Once we recognize the pursuit of well-being as an objective for our policy formulation problem (of responding to Covid-19) our discussion naturally broadens well beyond virus containment and, presumably, even beyond physical health. Surely, it must include mental health? This is what many child psychologists were implying when invoking the importance of considering the possible harm of isolation measures, especially on young children (Loades et al. 2020). But, if either individual or societal well-being is a fundamental objective, it is implausible that economic well-being is not a valid sub-objective. A wealth of empirical evidence shows poverty to be a major source of stress acting through a variety of mechanisms including a perception of a lack of control over one's life (Simandan 2018).

A critical issue that emerges from this discussion is: would those who advocate lockdowns and strong isolation measures accept well-being as an objective? If so, then there is probably no credible OH in which it is not a fundamental objective. But, so long as it is a fundamental objective, even if there are others (and we earlier saw a case in which it was the sole fundamental objective and a case in which it was not), we have to consider the extent to which it should be satisfied. This chain of reasoning strongly suggests (though perhaps not strictly requires) that these advocates of extreme isolation measures must be willing to accept some tradeoffs and make compromises. These tradeoffs would include relaxing isolation measures to allow some interactions, most likely, including those that would allow more economic activity.

Similarly, the deliberative process would also focus on advocates of unfettered economic activity and ask them if that were an end-in-itself. Some of these stakeholders may—*e.g.*, many free market fundamentalists— may well hold such a view. But, then, they would also face the question whether well-being is an objective at all. If they accept well-being as an objective, once again we are in a situation to negotiate tradeoffs. If unfettered economic activity is not an end-in-itself, it would be a sub-objective in some other OH which, most likely, would include well-being and require tradeoffs.

This discussion shows that a public deliberative use of MCA inexorably leads to a recognition that tradeoffs between incompatible values are necessary in framing Covid-19 response policy in such a way that the divergent values of stakeholders are accommodated. It does not show that there will be any agreement on what these tradeoffs should be. While recognition of the need to compromise is itself conducive to rational policy making—and that is the main point of this paper—it would be much better if there could be more agreement on policy particulars.

There are at least two impediments to achieving such agreement. The first, which will be discussed in some detail in the concluding section, is that the divergences in values in deeply divided contexts may simply be too extreme to bridge through rational decisions. The second, which is also a normative issue, is that different stakeholders even with the same value structure (as formalized in the OH) may have differences about acceptable risk. This could lead them to ascribe different weights to the same policy option depending on its associated risk.

For instance, those who are risk tolerant may be willing to assign a high weight to a policy that accepts a risk of new infection of 10% for an individual. Someone who is risk averse may weight the same policy very poorly. Navigating these disputes will once again require deliberation. A the present time formal analysis does not seem capable of contributing much to the process. But this problem should not be taken as any indication that rational policy formulation is doomed from the outset. In the United States, there are a plethora of examples in which norms about risk acceptance have been incorporated into policy decisions.

For instance, the acceptability of radiation from nuclear facilities were hotly debated on normative grounds by geneticists on a policy advisory committee in the 1950s before finally coming to a partial consensus (Crow 1995). In the context of biodiversity conservation, the definitions of various threat levels such as "endangered" or "threatened" reflect normative attitudes towards risk (Maguire 1996).

4.6 Final Remarks

Let us take stock of where we are. Decisions about appropriate societal responses to the ongoing Covid19 have been fraught with controversy in a large number of countries and have varied between them in bewildering ways (Baldwin 2021). In many regional contexts, consensus has been impossible to achieve, for instance, between different states in the United States or between Sweden and the other Scandinavian countries.

The MCA process outlined earlier recognizes that stakeholders diverge in their values. It does not try to enforce value convergence though it is highly likely that the deliberative decision-making process outlined earlier would sometimes lead to value revision in the direction of convergence. However, what it does require is deliberation between stakeholders so as to make all values explicit. Moreover, these values are structured in an acceptable way through a public elicitation of stakeholder preferences. The deliberative process is designed to require engagement between stakeholders with value divergences.

Ideally, this deliberative process should continue until there is not only agreement about the structure of the objectives hierarchy but also about the weights to be assigned to the different objectives at each level of the hierarchy. Is there any reason to believe than such agreement would have been achieved if this process had been played out, say, in the early stages of the pandemic in 2021? There are ample grounds for pessimism in some contexts. For instance, in deeply divided societies such as Brazil and the United States, due to the flawed political leadership at the national level in the form of Bolsonaro and Trump, it is even unlikely that beginning a deliberative process would have been possible at the national level. There is some reason for more optimism at the state and local levels at which policies with broad social support have sometimes been implemented.

Some putative democracies such as India did not carry out public deliberation between stakeholders at all, introducing a national shutdown with no consultation (Baldwin 2021). It is possible that a public discussion of policy objectives may have not only led to decisions with more public support but even to better decisions in the case of India and other South Asian countries. For instance, if Indian stakeholders had even recognized well-being as a high level objective, that would have precluded an unplanned sudden shutdown that left hundreds of millions of migrant and other impoverished workers without food and shelter. In countries of the European Union, especially those not ruled by populist strongmen, the most serious problem with using this type of deliberative process would have been the time it requires. Because of the rapid onset of the pandemic in Europe in early 2020, these countries required a rapid response that was entirely uncoordinated (Baldwin 2021).

This paper has defended the use of formal epistemology as a resource for deliberation rather than as providing mechanical or algorithmic techniques for quantification of decisions. Sarkar (2018) has documented extensive skepticism about the use of formal decision analysis in public environmental and other policy contexts because it is supposed to discourage public deliberative processes. However, this is a misperception about how formal decision analysis can work even if many examples emphasize computation at the expense of deliberation (see below). The point that gets forgotten is that formal decision analysis is supposed to provide decision *support* to stakeholders, not make decisions for them.

The methodology for the construction of an objectives hierarchy illustrates the last point. The structure of the hierarchy is elicited from the stakeholders. The decision analyst's role is to elicit preferences and organize them in a public forum. Unless the decision analyst is also a stakeholder, the analyst's personal preferences play no role in the this process (though, of course, we do have the problem of possible implicit bias and must guard against it). Moreover, weights (if used) are also elicited from the stakeholders. In the process envisioned here, formal decision analysis facilitates deliberation.

Compared to other areas that require societal decisions, for instance, contexts of environmental management, formal decision analysus has been rarely used in epidemiology. Moreover, these uses tend to be computational, relying on quantitative analyses, but open to objections that were noted earlier, chiefly the use of parameter values that cannot credibly be ascertained.[10] One contribution of the present paper could be not only to encourage more use of formal decision analysis within epidemiology but to do so in more deliberative ways that prioritize stakeholder participation and engagement over computation.

Notes

1. Li was forced to sign a retraction and later died from Covid-19. In 2021 the Chinese authorities finally admitted their fault and apologized to his family (Cheng 2021).
2. The deliberative value of formal decision analysis has often not been recognized by critics of formal methodologies. Sarkar (2018) addresses this problem in the context of complex environmental decisions.
3. See the analysis of Baldwin (2021) who emphasizes the political acceptability of policy decisions.
4. Writing in June 2021, it is striking that, even after a year of intensive scientific focus on the disease few of the original uncertainties have been successfully resolved.
5. Note that the terminology here is not fully standardized. We have defined utility as expected value, following Keeney and Raiffa (1993). However, utility is sometimes used for "value" and our expected value then becomes expected utility.
6. In the language of operations research, they are NP-hard (Garey and Johnson 1979).
7. However, even non-arbitrary methods cannot always avoid the last problem—see Arrow and Raynaud (1986) and Sarkar (2012).
8. These policy options were the subject of some debate and the choice between them never scientifically settled—see Jones et al. (2020).
9. In practice, if we were carrying out a formal MCA, not only would we elicit the structure of the OH but we would also elicit relative weights for nodes at each level of a hierarchy. These weights would reflect the perceived value of each fundamental and sub-objective relative to others at that level of the OH. But, given that we do not think that a quantitative analysis would contribute anything new in the context of Covid-19 policy decisions, we do not consider weight elicitation here.
10. For recent examples, see Liu and Xia (2020).

References

Arrow, K.J., and H. Raynaud. 1986. *Social Choice and Multicriterion Decision-making*. Cambridge, MA: MIT Press.

Baldwin, P. 2021. *Fighting the First Wave: Why the Coronavirus Was Tackled so Differently across the Globe*. Cambridge, UK: Cambridge University Press.

Baraniuk, C. 2021. What Do We Know About China's Covid-19 Vaccines? *British Medical Journal* 373: n912. https://doi.org/10.1136/bmj.n912.

Bellman, R.E. 1961. *Adaptive Control Processes*. Princeton, NJ: Princeton University Press.

Cesta, A., G. Cortellessa, and R. de Benedictis. 2014. Training for Crisis Decision Making—An Approach Based on Plan Adaptation. *Knowledge-Based Systems* 58: 98–112.

Cheng, A. 2021. Chinese Authorities Admit Improper Response to Coronavirus Whistleblower. National Public Radio 19 March: https://www.npr.org/sections/coronavirus-live-updates/2020/03/19/818295972/chinese-authorities-admit-improper-response-to-coronavirus-whistleblower; last accessed 17-May-2021.

Crow, J.F. 1995. Quarreling Geneticists and a Diplomat. *Genetics* 140: 421–426.

Duddy, C., and Piggins, A. 2020. Arrow's Theorem. Oxford Research Encyclopedia of Politics. https://oxfordre.com/politics/view/10.1093/acrefore/9780190228637.001.0001/acrefore9780190228637-e-936; last accessed 18-June-2021.

Figuera, J., S. Greco, and M. Ehrgott, eds. 2005. *Multiple Criteria Decision Analysis: State of the Art Surveys*. Berlin: Springer.

Gardner, L., E. Dong, K. Khan, and S. Sarkar. 2020. Persistence of US Measles Risk Due to Vaccine Hesitancy and Outbreaks Abroad. *Lancet Infectious Diseases* 20: 1114–1115.

Garey, M., and D.S. Johnson. 1979. *Computers and Intractability; A Guide to the Theory of NP-Completeness*. New York: W. H. Freeman.

Green, A., 2020. Li Wenliang. Lancet 395: 682.

Greenberg, J. 1994. Coalition Structures. In *Handbook of Game Theory*, vol. 2, ed. R.J. Aumann and S. Hart, 1305–1337. Amsterdam: Elsevier Science.

Horton, R. 2020. *The Covid-19 Catastrophe: What's Gone Wrong and How to Stop It Happening Again*. Cambridge, UK: Polity Press.

Hussain, S., W. Xuetong, T. Hussain, A.H. Khoja, and M.Z. Zia. 2021. Assessing the impact of COVID19 and safety parameters on energy project performance with an Analytical Hierarchy Process. *Utilities Policy* 70: 101210.

Ioannidis, J.P., S. Cripps, and M.A. Tanner. 2020. Forecasting for COVID-19 has Failed. *International Journal of Forecasting*. https://doi.org/10.1016/j.ijforecast.2020.08.004.

Jones, N.R., Z.U. Qureshi, R.J. Temple, J.P. Larwood, T. Greenhalgh, and L. Bourouiba. 2020. Two Metres or One: What is the Evidence for Physical Distancing in Covid-19? *British Medical Journal* 370: 3223.

Keeney, R.L. 1992. *Value-Focused Thinking*. Cambridge, MA: Harvard University Press.

Keeney, R.L., and H. Raiffa. 1993. *Decisions with Multiple Objectives: Preferences and Value Tradeoffs*, 2nd ed. Cambridge, UK: Cambridge University Press.

Liu, J., and S. Xia. 2020. *Computational Epidemiology: From Disease Transmission Modeling to Vaccination Decision Making*. Cham, Switzerland: Springer.

Loades, M.E., E. Chatburn, N. Higson-Sweeney, S. Reynolds, R. Shafran, A. Brigden, C. Linney, M.N. McManus, C. Borwick, and E. Crawley. 2020. Rapid Systematic Review: The Impact of Social Isolation and Loneliness on the Mental Health of Children and Adolescents in the Context of COVID-19. *Journal of the American Academy of Child and Adolescent Psychiatry* 59: 1218-1239.e3.

Longino, H.E. 1990. *Science as Social Knowledge: Values and Objectivity in Scientific Inquiry*. Princeton: Princeton University Press.

Maguire, L.A. 1996. Making the Role of Values in Conservation Explicit. *Conservation Biology* 10: 914–916.

Mahato, R., G. Nimasow, O.D. Nimasow, and D. Bushi. 2020. Analytic Hierarchy Process Based Potential Risk Zonation of COVID-19 in India. *Journal of the Social Sciences* 48: 4223–4238.

Marti, L., and Puertas, R. 2021. European Countries' Vulnerability to COVID-19: Multicriteria Decisionmaking Techniques. Economic Research–Ekonomska Istra˘zivanja 2021: Doi: https://doi.org/10.1080/1331677X.2021.1874462.

Moffett, A., J.S. Dyer, and S. Sarkar. 2006. Integrating Biodiversity Representation with Multiple Criteria in North-Central Namibia Using Non-Dominated Alternatives and a Modified Analytic Hierarchy Process. *Biological Conservation* 129: 181–191.

Moffett, A., and S. Sarkar. 2006. Incorporating Multiple Criteria into the Design of Conservation Area Networks: A Minireview with Recommendations. *Diversity and Distributions* 12: 125–137.

Raboisson, D., and G. Lhermie. 2020. Living with COVID-19: A Systemic and Multi-Criteria Approach to Enact Evidence-Based Health Policy. *Frontiers in Public Health* 8: 294. https://doi.org/10.3389/fpubh.2020.00294.

Roselli, L.R.P., E.A. Frej, R.J.P. Ferreira, A.R. Alberti, and A.T. de Almeida. 2020. Utility Based Multicriteria Model for Screening Patients Under the COVID-19 Pandemic. *Computational and Mathematical Methods in Medicine* 2020: 9391251.

Sarkar, S. 2012. Complementarity and the Selection of Nature Reserves: Algorithms and the Origins of Conservation Planning, 1980–1995. *Archive for History of Exact Sciences* 66: 397–426.

Sarkar, S. 2018. Deliberative Decisions and Formal Multicriteria Analysis: Addressing Norton's Skepticism. In *A Sustainable Philosophy: The Work of Bryan Norton*, Sarkar, S. and Minteer, B. Eds. Cham, Switzerland: Springer, pp. 213–236.

Sarkar, S., and J. Garson. 2004. Multiple Criterion Synchronization for Conservation Area Network Design: The Use of Non-Dominated Alternative Sets. *Conservation and Society* 2: 433–448.

Sarkar, S., and T. Uebel. 2015. Formal Epistemology and the Legacy of Logical Empiricism. *Studies in History and Philosophy of Science Part A* 53: 1–2.

Sarkar, S., A. Zlojutro, K. Khan, and L. Gardner. 2019. Measles Resurgence in the USA: How International Travel Compounds Vaccine Resistance. *Lancet Infectious Diseases* 19: 684–686.

Simandan, D. 2018. Rethinking the Health Consequences of Social Class and Social Mobility. *Social Science and Medicine* 200: 258–261.

Stevens, A. 2020. Governments Cannot Just 'Follow the Science' on COVID-19. Nature Human Behavior 4: 560. https://doi.org/10.1038/s41562-020-0894-x.

World Health Organization [WHO]. 2005. Strengthening health security by implementing the International Health Regulations. https://www.who.int/ihr/procedures/pheic/en/; last accessed 17-May 2021.

World Health Organization [WHO]. 2020. WHO Director-General's opening remarks at the media briefing on COVID-19, 11 March 2020. https://www.who.int/director-general/speeches/detail/whodirector-general-s-opening-remarks-at-the-media-briefing-on-covid-19---11-march-2020; last accessed 17-May-2021.

Chapter 5
Reevaluating Value in Public Health Policy: Values as Iterative Rational Inquiry

Peter Tagore Tan

Abstract Values are understood to be the guiding principles by which any one person can determine how to conduct themselves throughout their life. In that they are foundational, values are taken to be fixed; and in that they are personal, they are understood to be subjective. As such, values are taken to be beyond the reach of objective critique. In contrast, public health policy is meant to deliver recommendations based on empirical evidence to arrive at a rational strategy during pandemics, and as a way of separating an objective policy from subjective beliefs, such policies are presented free from values. This allows contrarian voices in the public forum to claim values as their own such that what values are present in public debate are often those that openly question pandemic protocols and promote vaccine resistance. Paradoxically, public health policies that were meant to protect the public with science-based and value-free recommendations may have the effect of harming significant portions of it. This is predicated on the understanding that values are more basic and important than empirically based strategies developed to combat the spread of COVID-19. Values as fixed is, however, unable to account for the entirety of what values are. Values are static, but they are also actively made and always in the making. A more descriptively accurate account of value is derived using Charles Peirce's analysis of belief formation, where values are iterative and share the same structure as human inquiry. Values can thus be judged according to a measure of pragmatic rationality developed by Jürgen Habermas's concept of the performative contradiction in public discourse. This standard of reason can be used to both critique contrarian values found to be performatively contradictory, and guide the process of developing public health policies that satisfy the internal need to be logically consistent and the public's need to find value in things.

Keywords Axiology · Iteration · Peirce · Habermas · Performative contradiction

P. T. Tan (✉)
Department of Philosophy, Mount Saint Mary's University, Los Angeles, CA 90049, USA
e-mail: ptan@msmu.edu

5.1 Introduction

While COVID-19 has elicited responses from the medical, political, and social fields, philosophy's response to the pandemic has been generally uniform. The great majority of philosophers have appealed to using our civically minded critical thinking skills to follow empirically driven medical advice, but this has by no means shared by all philosophers. The most outspoken has been Italian philosopher Giorgio Agamben, whose screed written in the early days of COVID-19 in Italy warned that a governmental abuse of power was unfolding exactly as Michel Foucault had feared, with the invention of a biological foe that justifies exceptional measures of public control. "[W]hat is once manifest," Agamben writes, "is the tendency to use a state of exception as a normal paradigm for government. The legislative decree immediately approved by the government 'for hygiene and public safety reasons' actually produces an authentic militarization" (Agamben 2020a). This has become the intellectual heart of the argument raised by the COVID-19 skeptic and the vaccine resister. It is shared with many neoliberals/libertarians.[1] Philosophy thus bleeds into the public sphere, this time reflecting a contrarianism. Binoy Kampmark succinctly states this position: "One enduring legacy of the novel coronavirus is the incremental development of surveillance technologies, ostensibly purposed to identify the threat and spread of a pandemic, giving birth to what amounts to the pandemic surveillance state" (Kampmark 2020).

This book combines ethics, public policy, and pandemics in its title. Philosophically speaking, it thus contains elements of moral theory, political philosophy, and bioethics, but in this article I want to explore proper pandemic response in terms of value. The reason for doing so is simple: values are misunderstood and has resulted in any talk of values being conspicuously absent in official attempts to control COVID-19.

We can of course surmise the reason for this. Values are understood to be the guiding principles by which an entity (be it a person, corporation, or country) can determine how to act. They are fixed core beliefs that are central to that entity's identity, and as such they are inherently subjective by nature. Public policy during a pandemic, on the other hand, are objective statements based on empirically derived medical data, and thus a pandemic response cannot even have the appearance of subjective bias. Official pandemic policy is thus scrubbed of any talk of values, but this is mistaken on three major fronts:

1. The first is that the official pandemic response is of course based on a value (the value, say, of saving human lives, or of reducing suffering), so not stating the value in the pandemic response is to either blithely think that everyone shares this intuitively obvious value, or to inauthentically claim a bias-free pronouncement that must be believed because it is scientifically based;
2. Not appealing to the values behind official COVID-19 strategies means that the proper pandemic response no longer controls the value narrative. Values are the common currency of public forums; where no value in public health policy is

stated, the public will assign values to it, including those from contrarian voices opposed to proper health protocols;

3. The third is that the obstacle in crafting a proper public policy isn't really about the content of what such policies should include. We intuitively know the rough outlines—that the findings of medical science must be openly and transparently presented and then efficiently operationalized according to need. But widespread acceptance of public policy can be hard to come by not because there is a dearth of rational debate or democratic opportunities, but because reasoned debate and open communal discourse may not be valued by significant and vocal portions of the population.

I want to take a closer look at value because they are more important for the formation of public policies than we think. Values are treated as if they are fixed beliefs that have deep subjective meaning. We create our identities in part with the values we choose, and since they are constitutive of our very being, they resist objective critique. This is not to say that we cannot objectively critique a person's values: it is just that when we do, that person is likely to ignore it and keep valuing what they will, irrational as it may be.

As different as pandemic protocols and Agamben's[2] argument are, they do share a point in common: both are based on an incomplete account of value. Values are not only fixed, and their subjective importance does not mean that they are resistant to objective critique. I will argue that values have a structure, one shared with rational inquiry such that it becomes possible to analyze values objectively. This will necessitate a very different analysis of not just values, but of rationality as well. I will be using Charles Sanders Peirce's pragmatic analysis of human inquiry and Jürgen Habermas's analysis of the performative contradiction that serves as the heart of his theory of communicative action. The goal of this article is to establish the structure of value in part to address the contrarian argument, but also to highlight just how this structure is patterned after that of human inquiry and rationality in general. The hope is to rehabilitate value formation through pragmatic means such that it can serve as a prescriptive basis to argue for what ought to be included in a proper response to a pandemic.

5.2 Value in General

Axiology is the study of ἀξία, or value. As used by philosophy, it refers to the theory of values. Etymologically, 'value' comes from the Proto-Indo-European prefix, *wal-*, which means 'to be strong or worthy'. The source and nature of this strength is not the subject of this article; it is rather the practical sense of what effect such strength has in our lived experience. Understood as such, what we value is important enough that it has the power to make us do things that we otherwise would not be able to do.

There are two ways to understand value. The first is how it is used in the analysis above—as a fixed measure by which we derive all serious judgments. Agamben's value of autonomy, for example, gives him the ability to issue a scathing retort to any governmental program that would limit personal freedoms. But then there is the fact that values are made and, given the proper conditions, in the process of being made. This act of *forming* values as a way to respond to a novel situation introduces the activity present in valu*ing*. The complete process of valuation thus requires both the fixed and the active, and to argue one against the other is to have an incomplete grasp of what value is in general.

5.2.1 Value as Fixed

Agamben's position exhibits a classic fixed axiology. As with his intellectual mentor Foucault, ultimate value is placed on individual freedoms, and the disciplinary mechanisms enacted by the State of Italy during COVID-19 are arbitrary exercises in power meant to control and, if need be, punish. Yet there is something even more furtive for Agamben: whereas Foucault cites the plague-ridden states of 17th C Europe where state control was instituted in the face of widespread death, Agamben states that the present fear of pandemic is engineered from something "not too different from the normal flus that affect us every year" (Agamben 2020a). These pieces are from the early days of the pandemic, and his viewpoint may have evolved since late February and March of 2020, but he introduces the notion that COVID-19 is the invention of governments interested in amassing power and control over their subjects so that they could declare states of emergencies, making citizens "so used to living in conditions of permanent crisis and emergency that they don't seem to notice that their lives have been reduced to a purely biological condition, one that has lost not only any social and political dimension, but even any compassionate and emotional one" (Agamben 2020b). Agamben continues: "The state of fear translates into an authentic need for situations of collective panic for which the epidemic provides once again the ideal pretext" (Agamben 2020a). The entire goal is to strip self-determination from social subjects.

Lee Seung-Hwan succinctly states the particularly modern rendition of freedom and liberty that Agamben values. "Liberty is the condition in which an individual is able to determine her/his own actions autonomously without interference from others. One can do anything one wants to do, as long as one does not interfere with the liberty of others" (Lee 2018, 30). Because liberty pertains to individuals from having their freedom forcibly impinged upon by a central governing body, "the liberty pursued by liberalism is not a positive liberty, but a negative one that seeks only to avoid external interference" (Lee 2018, 30).

The individual freedom to pursue whatever goals one wants is understood by Foucault, Agamben, and libertarianism to be the value that supersedes all other values. To cite Lee again, "individual liberty is set above any other normative value, to the extent that laws and norms are founded upon the principle of noninterference" (Lee 2018, 30). The goal of society is to attain such freedom, and everything that frustrates its realization is considered an illicit use of power to make the individual succumb to the will of the governing body in power.

There is a stark either/or dichotomy inherent in this approach. When values are stubbornly fixed, anything that falls short of them are necessarily a compromise that is understood to be a moral failing as well. To be rational and universal is to stand with the side of rightness, no matter how easy or practical a compromise to the ideal is, how fraught with danger it is to stand firm. Certain key values must be defended even unto death. Witness a popular slogan during the French Revolution—*Vivre Libre ou Mourir*, the English translation of which happens to be New Hampshire's state motto: Live Free or Die. Deference to a fixed value shows an unbending extremism that underlies Agamben's suspicions of any civic power trying to govern during COVID-19. In Agamben's case, even the prevention of suffering and death are all somehow of less importance than individual autonomy.

5.2.2 Axiology in the Making

Those assiduously holding to a fixed value do so because that value forms the magnetic pole around which all events and situations are oriented. What is valued has the feeling of being unchanging and ever present, but of course nothing could be further from the truth. Values do not appear on one's horizon fully formed. They are made, and they are in a constant and complex interplay with the events experienced. While it is correct to say that events are interpreted according to a fixed value, it is incorrect to claim that this is the only way the interaction occurs. Values and events are together in the process of altering each other at the same time. Values can filter certain events as being unimportant, or they can highlight others as vital. But even more important is how events can alter values. Events may reinforce values, or they may refine them, or they may overturn them. In short, the interplay between value and event indicates that values are not fixed. They advance according to how well they allow the value holder to adjust to novel experiences.

Agamben's understanding of value as static and fixed is by no means unique to him. It reflects his European background that traditionally holds for the human being as the subject of philosophical inquiry. Value as activity comes from a different source. It is biological in origin, and it is freely patterned after American Pragmatism's recasting of philosophy in terms of the complex relationship between an organism and its environment.

One of the earliest texts in Pragmatism, Peirce's "The Fixation of Belief" is best known for his 4 methods by which to posit belief, but it is really more than that. It presents a Darwinian schematic by which humans, like all other organisms, seek equanimity in a changing environment that does not at all times favor its survival. Organisms are comfortable in their environment when their survival is secure and enjoyment becomes possible. All organisms seek just this sort of existence, and they will expend considerable individual and cultural energies to achieve it. This cessation of doubt—that feeling of existential uncertainty that disturbs our equanimity—is what Peirce calls belief. Axiologically, the belief that removes this irritation of doubt is valued because it allows us to attain, in William James's words, "a strong feeling of ease, peace, [and] rest". James reminds us that "The transition from a state of puzzle and perplexity to rational comprehension is full of lively relief and pleasure" (James 1896).

When conditions are in flux and previously held values can no longer address the challenges presented before us, they must be re-evaluated and recast accordingly. This search for value describes axiology's inherent activity. What ought our values be? How do we determine them? What obstacles are they meant to overcome? Once evaluated anew according to how well it addresses a social stressor, the determined value becomes something more—it becomes *valuable*. It has allowed us to settle a challenge to our collective experience, but once settled, it becomes a supervening value that we place above all others.

The process of forming values of course does not end there. It is cyclical in nature and reflects pragmatism's emphasis on iterative amelioration. A supervening value lasts only until the organism's environment changes. What does it take to overcome a settled value? In Peirce's analysis, only a state of doubt can do this. We doubt our previously held values when they fail to properly address an event the magnitude of which they cannot satisfactorily handle. Peirce calls this "the irritation of doubt [that] causes a struggle to attain a state of belief. I shall term this struggle inquiry", where "the settlement of opinion is the sole end of inquiry" (Peirce 1877, 5). This struggle to attain axiological belief out of a state of doubt describes the axiological process. It is the search for new values, perhaps created from old ones, that must be formed from the active balancing of opposing alternatives until we reach a value that stops the irritation of doubt. That new horizontally determined value can now stand as the ultimate value in the Vertical scheme until such a time that novel events erode our satisfaction with the value and begin to irritate us into a state of doubt.

Pragmatism allows for a far more complex and nuanced appreciation of what value is in both its fixedness and its activity. Fully absent one half of the axiological equation, Agamben must press for a singular understanding of value. His contrarianism may not be caused by shear stubbornness alone—it may also be caused by a lack of options. Stubbornly holding on to a value that no longer addresses a novel situation leaves the holder of that fixed value unable to evolve different axiological strategies to counter existential threats. He has no other choice but to reiterate his chosen value.

Axiology is iterative because values develop as responses to environmental pressures. From time to time values require re-evaluation to test whether they can still serve our best interests, or whether they prevent us from properly addressing a crisis situation. COVID-19 certainly satisfies the criteria for being a disruptor of social values. It has made us question the type of freedom that we in the West take to be our guiding political principle. When our autonomous actions no longer guarantee maximum safety and our individuality prevents us from collectively curtailing an existential threat, then we are forced to seek a deeper meaning of what it means to be free. And then we can finally partake in that part of the axiological process that seeks to negotiate a proper communal value that maximizes our survival.

5.3 Iterative Axiology and Rationality

The iterative nature of belief describes not just the process of value formation. Peirce develops it to track how human reason operates in general, and axiology here is identified as a sub-type of human reasoning. We can even borrow Peirce's categories of fixing belief: there is the method of authority, where value is fixed by a vaunted figure (Foucault perhaps); the method of tenacity, where we value that which we have always valued; and the a priori method, where values are what are to us intuitively obvious. What they all have in common is that none have undergone the full iterative process of amelioration. Any accepted value must undergo the entire process for it to be rationally proper. This biologized rendering of reason is a very different type of rationality than Modernity is used to, but at the outset it gives us a standard by which to judge whether a value claim is rational or not.

The subtext of the iterative model is that the methods of authority, tenacity, and the a priori describe incomplete processes of rational human inquiry. Does Agamben follow the method of authority in his deference to his intellectual mentor, Foucault? Or does he exhibit the method of tenacity for his absolute insistence on a static value despite the best medical evidence? It may be a combination, but whichever the case is not the issue. What is important is that while it is possible to hold to these other methods of fixing belief or value, doing so will not result in a reason-based belief or value. This is not to say that, for example, individual freedom is not a reasoned solution to a problem in political philosophy. It most definitely was—but only when such freedom was the active product of inquiry that addressed the particular intellectual challenges during political and social unrest. When those stressors that gave rise to it no longer exist or change and we insist on the repeated use of freedom as the master value by which to resolve all social problems (and in the context of this book that includes the social response to pandemics), then we are acting at cross-purposes with our own survival. We are, in other words, acting irrationally.

We can finally understand what type of rationality is involved in iterative processes. The pragmatic claim is that iterative processes are rational in the sense that iteration cannot work if the product of such amelioration ends up in an incoherent practice. The process of iteration tends towards freeing itself from such inconsistencies and is in that sense self-corrective according to its specific situation. It is also an inherently communal activity. The process becomes more self-corrective when it includes diverse points of view from which a value can be determined. Because the concept of reason is participatory and discourse based, the rationality present in iterative processes operates according to Habermas's detailed analysis of performative contradictions.

The concept of the performative contradiction is central to Habermas's larger theory of communicative action. Because such discourse depends on what Martin Matustik calls "the non-coercive force of the 'better argument'" that participants collectively agree upon or reject, Habermas has strong sympathies with the Modern project of rationally arriving at solutions to social problems. But because this non-coercive use of reason is at the heart of his critique of Modernity's instrumental and totalizing use of reason, Habermas is sometimes referred to (incorrectly) in the same sentence as postmodernists. The truth is somewhere in between: unlike the postmodernists, he is attempting to resuscitate modernity from its crisis of rationality. But unlike much of 20th C philosophy, Habermas is well aware of the totalizing effects of logical positivism that would decimate the richness of the experienced lifeworld. Habermas's project is the result of this difference-splitting. He is arguing for a rationalism, but a Pragmatic rationalism; he is criticizing Modernity, but refusing to partake in the postmodern critique of it that emphasize negative hermeneutics, or genealogies of power structures, or the dissolution of discourse into *différance*.

Performative contradictions occur when what one says is in direct violation of how one behaves, or, writes Matustik, "whenever one shifts from being engaged in discourse into evading one's own stance, when what I say is undermined by my saying it" (Matustik 146). Habermas levels this critique against postmodern figures, and it is the central theme of his position in the Foucault-Habermas debates of the mid-80s. There is no need to revisit them here, but we can follow the issue in Agamben's pieces. When, for example, Agamben claims that governments are seeking to "use a state of exception as a normal paradigm for government" (Agamben 2020a), where such a state is predicated on "such a vague and undetermined definition" (Agamben 2020a), he himself is resorting to making the medical and historical record seem vague and undetermined by selectively choosing which official reports to include in his analysis. The timing of his articles is important. On February 26th, 2020, when Agamben published his first piece, Italy was just beginning to notice the virus. Italy recorded its first case of COVID-19 only on February 21 (Capalbo et al. 2020), so it is understandable that Italy's National Research Council claimed a day later on the 22nd that the country at that time had no COVID-19 epidemic. His second piece, published in response to public criticism, is dated March 17, two days after Italy instituted a national lockdown policy, and during the time COVID-19 cases began its inevitable climb. This would have been the time for a to reassess our values with a horizontalism, and yet Agamben reaffirms his claim: "there have been more serious epidemics in the past, but no one ever thought of declaring a state of emergency like today" (Agamben 2020b). That there have been worse outbreaks in the past is historically accurate, but that seriously undermines the lethality of COVID-19. That such a state of emergency was never declared before is dubious, and Foucault, Agamben's intellectual mentor, even gives an example of even more restrictive response to outbreaks. His argument is using vagueness and indeterminateness even as his critique against government action is based on vagueness and indeterminacy.

The performative contradiction is also operative in the Foucauldian claim to freedom. "A society that lives in a permanent state of emergency cannot be a free one," states Agamben. "We effectively live in a society that has sacrificed freedom to so-called "security reasons" and as a consequence has condemned itself to living in a permanent state of fear and insecurity" (Agamben 2020b). Again, the stated appeal to freedom is offset by any performative action on Agamben's part that would make the population more vulnerable to, and less free from, COVID-19 related suffering and death. If freedom from the pandemic is the end goal of state action, the argument that respecting our freedom would result in the performative loss of freedom is patently contradictory and incoherent.

This critique is not unique to Agamben or Foucault: it is equally applicable to the hardline libertarianism response to the virus. Freedom to go unmasked does not mean freedom to force others to unnecessarily be exposed to disease. The autonomous choice to go unvaccinated does not mean forcing others to live amongst disease vectors. Acceptance of a governmental strategy to manage a pandemic is not an acceptance of biopower. There are times, as the iterative model shows, when our values need to adjust to the medical and scientific facts on the ground.

The connection between axiology and rationality is important because it allows for the introduction of non-contradictory values into policy development. That such values are not presented in policy matters can, I believe, be detrimental to the policy's outcome. Health policy is comfortably developed in the language of medical research, empirical evidence, and social statistics: it doesn't deal with values, even though basing policy on these very issues reflects a value of its own. Policies are meant to be universally applicable, as if universality meant being value-free, and I suspect that one of the results of excising value from health policy is hesitancy to follow policy recommendations. In the absence of a stated axiology in policy matters, those who hold fast to values are tacitly invited to furnish their own and claim superiority by dint of at least talking in the language of values with which people are familiar rather than the specialized language of public policy. In this way, policies meant to secure a strategy against a pandemic may in fact contribute to the frustration of those goals. There is no good reason for this. Values are not irrational or statements of blind belief or feeling, and the performative contradiction gives us a very good measure of how to be rational. If the presence of a performative contradiction in an argument results in an irrational argument, a rational argument is one that is free from performative contradictions.[3] Incorporating values in public policy sends the message that a reasonable and defensible solution that requires us to act as a community is indeed a value worth having.

5.4 Towards a Rational Public Health Policy During Pandemic

We are now free to consider how to construct public health policy during a pandemic. These are not specific elements, but are instead general markers that any public health policy regarding pandemics must include in accordance to the iterative model of rational inquiry.

The first claim is that public health policy must be the product of an iterative process. Engage the public with the language of values and what that entails in times of social crises. Letting policy be led by medical science seems intuitively obvious in a time of pandemic, but it is by no means universally held, much less practiced: witness the Trump administration's politicization of the CDC; Hungary's use of the pandemic to foment anti-immigrant rhetoric; China's initial cover-up of the virus to save political face; India's ruling party's decision to hold political rallies for Assembly Elections that led to its second wave; Brazil's denial of medical science in order to prop up at least the appearance of economic populism. These are unfortunately just a few examples of countries behaving badly. The issue is not just reserved for political leaders. Traditional and social media have advanced COVID-19 and vaccine skepticism and/or hesitancy, whether out of earnestness or monetized ratings or contrarianism. Whichever the case, the values behind this view have never evolved to complete a fully developed axiological process. We cannot expect a political or social value to prevail during a medical crisis, and yet we note that the value Agamben and libertarianism want to uphold is political in nature. Negative liberty was at one point in history determined to address the pressing crisis for which philosophical Modernity was the answer. The pandemic is another such crisis, different in character because it is biologically based. Agamben is in effect insisting that the values established from the social and intellectual crises refer exactly to the crisis of survival that is biological. A reasoned public health policy cannot afford to make a similar mistake.

Secondly, any public health policy must be free from any performative contradictions in practice. Given that these contradictions may not be apparent at the outset, there is an amount of ameliorative flexibility necessary in this requirement, and when such an inconsistency is noted, policy must be able to rectify the issue. The stated policy must never run counter to the effect of the policy. This is yet another way to make sure that the policy is itself rationally binding. We've seen that the hard line libertarian message fails this test, and it is an invitation for us to determine how any resulting policy measures up to this rational standard. Is it logically coherent to forward health policies that, for example, relax restrictions without proof of vaccination, or allow de-masking on public transportation? What would the effects of those policies have in the public sphere? Much of this needs to be driven by empirical study, but the general question that should guide any policy is the following: Is that which is claimed consistent with the performance of an act based on that claim? Proper public health policy must not just present a non-contradictory position: it must also anticipate and properly respond to performatively contradictory values. Policy is not responsible for actively dismissing them—leave it to the public to decide which axiological claim is preferable, and trust the outcome of the debate. There is very good reason to be confident that the better argument will be the accepted one as avoiding performative contradictions are universal. It is the central concept in rationality. It is one way Plato disarms opposing arguments via the *elenchus*; it is expressed in the elements of logic found in the Mohist *Canons*, developed formally in the west by Aristotle's and Leibniz's Principle of Non-Contradiction, and in the east by the Indian concept of the Law of the Excluded Middle. These are formal ways of saying a basic truth of public discourse: no one likes a hypocrite.

And finally, any public health policy must be developed and reviewed openly and transparently. This is not just a political reality that has to be tolerated by policy makers, and it is more than just an aspirational claim or a proviso added because it is expected to be part of every public policy statement. It is necessitated because the structure of rational inquiry is involved in any effective form of public discourse. The iterative process means that policy makers must fully engage with public discourse and properly entertain good-faith feedback, especially criticism, instead of dismissing them *pro forma*. This again sounds obvious, but what we say as the ideal democratic goal of a transparently derived policy is often at odds with the consequences when those policies are firmly established. Because policy is disseminated from the top down, it is vulnerable to resistance at the street level. While the policy of accessible and free vaccination, for example, is openly agreed upon and accepted by experts and large swaths of the public, the actual vaccination campaign can be perceived as heavy handed to those not paying attention. When policies are operationalized outside of public view and critics are summarily discounted, public perception easily swings towards populist skepticism, oftentimes entertaining absurd claims. Public policy needs to get in front of the perception issue to prevent this, and it needs to actively address it when it occurs. The importance of underscoring communal discursive practice is for the policy itself to not fall prey to the very charge of the performative contradiction on which it is based. It is incoherent to author a public health policy that has the practical effect of stalling public health efforts.

Iteration, rationality, and communal discourse are of course not to be understood as separate from one another. To be iterative is to be rational is to be communal. Proper public health policy must exhibit all possible permutations of this triadic combination. It needs to appeal to the general value of human flourishing as determined by pandemic, and it needs to engage with critics on the basis of discursive rationality. Invite good faith criticisms and subject them to the test of performative contradiction, and offer only those reasons and directives that are free from dogmatic and non-transparent appeals to performatively contradictory statements. If the process of discursive rationality is the best way to sustain our flourishing, iteration, rationality, and communal discourse become valuable to us and we need to develop public health policy that has those values at the outset.

5.5 Conclusion

Values are far more plastic than we may like for something so fundamental to our ability to navigate the world, more stubborn than we may want for something that demands axiological nimbleness to ensure survival. They are products of inquiry that must be continuously made, unmade, remade in a process that unfolds in accordance to the environmental challenges humans face. They are not mere "feelings" or "beliefs" that inform our decision-making process by non- or irrational means. They are instead uniquely intertwined with reasoning, and they can be assessed for rational content.

It is thus important that values figure into the proper development of public health policies, especially during times of crises such as COVID-19. Every policy reflects a value, but no public health policy should be made using already established values that have never been iteratively determined. Policies are operationizable solutions meant to address an issue that spurs us into action. To not acknowledge values in their creation and dissemination only serves to invite the public to impute values that may reflect a contrarianism harmful to public health.

Understanding the structure of value also allows us to identify just how iteration, discursive rationality, and publicity are central to the development of public health policy. It gives an important measure of how to judge the rational content of value claims, and it gives us a map of how to make our policies better able to be as effective in practice as we say they can be.

Notes

1. Like all other groups, libertarianism includes a wide range of opinions. Many of them agree with government-set pandemic protocols, but there are those who do not. The libertarian position in this article refers to the latter.
2. I will be using Agamben's argument as a readymade exemplar of the hardline contrarian libertarian position throughout this article.
3. We note a curious outcome of this analysis: the postmodern claim that irrationality is a value can itself be rational—if it does not result in a performative contradiction in practice. This is not the case with Agamben, and there is thus good reason to dismiss his contrarian value claims. If Agamben were true to his Foucauldian roots, he might well not really care that his arguments are irrational, but a proper public health policy does not have the leisure of partaking in postmodernity's evasion of reason.

Works Cited

Agamben, Giorgio. 2020a. The Invention of an Epidemic. February 26, 2021. https://www.journal-psychoanalysis.eu/pandemics-and-philosophy/. Accessed June 28, 2021.

―――. 2020b. Clarifications. March 17, 2021. https://www.journal-psychoanalysis.eu/pandemics-and-philosophy/. Accessed June 28, 2021.

Capalbo, C., E. Bertamino, A. Zerbetto, I. Santino, A. Petrucca, R. Mancini, R. Bonfini, V. Alfonsi, S. Ferracuti, P. Marchetti, M. Simmaco, G.B. Orsi, and C. Napoli. 2020, November 16. No Evidence of SARS-CoV-2 Circulation in Rome (Italy) During the Pre-Pandemic Period: Results of a Retrospective Surveillance. *International Journal of Environmental Research and Public Health* 17 (22): 8461. doi: https://doi.org/10.3390/ijerph17228461. PMID: 33207548; PMCID: PMC7696939. https://pubmed.ncbi.nlm.nih.gov/33207548/.

James, William. 1896. The Sentiment of Rationality. *The Will to Believe and Other Essays in Popular Philosophy.* https://www.gutenberg.org/files/26659/26659-h/26659-h.htm#P63. Accessed July 3, 2021.

Kampmark, Binoy. 2020. The Pandemic Surveillance State: An Enduring Legacy of COVID-19. *Journal of Global Faultlines,* 7 (1): 59–70. *Gale Academic OneFile.* link.gale.com/apps/doc/A642349602/AONE?u=oregon_oweb&sid=googleScholar&xid=3c7c77c5. Accessed July 7, 2021.

Lee, Seung-Hwan. 2018. Confucianism as an Antidote for Liberal Self-Centeredness: A Dialogue Between Confucianism and Liberalism. In *Confucianisms for a Changing World Cultural Order,* ed. Roger Ames and Peter Hershock, 29–42. Honolulu: University of Hawai'i Press, *JSTOR,* www.jstor.org/stable/j.ctv3zp05k.5. Accessed July 2, 2021.

Matustik, Martin J. 1989. Habermas on Communicative Reason and Performative Contradiction. *New German Critique* 47. Duke University Press. https://www.jstor.org/stable/488111.

Peirce, Charles S. 1877. The Fixation of Belief. http://www.bocc.ubi.pt/pag/peirce-charles-fixation-belief.html. Accessed June 21, 2021.

Chapter 6
Pandemics and Race

Takunda Matose and Paul C. Taylor

Abstract In this chapter, we identify three ways in which pandemics function as both racialized and racializing phenomena. First, invidious racial ideologies often inform attempts to explain and respond to pandemics. Second, critical and diagnostic forms of race-thinking pick out the clusters of conditions that increase the risk of vulnerability to pandemic diseases. And third, racist practices are often causally related to disease incidence. In light of these three ways in which pandemics are both racialized and racializing, we explore how the racialization of the COVID-19 crisis compares with historic patterns of pandemic racialization.

Keywords COVID-19 · Pandemics · Public health ethics · Necropolitics · Race · Racial projects · Racism · Racialization · Critical race theory

6.1 Introduction

Five months after the World Health Organization (WHO) declared that the COVID-19 crisis met the criteria for a pandemic, a researcher in the United States (US) described the disease as "another unwelcome addition to the long list of health conditions that disproportionately affect black and brown lives in the United States."[1] If anything, this description did not go far enough. The COVID-19 pandemic has had racially disparate impacts across the globe, and the racial dimensions of the crisis go beyond the sheer fact of disproportionate impact. It is, in this respect, quite representative of pandemics throughout history.

In this chapter, we identify three ways in which pandemics function as both racialized and racializing phenomena. First, invidious racial ideologies often inform attempts to explain and respond to pandemics. Second, critical and diagnostic forms

---

T. Matose (✉)
Edmond J. Safra Center for Ethics, Harvard University, Cambridge, MA, USA
e-mail: tmatose@luc.edu

P. C. Taylor
Department of Philosophy, Vanderbilt University, Nashville, TN, USA
e-mail: paulc.taylor@vanderbilt.edu

© The Author(s), under exclusive license to Springer Nature Switzerland AG 2022
M. Boylan (ed.), *Ethical Public Health Policy Within Pandemics*, The International Library of Bioethics 95, https://doi.org/10.1007/978-3-030-99692-5_5

of race-thinking can perspicuously pick out the clusters of conditions that increase the risk of vulnerability to pandemic diseases. And third, racist practices are often causally related to disease incidence.

The remainder of the chapter proceeds in five sections. The second section explores the meaning of race and explains how we propose to talk about it. Section three explores the modern emergence of public health and (the most familiar forms of) race-thinking, thereby setting the stage for the discussion in section four of some historical examples of pandemics and the three broad modes of racialization at work in each case. Then section five compares the racialization of the COVID-19 crisis with historic patterns of pandemic racialization.

6.2 A Consensus Conception of Race

Race is a notoriously slippery and controversial subject. Because of this slipperiness and because of the dynamics that routinely emerge in vibrant sub-fields of philosophy, race theorists have staked out a variety of distinct positions on various aspects of the subject. Some think the vernacular conception of race (if there is just one) is indefensible, while some think it's salvageable. Some are interested in race as a political tool that governments and societies use to contain unruly populations, while others regard it as a conceptual tool that theorists can use to capture the way human social practices have created porous but identifiable breeding populations. Some attach a great deal of importance to the fact that race-thinking works differently in different places, while others are content to focus primarily on the color-coded US-style approach. Finally, some think race-talk does more harm than good and should be abolished, while others think some refined, critical forms of it do useful anti-racist work.

Let's say that these differences mark the boundaries between different conceptions of race, and then note that a handful of basic commitments have won wide assent from people otherwise committed to widely divergent views. These basic commitments reveal the shape of a viable contemporary concept of race, a concept that the various conceptions aim to refine and operationalize. This outline of a concept can serve as the ground for our inquiry here into the relationship between race and pandemics. Once one sets aside the more divisive questions about what the outline contains, a handful of guiding principles for race-theoretic inquiry come into view.

The first principle is that one should take race seriously, which means accepting that it is important to examine the practices and populations that words like "race" denote. There are different ideas about how the practices work and what the populations are and how to use the words properly, but the shared starting point typically involves attending to the vernacular practices of race-thinking in places like the US. In these places it is common to sort humans into five or so color-coded populations (brown, black, red, white, and yellow), and to think of these populations as interestingly (if not always directly) descended from the premodern inhabitants of the world's major land masses.

The remaining principles explain what it means to take race seriously. One should, at a minimum, approach race *critically*, with an eye toward contesting the mechanisms of racial oppression and injustice and questioning the racial discourses that support, sustain, and emerge from these mechanisms; as an *artifact*, accepting that words like "race" pick out products not (just) of natural forces but of the meaning-laden, historically evolving exercise of human agency (even if those products still implicate human biology or psychology); as an importantly *modern* invention, with its most influential forms emerging during the modern period (even if those forms have important premodern roots, and even if other forms reward study); as a *political* phenomenon, or as something that matters in part because of its role in distributing social goods, in formulating and applying ethico-political norms, and in advancing—and contesting—schemes for human exploitation, oppression, and extermination; and, finally, as a *social* phenomenon, one that locates individual choices about which cultures and ideologies to choose in the wider social contexts that set the choice parameters and that, in the limit case, and with the threat of deadly force, set those parameters quite narrowly (all of which is to say that one can't simply decide what race one will be; society has some say in this).

This consensus race theory is a critical, revisionary alternative to the classical race theories that have done so much to shape the modern world. The classical race theories that informed the US slavocracy, the Holocaust, South African apartheid, the life and long afterlife of the Confederate States of America, and much else besides, took race seriously, but (usually) as a natural aspect of the human condition and as an occasion and resource for oppression and exploitation. This newly (in the grand sweep of human history) assertive *critical* racialism attempts to use ethically and scientifically responsible modes of race-thinking to grapple with the world that classical racialism helped make. On these revisionary, critical approaches, racial identities are ways of registering an individual's location relative to societal patterns of advantage and disadvantage, in part by noting the way superficial (and often physiognomic) traits link to variations in life chances, social holdings, and other markers of well-being.

It is important to note that on the provisional, broadly methodological approach laid out here, races are not necessarily self-aware culture groups or political collectives with shared we-intentions, nor are they necessarily coterminous with the things that the Modern West decided to call races. They may be those things (depending on which conception one endorses), but they are also, and at a minimum, sets of human persons who are similarly situated with respect to some social condition or mechanism. To invoke a distinction that we will note but not insist on in what follows, races often function more saliently as populations than as groups.

Similarly, for social theoretic purposes, to belong to a race is, at a minimum and perhaps most saliently, to be similarly situated with respect to the social forces and distributions that, in places like the US, distribute social goods in ways that track the possession of superficial traits like hair texture and skin color. To be white is, for example, to be more likely than members of other races to enjoy certain social advantages and avoid certain risks of harm and ill-treatment, with this increased likelihood of risk-avoidance and reward-conferral both generalizing across income strata, age groups, geographic regions, and so on, *and* reliably varying what Ron Mallon helpfully refers to as the "thin racial endowment"—the collection of superficial traits (like physiognomy and ancestry) that societies use to assign racial identities.[2] These racialized social locations are in some ways easiest to discern in relation to modern mechanisms of socioeconomic stratification—income levels vary by race within occupational niches, wealth levels vary by race within income strata, and so on—but they, of course, have implications for other markers of well-being, such as educational attainment and health care delivery. The risk-reward profile (like its link to the thin racial endowment) is not completely seamless or indefeasible, nor is it all there is to racial identity, but it is crucial in thinking about the way race intersects with public health.

6.3 History, Public Health, and Modern Racialism

Epidemiologists trace modern-day public health to Edward Jenner's discovery of the smallpox vaccine in the eighteenth century.[3] Further advancements in public health were made in the twentieth century when changing material and conceptual conditions forced a re-envisioning of health and its requirements. These changes meant that medical practitioners had to start thinking about population-level and socially contingent factors to address the medical needs of patients. In other words, changes in material conditions forced a reconceptualization of the connection between health, disease, and health care. Attending to human well-being came to mean, in a way it had not before, caring for the health of populations and groups. As it happens, at nearly the same moment, new conceptual resources for thinking about populations were becoming available, for good and for ill.

Not long before Jenner introduced the smallpox vaccine, key shifts in European and Eurocentric racial discourse and practice signaled the transition from early modern to high modern approaches to racialization. One of the clearer markers of these shifts is Thomas Jefferson's *Notes on the State of Virginia* (1786), which offers its author's "suspicion" that varying degrees of capacity and worth attach to distinct racial types, and then models his conviction that suspicions like this can and should be at the heart of systematic scientific inquiries and rigid social hierarchies. This Jeffersonian sensibility supplanted ideas rooted in older and looser conceptions of human difference and marked the emergence of an episteme that spawned thriving research programs and far-reaching policies. The research programs included cornerstones of scientific racism like Samuel George Morton's biometric studies from the 1830s. The policy regimes included the Naturalization Act of 1790, which declared that only "free white persons" could become naturalized citizens of the new United States, and the refinements of racial capitalism that emerged in the US slave economy after the invention of the cotton gin in 1793.

As the epistemic and political projects of high modern racialism matured and evolved, they combined with increasingly assertive and ambitious state bureaucracies to create a toxically racist orientation to the prospects for medical and public health interventions. In the age of what Foucault encourages us to call bio-power, in which states grow ever more comfortable actively attempting to promote something like the health of their populations, a commitment to inherited and rankable differences between human types leads directly to a variety of outcomes that now seem grotesque. The eugenics movement, a policy regime aimed at improving the genetic stock of the citizenry by manipulating the production and reproduction of more or less desirable human types (using, among other means, forced sterilization), may be the clearest emblem and example of this worrisome convergence of social forces. But it is evident also in the pathologization and demonization of racialized populations and spaces as somehow inherently prone to vice, crime, and disease. For example, one of the founding texts of American sociology, W.E.B. Du Bois's *The Philadelphia Negro* (1899) aims in part to contest the then-popular idea that "Negro" slums were unsanitary and unhealthy because of the character of the people who lived in them, instead of, as Du Bois (a trifle unevenly) suggested, because of the way society deigned to treat the people who lived in them.

6.4 Racializing Pandemics

This historical perspective highlights the broad convergences linking public health practices to racialization processes. A closer look at pandemics in particular reveals three striking connections between race and public health crises. First, invidious race-thinking often informs pandemic analysis and response. Second, critical race-thinking can highlight certain conditions that increase the risk of vulnerability to disease. And third, racism is often causally related to disease incidence. This section will explore the three modes of pandemic racialization in seven historical cases: the plague, smallpox, malaria, cholera, tuberculosis, influenza, and HIV/AIDS.

6.4.1 Pandemics, Ideology, and Explanation

Societies facing novel diseases often mobilize invidious racial ideologies as resources for explanation and response. Examples of this abound throughout history, from centuries-old plague and cholera pandemics to more recent bouts with HIV/AIDS and smallpox. The mechanisms of epistemic distortion in these faux-explanations are repetitive and produce distressing patterns of societal response.

The plague provides an instructive set of early instances of the link between pandemic explanation and response and racial stereotypes and oppression. The arrival of the plague in fourteenth century Europe led to anti-Jewish pogroms, during which approximately one thousand Jewish communities were wiped out across Europe.[4] But even as early as 430 BC, Athenians blamed the plague on poisons administered by the Peloponnesians.[5] During later episodes of the plague, people and goods traveling from Asia to Europe were detained because the plague originated in the East.[6] Elsewhere, efforts to combat the plague through quarantine were used to justify racial policies designed to manage the black African in Cape Town and Chinese populations in Sydney, San Francisco, and Honolulu.[7]

By the time of the first cholera epidemic in the early nineteenth century, the link between disease and race-thinking was solidified. Europeans believed that cholera, like the plague, originated in the East. As a result, they attributed the emergence of cholera to racialized others from the Indian subcontinent.[8] Cholera was associated with the urban poor, particularly Indian immigrants, so Europeans took the disease to signify filth and primitivism.[9] The fact that subsequent cholera epidemics were linked to other places in the East failed to diminish this association. One writer suggested that:

> The actual danger for Europe lies in the international [Islamic] places of pilgrimage Mecca, Medina, Kerbalah, Damascus, Jerusalem, the different places in Persia and the large places of rendezvous of the processions of pilgrims... Oriental squalor and the absence of any, or any serious sanitary police at the great places of pilgrimage encourage the disease whose germ finds a fertile soil in the bodies of the pilgrims, weakened by all kinds of deprivations.[10]

As this quote suggests, Europeans quickly conflated disease with persons, race, religion, and sanitary practices. Because of these conflations, Europeans took the spread of cholera to non-whites to be evidence of their superiority. Race and ethnicity became ready proxies for these conflations.

Nor was the conflation of race, practices, persons, and disease restricted to cholera and the plague. Colonists in seventeenth-century New England thought smallpox was punishment for the heathen ways of the Indians and was God's way of confirming manifest destiny.[11] In Western Samoa, the spread of pandemic influenza and its effects were attributed to the moral failings of the Tongan people, who were blamed for being apathetic and indifferent to the outbreak and being lazy when they were afflicted.[12] In both these cases, the spread of disease was taken to signify something about the racialized peoples suffering its effects instead of merely pathogenic events.

The HIV/AIDS pandemic also involved racialized conflations of persons, meanings, and pathogens. One prominent example is the quarantine of Haitians at Camp Bulkeley in Guantanamo Bay in the early nineties. Haitians suspected of having HIV or AIDS and those related to someone with HIV were held at the camp, sometimes for years, to control the pandemic. This quarantine was part of a historical practice initiated by the US Centers for disease control, of designating the mere fact of being Haitian as a risk factor for HIV.[13] Because of this designation, HIV came to be known as the "4H Disease," supposedly afflicting Haitians alongside "hemophiliacs," "heroin users," and "homosexuals."[14] The inclusion of Haitians in this list had racial undertones. According to Paul Farmer, this designation "invoked reference to the Haitians' poverty, their race, and their 'foreignness.'"[15]

If these invocations were present in the association of Haitians with HIV, they dominated the thinking around HIV/AIDS and Africans. For example, Andrew Natsios, then head of USAID, told members of Congress that Africans were incapable of taking antiretroviral drugs because they don't wear watches and would not be able to follow the treatment schedule.[16] In other words, for Natsios and like-minded folks, the mere fact that the target population consisted of Africans was enough to predict the failure of what was already known to be the most effective treatment and prevention regimen for HIV.

In contrast to the perceptions of non-white people exhibited in the preceding examples, people of European descent have historically seen themselves as cleaner, more civilized, and intellectually, technologically, and morally superior. For example, the discovery that mosquitos were the vectors for malaria meant that controlling mosquitoes would control the disease. Europeans then took this mastery of malaria, and therefore the tropics, to affirm their superiority over other races. A similar story can be told about Tuberculosis (TB). Although Europe and the United States had long histories with the disease, they experienced a steep decline in cases starting in the mid-nineteenth century. Still, TB continued to affect non-whites disproportionately.[17] However, as TB incidence declined in Europe and the United States for people of European descent, it increased in other places globally and for those who were racialized as non-white. This increased incidence led to racially charged explanations where black South Africans, American Indians, and African Americans were taken to be more susceptible to TB because of their race, while white Europeans were assumed to be genetically better equipped to fight the infection.[18] In other words, there was an idea, especially in the early twentieth century, that the different stages of the TB pandemic could be explained by racially indexed genetics.

These examples suggest a few ways in which race-thinking functions as an explanatory tool during pandemics. First, race is sometimes taken to be a cause of pandemics. That is, the mere fact of place or of being a racialized person from a particular place is taken to be itself pathogenic. This line of thought helps explain why pandemics have often coincided with travel restrictions and the banning of goods, predominantly those involving Asian countries or countries in the global South. It also helps explain the rationale, albeit mistaken, behind the HIV quarantine at Camp Bulkeley.

Second, the social practices of racialized others are taken to explain the emergence and spread of pathogens during pandemics. This type of explanation often relies on the presumed inferiority and primitiveness of the racialized others and takes the form of accusations of uncleanliness or participation in uncultured, that is, non-Western/European social practices. The suggestion being that if the racialized others were to participate in more cultured social practices, the pandemic might not arise. Additionally, race is sometimes used as the basis of moralized explanations of the inferiority of the racialized others. In this sense, pandemics are taken to be the result of more than just backward social practices. Instead, pandemics are seen as the result of the moral inferiority of racialized others.

Finally, race is taken to provide a biological/genetic explanation for disease susceptibility. In this way, race and ethnicity are taken to denote inherent genetic differences that explain differences in disease incidence and prevalence. These differences can be direct, as in the sense of one's susceptibility to particular pathogens, or indirect, as in one's ability to develop solutions to these pathogens. In either case, race is supposed to pick out objective and medically significant differences between people.

As the examples discussed in this section suggest, these three ways in which race can function as an explanatory tool have negative consequences for people racialized as non-white. These consequences include quarantine, ostracization, and dehumanization. Through these practices, pandemics often serve as an opportunity to reaffirm the racial project or otherwise exclude or subjugate racialized others.

6.4.2 Race, Epidemiology, and Risk

In addition to providing a field for invidious racial ideologies to prop up flawed explanations and heinous social practices, pandemics also reveal the epidemiological utility of a critical orientation to race-thinking. As with the previously discussed example of TB, pandemics afflict non-whites at higher rates that outstrip the non-white share of the population. This disproportionality might be attributed to two key factors used to track a post-classical conception of race within social theories rooted in critical race thinking.

First, non-whites tend to have lower socioeconomic statuses than whites, partly because of the legacies of colonialism. In particular, pandemics tend to disproportionately afflict the poor who are forced to live in higher density, less sanitary conditions that are fertile breeding grounds for communicable diseases. Additionally, the poor often have less access to the best treatment and protective resources than people from higher socioeconomic strata. For example, the rich in the US not only had access to the best available TB treatment during the late nineteenth century, but they also had the resources to escape places like New York City, where the risk of transmission was the greatest.[19] The effect of these kinds of socioeconomic factors on disease experience is often that the socioeconomic profile skews poorer as pandemics progress.[20]

Pandemics also tend to disproportionally affect non-whites due to co-morbidities, immunological profiles, endemic cultural practices, geographic factors, and societal arrangements, all of which join socioeconomic status in the "homeostatic property clusters" that critical race theorists often use race-talk to denote.[21] These factors increase the risk of exposure and transmission of the relevant disease vector while also leading to disparate levels of the burden of disease within each racial population. For example, although blacks had lower rates of infection during the 1918 Influenza pandemic, they experienced significantly higher rates of mortality, likely due to co-infections with a variety of other diseases, including pneumonia and TB.[22] But, as discussed in the earlier examples of smallpox and cholera, pandemic vulnerability can also result from immunological naivete. In each case, the result is that pandemics tend to afflict non-white racial groups at greater rates as pandemics progress.

These two ways in which pandemics tend to afflict non-white racial groups disproportionately suggest another reason why race has been taken to explain disease susceptibility. In the eighteenth century, medical researchers like James Lind, who famously recognized the benefit of citrus juice in preventing scurvy, theorized that humans were equally adaptable to different climates. But colonizing Europeans found themselves succumbing to "tropical" diseases like malaria at rates far greater than some of the peoples they were colonizing, leading Europeans to believe that race could explain different susceptibilities to disease.[23]

Improved understanding of how diseases work and the factors that impact their transmission have led most epidemiologists to dismiss this assumption of race-linked disease susceptibility. As the earlier examples suggest, evidence shows that in addition to socioeconomic factors, the disproportionate impact of pandemics on racial and ethnic minorities stems in part from pre-existing or co-morbid, generally chronic conditions like diabetes and heart disease. Nonetheless, because of these factors, membership in racial groups is a useful marker for tracking the impact of pandemic disease in a population. In other words, although epidemiologists have largely dismissed the notion that there are inherent race-based differences in disease susceptibility, there are still appreciable differences in the pandemic experiences of members of different racial groups.

Given this type of evidence, there are at least two ways in which conceptions of race have historically had epidemiological import. First, race has been used to identify the incidence of pandemic disease in different communities. That is, even when problematic assumptions were drawn about the meaning of disease prevalence in people from different racial and ethnic groups, these categories nonetheless were instructive as to the disparate impact of pandemics. Second, because of its utility as a marker for the prevalence of pandemic disease in different health groups, race has also served as a useful proxy for diagnosing existing inequalities in health. Again, these links between race and pandemics can exist even if claims about race-based susceptibility to disease are misguided or if the mechanisms that underwrite the links are misunderstood.

6.4.3 *Racism, Oppression, and Causality*

The third way pandemics have historically had a racial dimension is that they have often been the direct consequence of racist practices. The prime example is the introduction of smallpox and malaria to the Americas. With smallpox, an initial strain was brought to the Americas from Europe through settler colonialism before a second strain from Africa was brought to the Americas through the trans-Atlantic slave trade. In both cases, the smallpox virus spread rapidly because it was entering an immunologically naïve population. The impact of this two-pronged smallpox attack was devastating, reducing the indigenous population by as much as 90%.[24] In addition to directly eradicating some smaller indigenous groups, smallpox also led larger groups like the Iroquois to initiate "mourning wars" to replace their dead. The result was pandemic-induced migration and mixing, which caused the forging of new ethnic identities and new demographic profiles of the different regions of North America.[25]

In addition to smallpox, the transatlantic slave trade also brought the *Plasmodium Falciparum* strain of malaria to North America in the seventeenth century.[26] As with the introduction of smallpox, the rampant spread of disease was partly driven by the availability of an immunologically naïve population who seemed less able to fight it. These conditions resulted in a harmful cycle where indigenous Africans kept being enslaved to replace the indigenous Americans who succumbed to a strain of malaria that kept being reintroduced with each arrival of the enslaved, all to keep plantations working.

Colonialism's pandemic effects also impacted colonizing Europeans and those who remained in Europe, leading to public health efforts that were initially Eurocentric. While the presence of pandemic disease in colonial settings was used to justify the pursuit of manifest destiny, this pursuit also directly led to Europeans being adversely affected by pandemic disease. As stated earlier, Europeans found themselves succumbing to malaria because of colonization. Europeans were also exposed to yellow fever in addition to malaria and the plague through colonization. The transmission of pandemic diseases to Europe because of colonization led to the International Sanitary Conventions that were convened starting in 1851. However, the first iterations of these conventions were focused on preventing pandemic diseases from entering Europe from the colonies, not on preventing the reverse transmission that was arguably just as big a problem.[27]

A similar focus can be found in HIV/AIDS pandemic responses. Despite a robust response to HIV/AIDS in Europe and North America since the eighties, there was a slow global response to the pandemic in Africa, even though it was thought to be the origin point and epicenter of the pandemic.[28] This inaction has likely exacerbated and perpetuated the HIV/AIDS crisis in Africa and other resource-limited settings. Additionally, evidence suggests that one of the key drivers of the HIV/AIDS pandemic has been urbanization and the strains of migration in post-colonial African countries. These factors help explain not only the persistence of the HIV/AIDS pandemic in these settings but also the different demographic profile of the disease from region to region.

These examples show that modernity's colonialist racial projects have historically played a causal role in the proliferation of pandemic disease to both the colonized and the colonizers. These racial projects can create the conditions that allow pandemics to spread, whether because of forced migration, global economic activities, or racially circumscribed disease mitigation strategies. These activities take diseases endemic to particular regions, introduce them to immunologically naïve populations, and facilitate rapid transmission in regions far beyond their origins. We contend, then, that pandemics are at least in part a result of race-thinking and its projects. Our view is that racialized modes of thinking and their projects help create the conditions that allow the proliferation of pandemic disease.

6.5 COVID-19 and Race

Despite repeated messaging about the "unprecedented" nature of COVID-19, race functions in this pandemic in quite predictable ways. We have argued that race-thinking and racial practices routinely play definite roles during pandemics. Ideological conceptions of race help motivate and justify crude explanations and short-sighted inquiries; critical conceptions of race function as resources for tracking patterned variations in vulnerability to pandemic risk factors; oppressive racial projects work directly to spread disease and vulnerability to disease. Unsurprisingly, the COVID-19 pandemic fits neatly into this pattern.

6.5.1 COVID-19 and Racial-Ideological Explanation

As in prior pandemics, invidious racial ideologies shaped attempts to understand, explain, and address the emergence and spread of COVID-19. Donald Trump, the US president during the onset of the pandemic, exemplified this tendency with his frequent references to COVID-19 disease as the "Kung Flu" and SARS-CoV-2 as the "China Virus."[29] This racially tinged nomenclature accompanied calls for people who looked even vaguely Asian to "go back home to China" and accusations that these persons were in some way responsible for the spread of the disease.[30]

Another trope at the beginning of the pandemic was the claim that the SARS-CoV-2 zoonosis originated in the Huanan wet market in Wuhan, China.[31] In particular, there was oft-repeated speculation that SARS-CoV-2 jumped from bats—the largest animal reservoirs of coronaviruses[32]—to humans because people in Wuhan consumed bat meat. Scientific exploration into the origin of zoonosis quickly led to xenophobic rhetoric concerning the dietary practices of people in Wuhan, including one Fox News anchor insisting that the Chinese are desperate and eat uncooked, unsafe animals.[33] Other public figures echoed the sentiment, including popular musicians Bryan Adams, Brian May, and the Beatles' Paul McCartney, the last of whom referred to the eating practices as "medieval."[34]

The epistemic distortions in this trope are not far to seek. While studies suggest that the virus might have started in bats, there was no direct evidence that the virus was circulating in animals and animal products tied to the market.[35] Attempts at explanation quickly homed in on non-Western cultural practices while marking those who participated in those practices as backward and unclean and ignoring other possible causal explanations, such as habitat destruction.[36] It is noteworthy that this rhetoric has persisted despite the central claim that these dietary practices are to blame for the pandemic being repeatedly disproven.

Responding to a public health crisis with ill-informed prejudices would be problematic enough in a vacuum, but vacuums are hard to find in racialized social formations. Accordingly, the rhetoric about COVID-19 does not simply get the facts wrong; it also builds on and extends a long Euro-modern tradition of Sinophobic and more broadly anti-Asian animus and activity. Some have sought to read this rhetoric not as racist animus but as criticism of China as a geopolitical entity,[37] but putting the rhetoric in wider context makes this move hard to sustain. Approximately 3800 attacks against Asian Americans were reported in the year following the pandemic's beginning in the United States, increasing roughly a hundred and fifty percent over the previous year.[38] Notably, most of those attacks were against women—a pattern that highlights the importance of intersectional studies of the gendered and sexualized dimensions of anti-Asian racism[39]—and people racialized as Asian were equally subject to attack regardless of whether or how recently they came from China.

These attacks suggest a direct correlation between ideas about COVID-19 originating in China and an increase in anti-Asian racism. The cultural or associational logic of this correlation is straightforward, and familiar to students of racial ideologies. If a disease originates in a certain kind of place—a place populated primarily by racialized Others, or prominently defined by public meanings attached to certain modes of racialization—then the people who belong to or issue from that place fall under suspicion as potential vectors for transmission. Any interest in defining the place or the people with precision swiftly gets overwhelmed by moral and political panic, and hasty overgeneralizations turn into broad stereotypes and sweeping xenophobic claims. In the case of COVID-19, this suspicion fell not only on ethnic Chinese people either in the country or residing elsewhere, but also on people mistakenly thought to be Chinese or, more simply, on people who appear to be Asian, all of whom are deemed pathogenic by association. This means that the social practices of these racialized others become resources for assembling ideologically distorted explanations of the emergence and spread of COVID-19. These attempts at explanation then persist in the absence of supporting evidence and without regard for the possibility of alternative explanations, such as the possibility that SARS-CoV-2 zoonosis happened outside China before the first cases were reported in Wuhan.[40]

6.5.2 COVID-19 and Race as an Epidemiological Marker

While race-based attacks during the COVID-19 pandemic have predominantly been aimed at Asian Americans, the epidemiological profile of the pandemic shows a broader impact across a wide range of racial populations. Even in the early days of the pandemic, its racially disparate impacts were already becoming clear.

Researchers quickly identified racial disparities in the impact of COVID-19 on all-cause mortality. (There are a variety of ways to measure the health impacts of COVID-19, mortality links to other health metrics in ways that make it particularly useful for exploring the intersection between race and public health.) Roughly six months into the pandemic, the US Centers for Disease Control (CDC) reported approximately three hundred thousand excess deaths than would have been expected around October 2020. Strikingly, the increases in expected all-cause mortality differed by race, with increases of 11.9% for white persons, 28.9% for American Indians/ Alaskan Natives, 32.9% for black persons, 36.6% for Asian persons, and 53.6% for Hispanic persons.[41]

Additionally, in nursing homes, where roughly 40% of deaths occurred at one point in the pandemic, black and Hispanic persons experienced higher rates of mortality than white persons during the initial stages of the COVID-19 pandemic.[42]

While racially stratified health outcomes during the pandemic varied by ethnoracial group in more or less the way one would expect—whites tended to be least negatively affected, blacks tended to be most affected, and others tended to fall somewhere in between—several cross-cutting factors complicate the picture considerably. For example, as the authors of one study point out, "[a]djusting for age exacerbates differences in excess mortality between White people and people of each other race or Hispanic origin" because age distributions differ in each population; similarly, adjusting for state of residence "substantially increases estimated excess mortality for American Indian and Alaska Native people, as well as for Native Hawaiian and Pacific Islander people." The authors continue: "in several states Black and Hispanic people experienced an increase in mortality in April 2020, whereas White people did not."[43]

While these disparate results reflect a broader reality about how the data vary from place to place and study to study, they also consistently align with the patterned differences across US racial groups that we noted above. At one point, a study of California's population put the increase in mortality during the pandemic at 6% for white persons, 18% for Asians, 28% for black persons, and 36% for Hispanic persons.[44] Another study noted that black persons comprised 14% of the population in Michigan but represented 60% of COVID-19 cases and had higher risks of death and markers relevant to COVID-19. This pattern even held when adjusted for class, as lower socioeconomic status was a greater predictor of poor morbidity and mortality outcomes for black persons than white persons.[45] Although the precise picture varies with factors like geography and age, the general trend of patterned racial differences in pandemic-related health outcomes remains.

We take the persistence of this racial patterning to show that race is a marker for the different rates at which COVID-19 afflicts different social groups. It can, as a result, be a resource for tracking COVID-19 and non-COVID-19 health inequities. It is important to disaggregate the data to track the impact on particular populations, like Asian Americans,[46] and to credit the way factors like occupation and socioeconomic status affect the risk of exposure.[47] Nonetheless, membership in a racial group is epidemiologically significant since it correlates with varying degrees of risk for negative pandemic-related health outcomes, even after one adjusts for other factors.[48]

6.5.3 COVID-19 and Racism as a Causal Factor

Racial identity is a useful proxy for vulnerability to COVID-related harms and risks in part because oppressive racial practices have played a role in the emergence and spread of this disease. Perhaps most obviously, racial prejudices—perhaps better, racialized variations in estimates of human worth—appear to have shaped policies and proposals concerning the distribution of public health resources. In addition, modernity's racialized colonial projects shaped the world in ways that bear directly on the material prospects for effective and racially egalitarian pandemic response.

European modernity was both a racial project and a global and globalizing enterprise. Europe's empires and forced labor regimes systematically promoted global flows of goods, people, information, capital, and resources long before our contemporary ideas about globalization took root. These flows were of course organized to benefit some parts and inhabitants of the globe more than others, and this asymmetric allocation of benefit persists today in forms that impact the capacity to address global health crises.

To put the point more crudely than it deserves but with as much nuance as our available space allows: health care systems worldwide were ill-equipped to mount a truly global response to the COVID-19 crisis because those systems were built on foundations laid not to promote health but to facilitate exploitation. Some of those foundations are ideological and cultural, involving traditions of consciously or unconsciously regarding some lives as inherently worth less than others. Others, however, are economic and material, and firmly constrain the kinds of options that are available to policymakers and political leaders.[49]

With respect to the material foundations, it is important to note that the colonies represented pools of cheap labor, reservoirs of raw materials, markets for the sale of goods, and dumping grounds for excess or otherwise undesirable populations. They were not part of the empire's community, entitled to equal concern and respect and to equitable shares of resources; not even when imperial domination came with promises of assimilation and citizenship. Consequently, providing for the colonized subjects was not the primary driver of colonial policy, including policies related to infrastructure, such as where and whether to build roads, where to promote sustainable agriculture and urban planning and where to frustrate these things.

Against this historical backdrop it should be no surprise that providing for the former colonies is not a primary driver of policy or social organization in the postcolonial world. Global aid regimes have long been tilted against bolstering the internal capacities of the former colonies, for example by linking eligibility for aid to limits on public sector investment and by insisting that the now-independent former colonies use resources they might invest in their people to repay the debts incurred by the colonial regimes. (Similar points apply, *mutatis mutandis*, to emancipated settler colonial states like South Africa and Zimbabwe.)

These neocolonial and postcolonial arrangements set a variety of material limitations on the capacity to mount an adequate response to a truly global health crisis. Relevant factors here include the inadequate sourcing and production of essential equipment and medicines in formerly colonized nations,[50] the shift to just-in-time manufacturing practices in the global supply chain, the privatization of health care systems, the willingness to exploit and encroach upon non-human animal habitats in ways that may contribute to zoonosis,[51] and the weakening of the World Health Organization and similar multi-lateral institutions. There are also, of course, considerations like the ones noted in the previous section, related to the way societies structured in racial dominance increase health risks by declining to ameliorate social conditions that promote vulnerability, like overcrowding and poor nutrition. This dynamic affects the global South just as it does other regions, but on a wider scale. Nations in the global South have limited capacity to structure their relationships to the global economy to benefit their citizens, so they remain, to some degree, at the mercy of economic and political decisionmakers in other countries. This forces us to widen the analytical frame and consider the entire world as a society structured in racial dominance, and to see the vulnerability of the poorer nations as a legacy of longstanding racially oppressive arrangements.

The question of the global distribution of essential materials marks one point at which the world's neocolonial material arrangements dovetail with similarly neocolonial ideological formations. US and European states and corporations have been reluctant to facilitate the distribution of essential resources to the global South in ways that reflect and reinforce the race-based—or, at least, race-shaped—assumption that it is appropriate for social distributions to tilt in favor of European-descended peoples.[52] This reluctance exacerbated the disparate experience of the COVID-19 pandemic at a global level, with India and several South American countries experiencing high rates of COVID-19 disease and deaths as the US rates declined steeply.[53] In this context, it is telling that the US enjoyed a glut of vaccines while some countries struggled to procure any at all, all while the efficacy of vaccine distribution within the US varied by race and ethnicity.[54]

Widespread equanimity in the face of racially skewed distributions of the risk of death raises deeper ethical and social-theoretic questions. Variations in the rates of excess pandemic-related mortality result at least in part from the racialized distribution of co-morbid conditions and social risk factors (like occupation and density of living conditions). These racialized patterns of co-morbidity and risk result in turn from racialized maldistributions related to wider social conditions, conditions that predate and will outlast the pandemic, including unequal access to education,[55] food,[56] and shelter.[57] Without these antecedent conditions, the distribution of mortality during the COVID-19 pandemic might look very different.[58]

Despite their predictable consequences for all-cause mortality, the persistence of these social arrangements suggests that members of non-white racial groups in these societies are deemed more dispensable than members of white racial groups.[59] This suggestion might put one in mind of Achille Mbembe's account of necropolitics, which aspires to a systematic understanding of the way states mobilize "the power and the capacity to dictate who may live and who must die."[60] Mbembe argues that necropolitical forces run along racial and colonialist lines,[61] which suggests that racial differences in COVID-related excess mortality go beyond simple racism to something rougher, something like the production of race as a way of sorting humanity into those who are suited for death and those who are meant for something better.

6.6 Conclusion

We have argued that invidious racial ideologies often inform attempts to explain and respond to pandemics, that critical forms of race-thinking can help track the clusters of largely socioeconomic conditions that increase the risk of vulnerability to pandemic diseases, and that pandemics sometimes result from racially oppressive practices aimed at propping up Euromodernity's most influential and damaging racial projects. If this account of the racial dimensions of pandemics is correct, the moral goal of public health cannot simply be, as some authors have maintained, to create the greatest good for the greatest number.[62] This consequentialist framing fails to make confronting these (presumably) unjust racial patterns an obligatory feature of public health interventions. It instead makes the warrant for this confrontation contingent on calculations about the greater good, which, depending on the demographic profile of the society in question and on necropolitical judgments about whose good figures into the calculus, may be an extremely distressing prospect.

There is obviously much more to say in this spirit about the ethics of public health in general and of pandemic response in particular. We will have to leave those topics aside for now. Our aim has been simply to explore the plausible intuition that racial stratification and racial politics are interestingly connected to the emergence, management, and experience of pandemics like COVID-19. Something similar is surely true of public health crises more broadly, but exploring this larger claim falls beyond the scope of this chapter.

Notes

1. Boulware (2020, par. 1). Throughout the paper we primarily focus on COVID-19 disease and not the SARS-CoV-2 virus that causes the disease but where appropriate, we reference the virus and not the disease.
2. Mallon (2004, 654).
3. Tulchinsky et al. (2014, 71).
4. McMillen (2016, 12).
5. Cohn (2012, 544).
6. McMillen (2016, 21).
7. McMillen (2016, 24).
8. Hays (2005, 10–23).
9. McMillen (2016, 61–62).
10. McMillen (2016, 70–71).
11. McMillen (2016, 33).
12. McMillen (2016, 92).
13. Farmer (2006), Marc et al. (2010).
14. Koenig et al. (2010).
15. Farmer (2006, 237).
16. Herbert (2001).
17. McMillen (2016, 78, 81).
18. McMillen (2016, 5, 82–83).

19. McMillen (2016, 80).
20. Hutchins et al. (2009).
21. Mallon (2018, 1044).
22. Hutchins et al. (2009), Økland and Mamelund (2019).
23. McMillen (2016, 48).
24. McMillen (2016, 32).
25. McMillen (2016, 35).
26. McMillen (2016, 48), Curtin (1968).
27. White (2020).
28. McMillen (2016, 108).
29. Ome (2020), Litam (2020), Kuo (2020).
30. Gover et al. (2020), Litam (2020), Dang et al. (2020).
31. Rettner (2020), Walsh and Cotovio (2020).
32. Fan et al. (2019), Anthony et al. (2017), Briggs (2020).
33. Baragona (2020).
34. Beaumont-Thomas (2020).
35. World Health Organization (2021).
36. Walsh and Cotovio (2020).
37. Shen-Berro (2020).
38. Yam (2021), Lee (2021).
39. *See* de Silva de Alwis (2021) and Zheng (2021).
40. See World Health Organization (2021), although it is important to note that critics have expressed concerns about the independence of the WHO report. See Schifrin et al. (2021) for the critique.
41. Rossen et al. (2020).
42. Kumar et al.(2021).
43. Polyakova et al. (2021).
44. Chen et al. (2021).
45. Quan et al. (2021).
46. E.g., Young and Cho (2021).
47. E.g., Chen et al. (2021).
48. Laurencin and McClinton (2020).
49. Harell and Lieberman (2021).
50. E.g., van Barneveld et al. (2020).
51. Quinney (2020).
52. E.g., Twohey and Kulish (2020), Schlosser (2021).
53. Al-Arshani (2021), The New York Times (2021).
54. Walker et al. (2021).
55. E.g., Mountantonakis et al. (2021).
56. Quan et al. (2021).
57. E.g., Sundstrom (2003), Sandset (2021).
58. Lee (2020) and Valles (2020).
59. E.g., Lithwick (2020), Gidla (2020).
60. Mbembe (2003, 11).
61. Mbembe (2003, 17).

62. E.g., Childress et al. (2002), Cole (1995).

References

Al-Arshani, Sarah. 2021. As India and Other Countries Struggle to Acquire Enough COVID-19 Vaccines for Their Populations, Doses are Sitting on Shelves Across the US. *businessinsider.com*. May 24. Accessed June 3, 2021. https://www.businessinsider.com/us-excess-vaccines-rest-world-struggles-supply-2021-4.

Anthony, Simon J., Christine K. Johnson, Denise J. Greig, Sarah Kramer, Xiaoyu Che, Heather Wells, Allison L. Hicks et al. 2017. Global Patterns in Coronavirus Diversity. *Virus Evolution* 3 (1): vex012.

Baragona, Justin. 2020. Fox News Host Claims Chinese People Eating 'Raw Bats' to Blame for Coronavirus. *Thedailybeast.com*. March 02. Accessed May 13, 2021. https://www.thedailybeast.com/fox-news-host-jesse-watters-claims-chinese-people-eating-raw-bats-to-blame-for-coronavirus?ref=scroll.

Beaumont-Thomas, Ben. 2020. Coronavirus: Bryan Adams Attacks China as 'Bat Eating, Virus Making' Source. *theguardian.com*. May 12. Accessed May 13, 2021. https://www.theguardian.com/music/2020/may/12/bryan-adams-attacks-china-coronavirus.

Boulware, L. Ebony. 2020. Race Disparities in the COVID-19 Pandemic-Solutions Lie in Policy, Not Biology. *Journal of the Americal Medical Association* 3 (8): e2018696–e2018696.

Briggs, Helen. 2020. Coronavirus: Cracking the Secrets of How Bats Survive Viruses. *bbc.com*. July 22. Accessed May 12, 2021. https://www.bbc.com/news/science-environment-53494566.

Chen, Yea-Hung, Maria Glymour, Alicia Riley, John Balmes, Kate Duchowny, Robert Harrison, Ellicott Matthay, and Kirsten Bibbins-Domingo. 2021. *Excess Mortality Associated with the COVID-19 Pandemic Among Californians 18–65 Years of Age, by Occupational Sector and Occupation: March Through October 2020*. Preprint.

Childress, James E., Ruth R. Faden, Ruth D. Gaare, Lawrence O. Gostin, Jeffrey Kahn, RIchard J. Bonnie, Nancy E. Kass, Anna C. Mastroianni, Jonathan D. Moreno, and Phillip Nieburg. 2002. Public Health Ethics: Mapping the Terrain. *Journal of Law Medicine & Ethics* 30 (2): 170–178.

Cohn, Samuel K. 2012. Pandemics: Waves of Disease, Waves of Hate from the Plague of Athens to AIDS. *Historical Research* 85 (230): 535–555.

Cole, Philip. 1995. The Moral Bases for Public Health Interventions. *Epidemiology* 78–83.

Curtin, Philip D. 1968. Epidemiology and the Slave Trade. *Political Science Quarterly* 83 (2): 190–216.

Dang, Elain, Samual Huang, Adrian Kwok, Harrison Lung, Michael Park, and Emily Yueh. 2020. *COVID-19 and Advancing Asian American Recovery*. Public Sector Practice Analysis, New York: McKinsey & Company.

de Alwis, Rangita de Silva. 2021. An Intersectional Approach to Violence Against Asian Americans and Women. *Georgetown Institute for Women, Peace, and Security*. May 14. Accessed April 19, 2022. https://giwps.georgetown.edu/an-intersectional-approach-to-a-systemic-challenge-the-role-of-education-in-addressing-asian-american-hate-crimes-and-violence-against-women/.

Du Bois, W.E.B. 1899. *The Philadelphia Negro*. Philadelphia: University of Pennsylvania Press.

Fan, Yi, Kai Zhao, Zheng-Li Shi, and Peng Zhou. 2019. Bat Coronaviruses in China. *Viruses*. 11 (3): 210.

Farmer, Paul. 2006. *AIDS and Accusation: Haiti and the Geography of Blame*. Berkeley, CA: University of California Press.

Gidla, Sujatha. 2020. We Are Not Essential. We Are Sacrificial. www.nytimes.com. May 20. Accessed May 17, 2021. https://www-nytimes-com.proxy.library.vanderbilt.edu/2020/05/05/opinion/coronavirus-nyc-subway.html.

Gover, Angela R., Shannon B. Harper, and Lynn Langton. 2020. Anti-Asian Hate Crime During the COVID-19 Pandemic: Exploring the Reproduction of Inequality. *American Journal of Criminal Justice* 45 (4): 647–667.

Harrell, Allison, and Evan Lieberman. 2021. How Information About Race-Based Health Disparities Affects Policy Preferences: Evidence from a Survey Experiment About the COVID-19 Pandemic in the United States. *Social Science and Medicine* 277: 113884.

Hays, J. N. 2005. *Epidemics and Pandemics: Their Impacts on Human History*. Santa Barbara, CA: ABC-CLIO.

Herbert, Bob. 2001. In America; Refusing to Save Africans. *The New York Times*. June 11. Accessed April 14, 2021. https://www-nytimes-com.proxy.library.vanderbilt.edu/2001/06/11/opinion/in-america-refusing-to-save-africans.html.

Hutchins, Sonja S., Kevin Fiscella, Robert S. Levine, Danielle C. Ompad, and Marian McDonald. 2009. Protection of Racial/Ethnic Minority Populations During an Influenza Pandemic. *American Journal of Public Health* 99: 261–270.

Jefferson, Thomas. 1786. *Notes on the State of Virginia*. Richmond: The Federalist Papers Project.

Koenig, S., L.C. Ivers, S. Pace, R. Destine, F. Leandre, R. Grandpierre, J. Mukherjee, P.E. Farmer, and J.W. Pape. 2010. Successes and Challenges of HIV Treatment Programs in Haiti: Aftermath of the Earthquake. *HIV Therapy* 4 (2): 145–160.

Kumar, Amit, Indrakshi Roy, Amol M. Karmarkar, Kimberly S. Erler, James L. Rudolph, Julie A. Baldwin, and Maricruz Rivera-Hernandez. 2021. Shifting US Patterns of COVID-19 Mortality by Race and Ethnicity From June-December 2020. *Journal of Post-Acute and Long-term Care Medicine* 22 (5): 966–970.

Kuo, Lily. 2020. Trump Sparks Anger by Calling Coronavirus the 'Chinese Virus'. *theguardian.com*. March 17. Accessed September 27, 2020. https://www.theguardian.com/world/2020/mar/17/trump-calls-covid-19-the-chinese-virus-as-rift-with-coronavirus-beijing-escalates.

Laurencin, Cato T., and Aneesah McClinton. 2020. The COVID-19 Pandemic: A Call to Action to Identify and Address Racial and Ethnic Disparities. *Journal of Racial and Ethnic Health Disparities* 7 (3): 398–402.

Lee, Bruce Y. 2021. Rising Anti-Asian American Violence Didn't Start with the COVID-19 Pandemic. *Forbes.com*. March 21. Accessed May 12, 2021. https://www.forbes.com/sites/brucelee/2021/03/21/rising-anti-asian-american-violence-didnt-start-with-the-covid-19-pandemic/?sh=6defb8442ca0.

Lee, Christopher J. 2020. The Necropolitics of COVID-19. *Africasacountry.com*. April 1. Accessed May 17, 2021. https://africasacountry.com/2020/04/the-necropolitics-of-covid-19.

Litam, Stacey Diane A. 2020. "Take Your Kung-Flu Back to Wuhan": Counseling Asians, Asian Americans, and Pacific Islanders with Race-Based Trauma Related to COVID-19. *The Professional Counselor* 10 (2): 144–156.

Lithwick, Dahlia. 2020. America's Heroism Trap. *slate.com*. April 20. Accessed May 17, 2021. https://slate.com/news-and-politics/2020/04/coronavirus-humans-vs-heroes.html.

Mallon, Ron. 2004. Passing, Traveling, and Reality: Social Constructionism and the Metaphysics of Race. *Nous* 38 (4): 644–673.

Mallon, Ron. 2018. Constructing Race: Racialization, Causal Effects, or Both? *Philosophical Studies* 1039–1056.

Marc, Linda G., Alpa Patel-Larson, H. Irene Hall, Denise Hughes, Margarita Alegria, Georgette Jeanty, Yanick Sanon Eveillard, Eustache Jean-Louis, and National Haitian-American Health Alliance. 2010. HIV Among Haitian-Born Persons in the United States, 1985–2007. *AIDS* 24 (13): 2089–2097.

Mbembe, Achille. 2003. Necropolitics. *Public Culture* 15 (1): 11–40.

McMillen, Christian W. 2016. *Pandemics: A Very Short Introduction*. New York, NY: Oxford University Press.

Mountantonakis, Stavros E., Laurence M. Epstein, Kristie Coleman, Johanna Martinez, Moussa Saleh, Charlotte Kvasnovsky, Rachel-Maria Brown et al. 2021. The Association of Structural Inequities and Race with out-of-Hospital Sudden Death during the COVID-19 Pandemic. *Arrhythm Electrophysiology* 14 (5): e009646.

Økland, Helene, and Svenn-Erik Mamelund. 2019. Race and 1918 Influenza Pandemic in the United States: A Review of the Literature. *International Journal of Environmental Research and Public Health* 16 (14): 2487.

Ome, Morgan. 2020. Why This Wave of Anti-Asian Racism Feels Different. *theatlantic.com.* March 17. Accessed March 17, 2021.

Polyakova, Maria, Victoria Udalova, Geoffrey Kocks, Katie Genadek, Keith Finlay, and Amy N. Finkelstein. 2021. Racial Disparities In Excess All-Cause Mortality During the Early COVID-19 Pandemic Varied Substantially Across States. *Health Equity* 40 (2): 307–316.

Quan, Daniel, Lucia Luna Wong, Anita Shallal, Raghav Madan, Abel Hamdan, Heaveen Ahdi, Amir Daneshvar et al. 2021. Impact of Race and Socioeconomic Status on Outcomes in Patients Hospitalized with COVID-19. *Journal of General Internal Medicine* 36 (5): 1302–1309.

Quinney, Marie. 2020. COVID-19 and Nature are Linked. *weforum.org.* April 14. Accessed May 17, 2021. https://www.weforum.org/agenda/2020/04/covid-19-nature-deforestation-recovery/.

Rettner, Rachael. 2020. New Coronavirus May Have 'Jumped' to Humans from Snakes, Study Finds. *livescience.com.* January 23. Accessed May 12, 2021. https://www.livescience.com/new-coronavirus-origin-snakes.html.

Rossen, Lauren M., Amy M. Branum, Farida B. Ahmad, Paul Sutton, and Robert N. Anderson. 2020. *Excess Deaths Associated with COVID-19, by Age and Race and Ethnicity—United States, January 26-October 3,2020.* Morbidity and Mortality Weekly Report, Atlanta: US Department of Health and Human Services/Centers for Disease Control and Prevention.

Sandset, Tony. 2021. The Necropolitics of COVID-19: Race, Class and Slow Death in an Ongoing Pandemic. *Global Public Health* 16 (8–9): 1411–1423.

Schifrin, Nick, Dan Sagalyn, and Layla Quran. 2021. WHO Report Says COVID Originated in Bats, But Critics Claim the Study Was Biased. *PBS.org.* March 29. Accessed May 12, 2021. https://www.pbs.org/newshour/show/who-report-says-covid-originated-in-bats-but-critics-claim-the-study-was-biased.

Schlosser, Kurt. 2021. Gates Foundation Reverses Position on COVID Vaccine Patent Protections After Mounting Pressure. *msn.com.* May 7. Accessed May 18, 2021. https://www.msn.com/en-us/news/world/gates-foundation-reverses-position-on-covid-vaccine-patent-protections-after-mounting-pressure/ar-BB1gtUCL.

Shen-Berro. 2020. Sen. Cornyn: China to Blame for Coronavirus, Because People Eat Bats. *nbcnews.com.* March 18. Accessed May 13, 2021. https://www.nbcnews.com/news/asian-america/sen-cornyn-china-blame-coronavirus-because-people-eat-bats-n1163431.

Sundstrom, Ronald R. 2003. Race and Place: Social Space in the Production of Human Kinds. *Philosophy and Geography* 6 (1): 83–95.

The New York Times. 2021. What to Know About India's Coronavirus Crisis. *nytimes.com.* June 2. Accessed June 3, 2021. https://www.nytimes.com/article/india-coronavirus-cases-deaths.html.

Tulchinsky, Theodore H., Elena Varavikova, and Joan Bickford. 2014. *The New Public Health.* London: Elsevier.

Twohey, Megan, and Nicholas Kulish. 2020. Bill Gates, the Virus and the Quest to Vaccinate the World. *nytimes.com.* November 23. Accessed May 18, 2021. https://www.nytimes.com/2020/11/23/world/bill-gates-vaccine-coronavirus.html?smid=url-share.

Valles, Sean A. 2020. The Predictable Inequities of COVID-19 in the US: Fundamental Causes and Broken Institutions. *Kennedy Institute of Ethics Journal* 30 (3): 191–214.

van Barneveld, Kristin, Michael Quinlan, Peter Kriesler, Anne Junor, Fran Baum, Anis Chowdhury, PN Junankar et al. 2020. The COVID-19 Pandemic: Lessons on Building More Equal and Sustainable Societies. *The Economic and Labour Relations Review* 31 (2): 133–157.

Walker, Amy Schoenfeld, Albert Sun, Yuriria Avila, Laney Pope, and John Yoon. 2021. The Racial Gap in US Vaccinations Is Shrinking, but Work Remains. *Nytimes.com.* May 14. Accessed May 18, 2021. https://www.nytimes.com/interactive/2021/05/14/us/vaccine-race-gap.html.

Walsh, Nick Paton, and Vasco Cotovio. 2020. Bats Are Not to Blame for Coronavirus. Humans Are. *cnn.com.* March 20. Accessed May 12, 2021. https://www.cnn.com/2020/03/19/health/coronavirus-human-actions-intl/index.html.

White, Alexandre I.R. 2020. Historical Linkages: Epidemic Threat, Economic Risk, and Xenophobia. *The Lancet* 395 (10232): 1250–1251.

World Health Organization. 2021. *WHO-convened Global Study of Origins of SARS-CoV-2: China Part.* Joint WHO-China Study Team report, Geneva: World Health Organization.

Yam, Kimmy. 2021. There Were 3,800 Anti-Asian Racist Incidents, Mostly Against Women, in Past Year. *nbcnews.com.* March 16. Accessed May 13, 2021. https://www.nbcnews.com/news/asian-america/there-were-3-800-anti-asian-racist-incidents-mostly-against-n1261257.

Young, Jennifer L., and Mildred K. Cho. 2021. The Invisibility of Asian Americans in COVID-19 Data, Reporting, and Relief. *The American Journal of Bioethics* 21 (3): 100–102.

Zheng, Lily. 2021. To Dismantle Anti-Asian Racism, We Must Understand Its Roots. *Harvard Business Review.* May 27. Accessed May 30, 2021. https://hbr.org/2021/05/to-dismantle-anti-asian-racism-we-must-understand-its-roots.

Part II
Public Policy and Administration

Chapter 7
Is There a Duty to Treat in a Pandemic?

Wanda Teays

Abstract Do physicians, nurses, and other health workers have a moral obligation to care for infected patients in a pandemic? Or is there something that distinguishes it from other medical contexts? In this chapter we will get an overview of the issues and consider what limits, if any, should be set on the duty to treat.

A central concern is whether the greater number of those potentially at risk should be factored into the decision. The contagion factor coupled with mortality statistics suggest that there are boundaries on what we can expect. The risks to care for a patient in a pandemic could end up killing the caregiver—not to mention a host of others who might get infected. Consequently, health care workers should have the right to decide how much risk they are willing to take, particularly when protective equipment is in short supply. The chapter concludes with six foundational rights of health care workers.

Keywords Duty · Oaths · Pandemic · Moral obligations · Duty to treat · Professional responsibility · SARS · Covid-19 · AMA

7.1 Introduction

> I couldn't ask anyone else to do it if I wasn't going to step up to the plate with them. It's my job.
>
> —Linda Wildey, as noted by Gretchen Reynolds

> Doctors and nurses and other health care workers may be heroes in this pandemic, but we will not be martyrs.
>
> —Sandeep Jauhar

There's not a lot that makes health care workers want to run to the hills, but a pandemic must be near the top of the list. Smallpox, SARS, Ebola, Marburg hemorrhagic fever, H1n1, MERS, Covid-19, and so on test the courage and commitment to

W. Teays (✉)
Mount Saint Mary's University, Los Angeles, CA, USA
e-mail: wteays@msmu.edu

treat the infected victims. Some step forward, seeing their assistance as a duty; others weigh the risks and find their participation untenable. As for the general public—and potential victims of highly contagious diseases—the situation is truly a crisis. We understand the concern, but need qualified personnel to tend to our medical treatment. There's fear and trembling on all sides.

As the American Medical Association (2020) recognized, these are trying times. In addressing the issue of professional responsibility, they said in the Preamble to the *Declaration of Professional Responsibility:*

> Never in the history of human civilization has the well-being of each individual been so inextricably linked to that of every other. Plagues and pandemics respect no national borders in a world of global commerce and travel. Wars and acts of terrorism enlist innocents as combatants and mark civilians as targets. Advances in medical science and genetics, while promising great good, may also be harnessed as agents of evil. The unprecedented scope and immediacy of these universal challenges demand concerted action and response by all.

And so we are called to look closely at the responsibilities owed one another in a pandemic. We need to give careful consideration to what we are asking of health care workers. Simply put, "Is there a duty to treat in a pandemic?".

Consider the case of 10 year-old Rebecca McLester of Rockford, Illinois. In the summer of 2003 she came down with pus-filled sores after playing with her family's two pet prairie dogs. As it turns out, they got infected from a Gambian pouch rat at the pet store that sold exotic animals. The pouch rat, the prairie dogs, and some unsuspecting owners got monkeypox, a relative of smallpox. Rebecca ended up in the parking lot of Swedish American Hospital waiting to get into an ER isolation room.

As Gretchen Reynolds (2004) reports, over the course of the summer, 72 cases of monkeypox would be suspected in the Midwest, and 37 would be confirmed. Up to 10% of the infected die from the disease.

Who was going to treat Rebecca? How long was she going to be stuck in the hospital parking lot? What terror was unleashed? And what reluctance was set in motion?

> The word "pox" tends to focus the medical mind. [Dr. Michael] Anderson considered for an instant his own daughters, ages 6 and 2. It was most unlikely that he could carry infection home. But it wasn't impossible. They had no immunity against a pox. Still, Anderson agreed to get involved with the case. But he saw that his decision did not please his colleagues, None of them had been vaccinated. "My partners told me I had not needed to take the case and I should not have done it without consulting them," he remembered... "They were angry," Anderson said (Reynolds 2004).

Anderson's colleagues rightfully concluded that his exposure to monkeypox could just as easily be *their* exposure, that the disease can quickly spread given the right conditions. And, unfortunately, those treating the infected patients could become patients themselves. For example,

> "If you have an outbreak of, say, Ebola," said Dr. Daniel Bausch, ..."the last two or three people to catch the disease were health care workers, and they decide, quite logically, that it's not worth the risk." During an outbreak in 1995, an international team of doctors arrived

in Kikwit in Congo to find that Kikwit General Hospital was deserted and silent, except for a half dozen or so patients, including medical staff, lying unattended in a back room, dying of Ebola (Reynolds 2004).

The sight of both patients and caregivers being struck down by a disease would be enough to send shivers down anyone's spine and call into question any sense of duty. How much risk is too great? What are the limits of a doctor's or nurse's fiduciary obligations? In the midst of a pandemic, it's no wonder we seek answers.

Kenneth V. Iserson (2018) cuts to the quick: "The moral backbone of medical professionals—a duty to put the needs of patients first—may be tested as they weigh multiple factors to determine whether to stay and carry out their professional roles or to step back and decrease their personal risks."

The truth is that we can't count on all of the medical staff to hang in there. "Although 80% or more of physicians and nurses might respond to mass casualty incidents, only about half would remain to work during an epidemic or radiological disaster or after a terrorist incident involving a chemical, biological, radiological, or nuclear agent" (Iserson 2018). This was born out on August 7, 2020, when health caregivers in India went on strike, citing inadequate protections against the coronavirus.

> About 900,000 members of an all-female community health workforce began a two-day strike Friday, protesting that they were being roped in to help with contact tracing, personal hygiene drives and in quarantine centers, but were not being given personal protective equipment or additional pay (Associated Press 2020).

And don't forget, there's not an unlimited amount of time to decide where the boundaries lie. Given that the physician workforce is not an unlimited resource, the dilemma is how to address competing needs. When it comes to disaster responses, physicians should balance benefits to current patients with caring for future patients, Iserson suggests (2018). That means assessing risks and apportioning resources.

Decision-making tends to focus on the present—*this* patient at *this* time in *this* context. However, the application of a caregiver's skills extends beyond these constraints and into the foreseeable future. It is of pressing importance that organizations representing health care workers clearly indicate what standard of care is expected of their members in the event of a pandemic, observe Carly Ruderman et al. (2006). Their advice has merit.

Because expectations around the standard of care may have dire consequences, assessing limits is imperative. An examination of the role of medical personnel will help set guidelines regarding professional rights and responsibilities, as well as ethical duties and obligations (Shaul et al. 2006). In light of an inconsistent response in a pandemic on the part of governments, politicians, and the general public (as seen with Covid-19), a great deal follows from the role health workers play.

Keep in mind that a healthcare system requires the participation of all sorts of medical personnel. This includes anesthesiologists, paramedics, x-ray technicians and other staff, as well as physicians and nurses. In other words, it's an ever-widening circle as to which parties are affected and which ones may have a duty to treat.

Who should stay and who can walk away? "What is clear is that the issue of duty to care has emerged as a matter of paramount concern among health care professionals, hospital administrators, public policy makers, and bioethicists" (Shaul et al. 2006). It is an important and all-too timely matter. Let's see how.

A pandemic like the Bubonic Plague, SARS, Ebola or Covid-19 can strike down people of all ages on a global scale, and do so in a matter of days. Daily reports of new cases and death statistics bear this out. In what follows we will look at the debate and examine the pros and cons of the duty to treat—and if it is a *duty*. In so doing, we should remember that the range of those at risk includes many more people than the ones directly caring for patients. The risk-factor in a pandemic continues to expand.

Some infections are spread far beyond the doctor's office or hospital. Families, friends, coworkers, strangers sharing elevators and fellow passengers on an airplane get little say as to whether health care workers have a duty to treat. It is often too late for them to avoid exposure. Victims may have no idea who passed the infection on to them; the source of transmission could be a complete mystery.

Whereas SARS was primarily a disease within healthcare institutions, "an influenza outbreak [or other pandemic] would hit the community at large. The patient surge would be tremendous" (Malm et al. 2008, 5). The number affected would be on a vastly greater scale, as seen with Covid-19. World-wide cases run into the millions and deaths number in the hundreds of thousands. And, so, what are the ethical obligations of caregivers? Let us consider the extent to which the medical professions have offered guidance.

7.2 Oaths and Codes

The "duty" to treat may seem like an open-and-shut case settled by the Hippocratic Oath ("Do no harm") or other professional oaths and codes. However, the matter is not so easily put to rest.

First, it is not obvious that "Do no harm" entails a duty to treat *regardless of risk*. In fact, the proscription not to harm may apply to a greater population than patients; it may be sufficiently large to include physicians and other caregivers as well.

Secondly, if we examine doctors' and nurses' fiduciary duties to patients, one virtue that stands out is beneficence. Its importance rests on the fact that,

> The ethical foundations of the duty to provide care are grounded in several longstanding ethical principles. Foremost among these is the principle of beneficence, which recognizes and defines the special moral obligation on the part of HCPs [health care professionals] to further the welfare of patients and to advance patients' well-being. In modern health care, it is commonly understood and generally accepted that the principle of beneficence constitutes a foundational principle of the patient-provider relationship (Ruderman et al. 2006).

We might see the moral prescription as follows: Let beneficence be your guide, but at least do no harm. Failing possible benefits, non-maleficence should prevail. However, this prescription focuses on the *doctor-patient* relationship—which leaves out all others in the path of a pandemic. Surely they warrant consideration. Here's where a need to balance competing interests comes in.

Thirdly, as Judith Jarvis Thomson suggests in another context, if we cannot be Good Samaritans, we could at least strive to be Minimally Decent Samaritans. Doctors may stop short of taking all possible steps to help patients when personal sacrifice seems too great. But that doesn't mean they don't take risks in the care rendered. Basically, a degree of risk goes with the territory.

We find an acknowledgment of this in the AMA's *Declaration of Professional Responsibility*. The AMA (2020) recognizes that physicians may have to take risks and should not shirk from doing so. Adopted by the AMA in 2001, this declaration "is an oath by which twenty-first century physicians can publicly uphold and celebrate the ideals that have inspired individuals to enter medicine and earn society's trust in the healing profession." In particular,

> We, the members of the world community of physicians, solemnly commit ourselves to… treat the sick and injured with competence and compassion and without prejudice [and] apply our knowledge and skills when needed, *though doing so may put us at risk* (AMA 2020, my emphasis).

How much risk is too much? And how many professional oaths and codes settle the question? Contrary to an assumption that the duty to treat would be commonly prescribed, Heidi Malm et al. point out that,

> A review of 61 professional codes revealed that 29 had no mention of a duty to [treat], 23 had broad statements (such as the Declaration of Geneva: A physician shall give emergency care as a humanitarian duty unless he is assured that others are willing and able to give such care), and 8 had what could be construed as specific direction to members" (Upshur 2006, noted in Malm et al. 2008, 15).

In other words, less than than 15% of professional codes offer clear guidelines on the duty to treat. That means more than 85% fall short on guidance. Subsequently, "This casts doubt on the idea that the duty is part of the very nature of the professions" (Malm et al. 2008, 15).

Such doubts imply that, "Efforts to ground a professional's duty to treat on a code of ethics are fraught with problems." For instance,"The relevant codes of ethics often do not clearly assert a duty to treat, and even when they do, their scope of application and their correct interpretation is open to significant dispute,"notes Malm et al. (2008, 16).

If professional codes do not set clear guidelines, health care workers face a quandary. Where should they look for guidance or an ethical framework with which to justify their actions? They may then infer a right to decide for themselves as to what is an acceptable risk. May we then conclude that treating patients in a pandemic is an act of *altruism* rather than duty? Let's give it a closer look.

7.3 Maybe There Is a Duty to Treat: The Pro Argument

When we consider whether there's a duty to treat in a pandemic, it is important to acknowledge the various concerns factoring into the decision. There's more at work than we might realize. Just note the key parameters that come into play:

- Access to information—e.g., on treatment options
- Contagion factors and statistics
- Mortality statistics
- Risks to infected patients
- Risks to health caregivers
- Second order risks—Risks to others, families, colleagues, other patients, etc.
- Safety concerns—Access to protective equipment, masks, disinfectant
- Quarantine requirements with positive diagnosis or suspected exposure

We should keep these in mind when weighing the pros and cons of the duty to treat. That said, let's look at the two sides, starting with the affirmative argument.

A major benefit in assuming a duty to treat is the recognition and appreciation of health care workers from both patients and the greater community. Taking significant risks to help another person is an act of selflessness and heroism in the dire circumstances of a pandemic. The value in that should not be underestimated.

The American Medical Association (2020) shines its light on this pressing issue in stating that,

> As physicians, we are bound in our response by a common heritage of caring for the sick and the suffering. Through the centuries individual physicians have fulfilled this obligation by applying their skills and knowledge competently, selflessly, and at times heroically. Today, our profession must reaffirm its historical commitment to combat natural and man-made assaults on the health and well-being of humankind. Only by acting together across geographic and ideological divides can we overcome such powerful threats. Humanity is our patient.

Moreover, looking back at 1847, the AMA code affirms under the *Duties of The Profession To The Public*. "When pestilence prevails, it is their duty to face the danger, and to continue their labours for the alleviation of the suffering, even at the jeopardy of their own lives." In this proclamation, the AMA sets a high bar.

This standard of personal risk is backed up by societal expectations. Amy Solnica, Leonid Barski, and Alan Jotkowitz (2020) explain: "Regarding healthcare workers, there is agreement for ethical, professional and societal reasons that they are *required* to put themselves in harm's way to care for their patients" (my emphasis).

By this view, not to accept a duty to treat is to pass the buck. If not you then *who?* The risk refused by a physician or nurse must be assumed by someone else. Isn't it reasonable to expect health caregivers to tend to the sick, even in a pandemic? The rule of rescue prevents abandoning those in need of help and "prompts a certain minimal decency that is expected from all individuals who are in a position to render aid at a time of crisis." Specifically, "The greater the need, the greater is the responsibility to help" (Anantham et al. 2008).

As we have seen with Covid-19, when faced with a contagious disease in pandemic proportions, the need is likely to be tremendous. Resources, personnel, and facilities are stretched to the limits and the need for healthcare workers is crystal clear. In addition, "Unqualified personnel without medical capabilities cannot provide services such as diagnosis and treatment of disease" (Anantham et al. 2008).

The bottom line is that we rely on doctors and nurses in a medical emergency. That reliance may be a catalyst for a self-generated sense of duty on the part of doctors in a pandemic—even if the profession lets them off the hook. Plus, we should not overlook the rewards inherent to the medical profession; that the benefits offset the risks. Just think of the respect and prestige attached to the profession. Think also of the "guild-like powers of self-regulation" over and above the remuneration, observe Anantham et al.

It's like having a goose that lays golden eggs, though not without a cost.

> As members of a profession who have taken advantage of its contract with society to reap social rewards, it is then onerous on physicians to commit to the obligations of the profession when called upon to do so. This is the essence of John Rawls' 'no free rider' principle (Anantham et al. 2008).

Ezekiel J. Emanuel would agree. He asserts that the devotion to caring for the sick is what distinguishes health professionals from lawyers, teachers, and business people. It defines the core element of being a medical professional. "The obligation is not chosen," he contends, "It is inseparable from the choice to become a doctor. To reject this ethical ideal is to reject the profession" (2003, 590).

If doctors have a duty to treat, they are not alone; others have such duties as well. That has not been given sufficient attention. Looking at rescue-related professions, there is no escape from risk. Firefighters, paramedics, police, and medical personnel implicitly agree to accept a reasonable level of risk when they enter their profession, Malm et al. argue. They say, "No one has any moral obligation to enter any of those social roles" (2008, 8, citing Fleck 2003). The picture is this: Choosing the health profession => acceptance of reasonable risk => moral obligations => duty to treat.

So goes the argument—the links in the chain—that doctors and nurses know what they are getting into when they enter the profession. The duty to treat is part of the bargain. "That is a risk they incur by virtue of their calling," said Justice Robert Sharpe in 2009 when deciding the SARS nurses' lawsuit in Toronto Canada.

"Nurses were, by virtue of their profession, in the eye of the SARS storm, but they had no higher claim to have their health protected by Ontario than any other resident of the province," he argued. "When dealing with a crisis like SARS, governments must have to consider the public interest as a whole." Consequently, factoring in the economic repercussions to [such matters as] tourism is "not necessarily out of line during a communicable disease crisis," he asserted (Makin 2009).

Not all would agree with Justice Sharpe on the value of tourism in a health crisis. For example, Emanuel reminds us of the reciprocity of duties. In his view, "Affirming health care workers' ethical duty to care for the sick imposes a correlative duty on health care administrators and senior physicians to maximize the safety of frontline physicians and nurses" (2003, 591). In a pandemic this duty may fall short, as when the demands for masks and safety equipment exceed the supply, which was the case with both SARS and Covid-19.

Finally, one other reason supporting the moral obligation to care lies in a comparison of the various professions. No one else can step up to the plate and be trusted to provide medical care. It follows that the physician's expertise and greater skills increases the duty to treat.

7.4 On the Other Hand: The Con Argument

Daniel K. Sokol (2006) observes that, "Duty of care, in the medical context, is often invoked as a sort of quasi-biblical commandment, akin to "do not lie" or "do not murder." He continues, "The term 'duty of care' (which I take to be synonymous with duty *to* care) is, at best, too vague and, at worst, ethically dangerous" (1238).

For these reasons, we need to be more precise about the obligations of health care workers and figure out how far those obligations extend. A central issue turns on the term "reasonable" when asserting the duty to treat entails a reasonable, and acceptable, risk. Furthermore,

> Nowhere do the laws oblige a mere bystander to take significant risks to aid another. The duty is limited to minimal risk at best …The hallmark of special positive duties is the existence of.. a role-related relationship such as that between lifeguard and swimmer or between custodial parent and child [and, presumably, between doctor and patient] (Malm et al. 2008, 6).

However,

> The fact that the lifeguard can be obligated to incur greater risks does not mean that she can be obligated to incur any and all degree of risk. Lifeguards are not obligated to enter the surf to try to rescue a swimmer from the mouth of a great white shark, for example. Similarly, paramedics are not obligated to enter a building on the verge of collapse to aid someone inside. They can even be obligated not to do so (Malm et al. 2008, 7).

Caring for patients should not entail death-defying acts on the part of doctors and nurses. So too with other rescue workers, though examples of suicidal risk-taking come to mind. "We felt like members of the Tokkotai [the kamikaze pilots of the second world war] in that we were prepared to sacrifice everything," observed one of the rescue workers at Fukushima's nuclear disaster of 2011. "The people lined up outside never said as much, but I could tell by their expressions that they didn't think we would return" (McCurry 2013).

Consider also the case of the terrorist attacks on the World Trade Center on 9/11. It stands as the deadliest incident ever for firefighters and law enforcement officers in the U.S. Three hundred and forty-three firefighters, 23 police officers and 37 Port Authority officers died.The 9/11 FDNY deaths amounted to more than a third of the emergency personnel at the scene (Kiger 2019). These rescue workers risked—and lost—their lives. But we should not consider that part of the job.

The difficulty is that, in practice, the boundary separating good medicine from suicide is unmarked. Every doctor and nurse may locate it differently, noted Dr.

Mark Cheung, who ended up seriously infected with SARS. "I would never blame anybody who decided they couldn't treat infectious patients," he said. (Reynolds 2004). Should we blame doctors who balk at such risks?

In the wake of the 9/11 terrorist attacks, the AMA adopted several new ethics policies focused on the medical profession's obligations and responsibilities in a public health emergency. The AMA policy document *Physician Obligation in Disaster Preparedness and Response* states,

> National, regional, and local responses to epidemics, terrorist attacks, and other disasters require extensive involvement of physicians. Because of their commitment to care for the sick and injured, individual physicians have an obligation to provide urgent medical care during disasters. This ethical obligation holds even in the face of greater than usual risks to their own safety, health or life.
>
> The physician workforce, however, is not an unlimited resource; therefore, when participating in disaster responses, physicians should balance immediate benefits to individual patients with ability to care for patients in the future (AMA 2016).

Bioethicist Peter Singer asks, "Do we in medicine have a higher obligation to treat the sick than do passersby on the street?" His answer is "Yes. We accept an added level of personal risk, just as policemen and firemen do." "But," he says, "that added risk has limits. We have an expectation that firemen will enter a burning building. We don't have an expectation that they'll jump into a burning pit and self-immolate" (Reynolds 2004).

There are limits to the degree of acceptable risk. As Anantham et al. point out,

> Physicians are not an inexhaustible resource, however, and should weigh the future benefits that a healthy doctor can provide against the good that can be done immediately. Consequently, ...expected standards of care may be lowered. Resuscitation codes may be even abandoned because the low probability of success may not justify the risk exposure to healthcare professionals (2008).

This is where the issue of widening the boundaries of "risk" comes in. Sokol puts it this way:

> In times of crisis, the duties deriving from doctors' multiple roles may come into conflict. Doctors, for instance, may have a duty to care for their SARS or avian influenza–infected patients as well as a duty to care for their own children by protecting them (and hence themselves) from infection. So a further problem with the duty to care, aside from its vagueness, is that it fails to consider the holder of the duty as a multiple agent belonging to a broader community (2006, 1239).

The reality is that a pandemic is on a much greater scale—and with a much wider range of risks and those put at risk—than in the case of *this* doctor caring for *that* patient. The parameters are vastly different. Therefore, the typical "duty to treat" arguments are stretched to the breaking point.

When caregivers and their circle of contacts may succumb to the very disease being treated, we might admire their dedication, but we ought not view that dedication as a duty. Their patients are not their only concern. They also have a moral obligation not to spread the infection to others with whom they come into contact and not to shut the door on future patients they may be called to serve.

Let us honor the fact that health workers tend to approach their profession as a calling. It's a special vocation, in *caring* for others whose needs require a host of specialized skills—and the compassion to apply them, even at personal risk. We ask a lot of doctors and nurses, whose dedication deserves our gratitude. Their service to the community calls for protections and limits on what we should expect of them.

7.5 Conclusion

Whether there is a duty to treat in a pandemic raises a number of questions, as we have seen in this chapter. Not all are easy to answer. Expectations are put to the test when the numbers are great and the risks considerable.

A central dilemma is what to expect in the event of conflicting duties involving multiple parties. It's not just a matter of what health care workers owe their patients. It's also a matter of what they owe a host of others—others who are also at risk in a pandemic. This includes families, coworkers, members of a church choir, attendees at a wedding, shoppers at the grocery store, and so on. Far more people factor into the decision than the patient and the caregiver.

Sokol (2006) observes that, "Defining the limits of the duty of care is a daunting task, strewn with philosophical and logistical difficulties." This duty "is not absolute but, rather, constrained by several factors. First, the limits of the duty should be a function of the normal risk level" (1238). We should not lose sight of that.

Clearly the risk levels vary depending upon the context of contagion potential, extent of the numbers possibly affected, as well as the mortality statistics. Reluctance to treat will take its toll.

> Pandemic influenza imposes foreseeable high risks to physicians with the potential consequence of mortality. Survey data suggest that 24% of physicians find it acceptable to abandon their workplace during such a pandemic in order to protect themselves and their families (Anantham et al. 2008).

Doctors and nurses are a treasured resource in a society facing a health crisis. They deserve to be protected from lethal risks. Health caregivers have foundational rights in a pandemic. Six stand out:

Foundational Rights of Health Care Workers

1. *The Right To Institutional Support*

   Although society may have the right to demand service in a pandemic, physicians have the reciprocal right to demand sufficient institutional support (such as protective equipment, staff assistance and, if available, vaccination) (Ehrenstein 2008, 165).

2. *The Right to Safeguards*

   Many who treated SARS patients raised concerns about the protections to safeguard their own health and that of their family members. Conflicting obligations were another significant concern. (Ruderman et al. 2006).

3. *The Right to Competing Duties*

> Health care workers have competing obligations to their families and friends, whom they feared infecting, in addition to obligations to their own health. During SARS, some questioned their choice of career; indicating an unwillingness or inability to care for patients in the face of risk (Shaul et al. 2006).

4. *The Right to Minimize—and Justify—Risk*

> It is unrealistic to expect that this obligation to treat should be burdened with unlimited risks. Some limits in the level of risk will be needed for these obligations to be practically binding, and society will need to question the extent to which doctors have to endanger their lives for public good (Anantham et al. 2008).

5. *The Right to Clear Communication*

> To improve individual response rates, disaster planners and managers must communicate the risks clearly to all members of the health care system and provide them with as much support and security as possible. "Clinicians need not assume suicidal risks to care for patients" (Iserson 2018).

6. *The Right to Set Limits on the Duty to Treat*

> As dramatic as it may sound, delineating the limits of the duty of care may prevent large numbers of doctors from abandoning their patients in a crisis. Such abandonment has happened in the past and may occur again (Sokol 2006, 1240).

We cannot assume that health workers will (or should) accept a greater occupational risk during a pandemic. We need to acknowledge the competing needs and interests. We need to acknowledge that our expectations of medical professionals should not be boundless. And we need to honor the fact that they are not just creatures of the present. Future patients factor into the equation as well. Otherwise we may incur a shortage of health workers farther down the road.

We need to trust physicians, nurses, and other caregivers to weigh the risks they are asked to take and decide where to draw the line in the sand. Too many lives figure into the decision for there to be a rigid duty constraining their actions.

References

American Medical Association. 1847, May. "1847 Code of Ethics of the American Medical Association," 105, Accessed August 10, 2020 at https://www.ama-assn.org/sites/ama-assn.org/files/corp/media-browser/public/ethics/1847code_0.pdf

American Medical Association, 2016, November 14. "Physician Obligation in Disaster Preparedness And Response." *American Medical Association*, Accessed August 10, 2020 at https://www.ama-assn.org/delivering-care/ethics/physicians-responsibilities-disaster-response-preparedness

AMA Council on Ethical and Judicial Affairs, 2020, March 11. "AMA Declaration of Professional Responsibility," *American Medical Association*, Accessed August 10, 2020 at https://www.ama-assn.org/delivering-care/public-health

Amy Solnica, Amy, Leonid Barski, and Alan Jotkowitz. 2020, May. "The Healthcare Worker At Risk During The COVID-19 Pandemic: A Jewish Ethical Perspective," *Journal of Medical Ethics*, Vol. 46 Issue. 7, Accessed August 10, 2020 at https://jme.bmj.com/content/46/7/441

Anantham, Devanand, Wendy McHugh, Stephen O'Neill, and Lachlan Forrow. 2008, Jun 24. "Clinical Review: Influenza Pandemic—Physicians And Their Obligations," *Critical Care*, Vol. 12, No. 3: 217. Accessed August 10, 2020 at https://www.ncbi.nlm.nih.gov/pmc/articles/PMC2481470/

Associated Press. 2020, August 7. "India Hits 2 Million Coronavirus Cases As Health Workers Go On Strike," *The Los Angeles Times*, Accessed August 7, 2020 at https://www.latimes.com/world-nation/story/2020-08-07/india-hits-2-million-coronavirus-cases

Ehrenstein, Boris P. 2008. "Pandemic Influenza: Are We Prepared To Face Our Obligations?" *Critical Care*. Vol. 12 No. 4: 165, Accessed August 10, 2020 at https://www.ncbi.nlm.nih.gov/pmc/articles/PMC2575555/

Emanuel, Ezekiel J. 2003, October 7. "The Lessons of SARS," *Annals of Internal Medicine*, Vol. 139 No. 7: 589–591, Accessed August 10, 2020 at https://pubmed.ncbi.nlm.nih.gov/14530230/

Iserson, Kenneth V. 2018, August. "Must I Respond if My Health is at Risk?" *The Journal of Emergency Medicine*, Vol. 55 No. 2: 288–293, Accessed August 10, 2020 at https://pubmed.ncbi.nlm.nih.gov/29773480/

Kiger, Patrick J. 2019, May 20. "How 9/11 Became the Deadliest Day in History for U.S. Firefighters," *History*, Accessed August 10, 2020 at https://www.history.com/news/9-11-world-trade-center-firefighters

Makin, Kirk, 2009, May 8. "Top Court Dismisses SARS Suits Against Ontario," *The Globe and Mail*, Accessed August 10, 2020 at https://www.theglobeandmail.com/news/national/top-court-dismisses-sars-suits-against-ontario/article1202719/

Malm, Heidi, Thomas May, Leslie P. Francis, Saad B. Omer, Daniel A. Salmon & Robert Hood. 2008. "Ethics, Pandemics, and the Duty to Treat," *The American Journal of Bioethics*, Vol. 8 No. 8: 4–19, Accessed August 10, 2020 at https://www.tandfonline.com/doi/full/10.1080/15265160802317974

McCurry, Justin. 2013, January 11. "Fukushima 50: 'We Felt Like Kamikaze Pilots Ready to Sacrifice Everything" *The Guardian* (UK), Accessed August 10, 2020 at https://www.theguardian.com/environment/2013/jan/11/fukushima-50-kamikaze-pilots-sacrifice

Reynolds, Gretchen. 2004, April 18. "Why Were Doctors Afraid to Treat Rebecca McLester?" *New York Times Magazine*, Accessed August 10, 2020 at https://www.nytimes.com/2004/04/18/magazine/why-were-doctors-afraid-to-treat-rebecca-mclester.html

Ruderman Carly, C Shawn Tracy, Cécile M Bensimon, Mark Bernstein, Laura Hawryluck, Randi Zlotnik Shaul & Ross EG Upshur. 2006, April 20. "On Pandemics and the Duty to Care: Whose Duty? Who Cares?" *BMC Medical Ethics*, Vol. 7 No. 5, Accessed August 10, 2020 at https://www.ncbi.nlm.nih.gov/pmc/articles/PMC1459179/

Sokol, Daniel K. 2006, August 12. "Virulent Epidemics and Scope of Healthcare Workers' Duty of Care," *Emerging Infectious Diseases*. Vol. 12 No. 8: 1238–1241, Accessed August 10, 2020 at https://wwwnc.cdc.gov/eid/article/12/8/06-0360_

Upshur, Ross. 2006. "The Role and Obligations of Healthcare Workers During a Pandemic Influenza Outbreak". *WHO Working Draft*, Accessed August 10, 2020 at https://www.who.int/ethics/PI_Ethics_draft_paper_WG3_14Sept06.pdf

Voo, T.C. and Benjamin James Capps. 2010, April. "Influenza Pandemic and the Duties of Health-Care Professionals," *Singapore Medical Journal*, Vol. 51 No. 4: 27–81, Accessed August 10, 2020 at https://pubmed.ncbi.nlm.nih.gov/20505904/

Chapter 8
Principlist Pandemics: On Fraud Ethical Guidelines, and the Importance of Procedural Transparency

Jonathan Lewis and Udo Schuklenk

Abstract The COVID-19 pandemic has coincided with the proliferation of ethical guidance documents to assist public health authorities, health care providers, practitioners and staff with responding to ethical challenges posed by the pandemic. Like ethical guidelines relating to infectious disease that have preceded them, what unites many COVID-19 guidance documents is their dependency on an under-developed approach to bioethical principlism, a normative framework that attempts to guide actions based on a list of *prima facie*, unranked ethical principles. In this chapter, we aim to explore the limits and limitations of pandemic ethical guidance documents as, specifically, *ethics* documents—documents that fulfil the functions of ethics as a fundamentally normative discipline. This means not only determining whether such ethical guidance documents can, in principle, provide adequate action guidance and action justification, but also, more importantly where pandemics are concerned, determining whether they support *consistent* decision making and *transparent* processes of justification. Having highlighted the problems with merely furnishing ethical guidelines with *substantive* ethical content in terms of principles and values, we argue that organizations that develop these documents should focus on the *procedural* dimensions of action guidance and action justification, which extend to questions regarding the make-up of the committees, panels and groups that develop such guidelines, the public transparency of justifications for specific pandemic-related advice or interventions and the development of explicit procedures for transparent and consistent decision making.

Keywords COVID-19 · Pandemic ethics · Principlism · Ethical guidelines · Ethics expert · Rawls · WHO · Public health ethics

---

The original version of this chapter was revised: Typo in the chapter title has been updated. The correction to this chapter is available at https://doi.org/10.1007/978-3-030-99692-5_14

J. Lewis (✉)
Centre for Social Ethics and Policy, University of Manchester, Manchester, UK
e-mail: Jonathan.lewis-2@manchester.ac.uk

U. Schuklenk
Department of Philosophy, Queen's University, Kingston, ON, Canada
e-mail: udo.schuklenk@protonmail.com

© The Author(s), under exclusive license to Springer Nature Switzerland AG 2022, corrected publication 2022
M. Boylan (ed.), *Ethical Public Health Policy Within Pandemics*, The International Library of Bioethics 95, https://doi.org/10.1007/978-3-030-99692-5_7

8.1 Introduction

The COVID-19 pandemic has generated a vast amount of bioethical research, particularly with regards to ICU triage, disparities in the impact of COVID-19 on different ethnic and social groups, the mental health effects of lockdowns, immunization priorities, the employment of challenge studies for vaccine development, immunity "passports", immunization incentives and the vaccination of children. In addition, there appears to have been a greater than usual demand for the involvement of bioethicists in the public sphere, particularly in print and broadcast media. However, it is in the development of so-called COVID-19 ethical guidance or other advisory documents that bioethicists have had their biggest impact during the pandemic.

Although ethical guidelines pertaining to COVID-19 clinical and public health policy have been produced by governments, state and federal agencies, health care providers and professional bodies across the globe to assist health care practitioners and staff with responding to the ethical challenges posed by the pandemic, it should be noted that the "ethical frameworks" and recommendations presented in these documents are not altogether new. For instance, in the UK, both the Royal College of Physicians and the British Medical Association ("BMA") acknowledge that their respective frameworks are derived from previous guidance issued by the UK government in relation to the pandemic flu in 2009.[1] Furthermore, in terms of specific advice, there is already a significant body of literature on, for example, the ethics of scarce ICU resources, and the actual ethical recommendations put forward in COVID-19 ethical guidelines regarding the triaging of patients largely reiterate what has already been said.[2]

Given that international, national and local organizations have responded to the pressing need for practical guidance and given the calls for the production of authoritative government guidance where none exists, in this chapter we seek to determine whether the kind of ethical guidelines that have been—and are still being—generated fulfil the functions of ethics as a fundamentally normative academic discipline. Secondly, we will address the question of whether the guidance they purportedly offer meets the needs of patients, practitioners and the public, which, as John McMillan notes, we might expect of "good bioethics".[3] Thirdly, in the light of these needs, we will outline what ethical expertise should offer for the purpose of developing ethical guidelines (in a pandemic).

Broadly speaking, the ethical basis of a large number of COVID-19 clinical and public health guidance documents runs counter to the methodological drift in mainstream, Anglo-American bioethical research away from philosophically oriented principlist and more theory-driven approaches. Specifically, the primary form of COVID-19 ethical guidance is bioethical "principlism", albeit an overly narrow application of that approach. According to DeGrazia, principlism denotes any "ethical theory that (1) emphasizes principles, (2) features more than one basic principle, and (3) leaves at least some of its principles unranked relative to each other".[4] If we take the COVID-19 ethical guidance documents issued by the devolved governments in Scotland and Northern Ireland, the Royal College of Physicians (supported by 15 other professional bodies) and the BMA as examples, we find sets of more or less overlapping and unranked "ethical principles" (e.g., autonomy, fairness, minimizing harm, accountability, respect, transparency and so on) together with varying specifications of those principles.[5] In these documents, the principles and their specifications are designated either as "ethical considerations" (to guide clinical decision making) or as an "ethical framework", which can also act as a kind of preface to more specific discussions regarding, for example, resource allocation, triage and risk management for health practitioners.

In the field of bioethics principlism arose in the 1970s in response to what its developers saw as a lack of a unifying theory to guide ethical decisions. Tom Beauchamp and James Childress led the development of a shared normative framework that sought to incorporate long-standing clinical duties to maximize benefits and minimize harms, while also addressing concerns about justice and respect for patient autonomy.[6] They proposed four *prima facie* principles: respect for autonomy, beneficence, non-maleficence and justice. What later came to be known as "principlism" claimed to provide a common source of ethical guidance to which bioethicists from a range of theoretical backgrounds could appeal in their deliberations.

8.2 Philosophical Debates on Principlism

Although we cannot do justice here to the intricacies of these debates or account for all of the issues discussed over the past decades, we can highlight the main criticisms levelled against principlism, particularly as they continue to be relevant to the use of principlist elements in COVID-19 and other infectious disease pandemic ethical guidance documents, and we can outline the ways in which principlists responded to those issues.

According to Beauchamp and Childress, their normative framework was intended not as an ethical theory but as a guide for action, with the four categories of principles functioning as "relatively general norms of conduct that describe obligations, permissible actions and ideals of action".[7] Responding to early editions of their book, critics raised concerns not only about the lack of justification for the choice of principles and the lack of a priority ranking among them, but also about the problems with filling the gap between abstract principles and concrete judgments and the absence of any specified procedure for resolving the conflicts between the principles.[8] Despite Beauchamp and Childress' attempts to deal with some of these issues in later editions, critics of principlism still call into question the ability of the four principles to function as adequate action guides in biomedical contexts.[9]

Firstly, in relation to early versions of Beauchamp and Childress' normative framework, it was suggested that it fails to provide genuine action guidance because, although each of the four principles embodies what is taken to be a key concern in bioethics, there is no account of whether or, indeed, how they are related to each other.[10] The problem is most clearly seen when two or more of the principles conflict with one another (take, for example, the principles of respect for autonomy and justice). Not only did there not appear to be an agreed-upon procedure for resolving conflicts, Beauchamp and Childress did not posit an underlying ethical theory to which one could appeal in order to understand or resolve such conflicts.[11] This led critics to suggest that principlism is merely "a sophisticated technique for dealing with problems ad hoc".[12]

Secondly, Beauchamp and Childress realized that the four categories of principles are too abstract to perform any substantial practical role in biomedical decision making. Consequently, they claimed that the development of principles requires "specification", a process of "judgment and decision making" with the aim of "reducing the indeterminacy of abstract norms and generating rules with action-guiding content".[13] Beginning with the fourth edition of their book, Beauchamp and Childress made use of principle specification, which, as Beauchamp claims (citing Henry Richardson), is achieved by "narrowing their scope...by 'spelling out where, when, why, how, by what means, to whom, or by whom the action is to be done or avoided'".[14] However, critics argued that although the spelling out of these questions does encompass some morally relevant features of a situation, it does not help us to understand why they are relevant nor does it help us to understand what weight should be accorded each morally relevant feature when making moral decisions.[15] More importantly, the continuing lack of an underlying ethical theory meant that, for critics of principlism, no explanation could be offered for how these principles might be applied in specific instances.[16]

Beauchamp and Childress acknowledged that in order for users to employ the method of specification in a way that could support some specifications and not others, and thereby could assist with the application of the principles to specific situations and moral problems, specification needed to be connected to a model of action justification.[17] Without it, not only would specification support an ad hoc approach to bioethical decision making, the user would not be "aware of the real grounds for his moral decision", that is, "what is really guiding his action".[18]

Beauchamp and Childress responded to these issues by developing a metaethical basis for action justification that, simultaneously, could function as a constraint on the specification and balancing of their principles in order to support action guidance.[19] This involves an "integrated model" that combines a coherentist methodology of "wide reflective equilibrium" with "considered judgments" regarding "the set of universal norms shared by all persons committed to morality".[20] Accordingly, Beauchamp and Childress claim that a sufficient account of action justification entails: (i) coherence between principles, broader theoretical considerations and moral judgments and intuitions in which we have the highest confidence and the least bias; (ii) the restriction of the starting points for the method of reflective equilibrium to considered judgments that are acceptable without the support of reasons; and (iii) the formation of those considered judgments under specific epistemic conditions.[21]

According to Norbert Paulo, moral problems are conceived in principlism as conflicts between principles that are part of the specific framework's set of principles.[22] As we have seen, in order to guide action, principlism requires the balancing and specification of principles. For Beauchamp, a specified principle "is acceptable in a system of norms if it heightens the mutual support of other norms in the system that have themselves survived in reflective equilibrium".[23] Furthermore, when attempting to deal with the conflicts between two or more principles, "which resolution is justified is, in principlism, ultimately a matter of coherence".[24] Consequently, as well as contributing to their approach to action justification, "coherence serves as a basic constraint on the specification and balancing of norms that guide actions".[25]

Whether Beauchamp and Childress' "integrated model" for action guidance and action justification has adequately addressed the three primary criticisms of principlism discussed above is still up for debate. However, as shall become clear in what follows, for the purpose of determining whether COVID-19 ethical guidelines fulfil the functions of ethics as a normative discipline, we need not consider these more recent debates here on the basis that no effort was made by the developers of ethical guidelines to deploy such an integrated model.[26]

8.3 Principlist Pandemic Guidelines and the Functions of Ethics

Ethics is a normative discipline, and this means that it has two primary functions: (1) to provide action guidance; (2) to provide action justification. While there are different views about how we should taxonomize bioethics and bioethically-informed public policy, it's reasonable to assume that, in virtue of being forms of ethics, they should share these functions and aim to provide guidance and justification for actions in normative matters related to health care and public and personal health in general.

Let us, for the sake of argument, assume that Beauchamp and Childress' "integrated" approach to principlism is able to deliver adequate action guidance and action justification. One of the problems with their normative framework is that it is solely dependent on the intuitions and/or judgments of the individual employing the method, whether that is, in an academic context, a bioethicist, legal scholar or theologian, or, in clinical circumstances, a health care practitioner or health care facility manager. There is no reason to believe that others will reach the same conclusion and, accordingly, act in the same way when they apply the same method to the same moral problem.[27] The result is that it is by no means clear whether such an approach can meet the needs of patients and the public in terms of, for instance, the consistency and predictability of particular policies in a given health care context. As McMillan argues, "good bioethics" should not only fulfil the functions of ethics, that is, action guidance and action justification, it should do so in a way that "connect[s] with the experiences of those impacted by, and making, decisions in health care".[28] In other words, bioethics should meet the needs of stakeholders, including patients, practitioners and the public.

It is a truism that patients, practitioners and the public will, particularly in pluralistic societies, have diverse and often conflicting needs where clinical or public health decision making is concerned. However, when it comes to national or global infectious disease, there are at least two types of need that members of these groups would reasonably be expected to share given their shared experiences of civil rights infringements, the prioritization of public health and its associated obligations and the statutory and normative demands for certain forms of collective action and responsibility. As the BMA has recognized, when it comes to specific pandemic-related clinical and public health decisions, the first concerns the need for citizens to be "informed beforehand of the anticipated response".[29] The BMA acknowledges the fact that this presupposes that clinical and public health decision makers have a shared understanding of what that response will be. What patients, practitioners and the public share is the need for *consistent* application of the relevant ethical guidelines. More importantly, there is also a need for "legitimate" decisions, that is, "transparent and accountable decision-making processes, including explicit discussion of the ethical principles and reasoning upon which decisions are made".[30] In other words, we are not just talking about ethical guidelines fulfilling the demands of action justification, what is required are *publicly transparent* processes of justification.

Given that the success of guidelines in dealing with ethical, pandemic-related issues depends on health practitioner and provider uptake and the cooperation of patients and the public, it is vital that these groups not only perceive the recommendations contained in these documents to be ethically justifiable (even if they are not normatively acceptable to everyone), but also are able to determine the ways in which ethical guidance will be consistently applied by those charged with protecting their health and wellbeing. These are just some of the reasons for calls during the early stages of the COVID-19 pandemic to consult patients, practitioners and the public on the proposed content of COVID-19 ethical guidance documents and to facilitate development processes that are publicly transparent and accessible—an issue we will explore in the final section of this chapter.[31]

This leads us to the first question we seek to answer in this chapter: can principlist approaches to pandemic ethical guidance fulfil the functions of ethics as a fundamentally normative discipline?

Although it may appear as if we have answered this question already, the issues are not clear-cut when we consider the appropriation of principlist elements in COVID-19 ethical guidance documents. The key concern is that these ethical guidelines rely upon an under-developed approach to bioethical principlism. This is not particular to COVID-19 ethical guidance documents, but something which, as Gert, Culver and Clouser noted in the 1990s, has resulted from "the widespread popularization of principlism throughout the biomedical world, where it is not dealt with as carefully as it is in the hands of Beauchamp and Childress".[32] They argue that, in biomedical contexts, "the principles of principlism primarily function as checklists, naming issues worth remembering when one is considering a biomedical moral issue. 'Consider this … consider that … remember to look for …' is what they tell the agent; they do not embody an articulated, established, and unified moral system capable of providing useful guidance".[33] For Gert, Culver and Clouser, the upshot of this critique for ethical guidelines inspired by certain elements of principlism is that, firstly, with regards to action guidance, the principles are too abstract and empty to provide any help, and, secondly, the use of principles "simply masks ad hoc and unreasoned decisions and judgments due to lack to a lack of adequate grounds for justification".[34] These criticisms resemble those made against Beauchamp and Childress' early iterations of their normative framework.

In order to demonstrate how these problems manifest in concrete guidelines, we will focus, firstly, on the World Health Organization's ("WHO") "Guidance for Managing Ethical Issues in Infectious Disease Outbreaks".[35] Responding to the Ebola outbreak in West Africa between 2014 and 2016, the WHO formed an Ethics Panel and, subsequently, an Ethics Working Group, which was charged with developing general guidance to address ethical concerns associated with global infectious disease outbreaks, including Ebola, severe acute respiratory syndrome ("SARS"), pandemic influenza and multidrug-resistant tuberculosis. The questions this guidance seeks to address are serious ones, such as state obligations, vulnerability, the allocation of scare resources, restrictions on freedom of movement, the rights and responsibilities of frontline workers and medical interventions for the diagnosis, treatment and prevention of infectious disease. The WHO experts preface specific guidelines relating to each of these issues with a list and specifications of "relevant ethical principles": justice, beneficence, utility, respect for persons, liberty, reciprocity and solidarity. They recognize that "the process of ethical analysis involves identifying relevant principles, applying them to a particular situation, and making judgements about how to weigh competing principles when it is not possible to satisfy them all".
[36]Furthermore, they acknowledge the needs of patients, practitioners and the public as detailed above, specifically, that the principle of solidarity commits the global community to apply principles "in a consistent manner, both within individual institutions and, to the extent possible, across geographic areas" with the development of "decision-making tools" to ensure that like cases are treated alike",[37] and that policymakers and providers should develop action guidance "with the genuine input of affected communities".[38] Despite these promising claims, the WHO guidance fails to facilitate or support these ends.

In terms of action guidance, the WHO experts claim that the application of the principles should be informed by "specific evidence" and ensure fairness and consistency.[39] If this evidence is not available, then "decisions should be based on reasoned, substantive arguments and informed by evidence from analogous situations, to the extent possible".[40] But these statements are question-begging. Without some sort of common procedure or theoretical framework that delineates "reasoned, substantive arguments" from those that aren't and that explains how "specific evidence" (whatever that may be) relates to each of the stated ethical principles, there is no reason to believe that the WHO's guidelines will deliver or, indeed, support *consistent* action guidance. In addition, when principles come into conflict (e.g., respect for persons and beneficence or utility and equity), the WHO's ethical guidelines merely state that when "balancing competing principles during infectious disease outbreaks, countries must respect their obligations under international human rights agreements".[41] Although this is an important and legitimate consideration where the infringement of people's civil liberties in a pandemic are concerned, it is by no means the only factor that can influence judgments about how conflicts between principles should be resolved. For instance, when offering guidance regarding the allocation of scare resources, the WHO experts state that although "resource allocation decisions should be guided by the ethical principles of utility and equity", "there is no single correct way to resolve potential tensions between utility and equity; what is important is that decisions are made through an inclusive and transparent process that takes into account local circumstances".[42] Not only does this ethical guidance document, therefore, fail to deliver adequate action guidance, it begs the question of how "inclusive and transparent" processes and "local circumstances" should contribute to principle balancing in practice.

The overarching issue is that there is no explicit connection between the WHO experts' "relevant ethical principles" and their more focused discussions and recommendations regarding pandemic-specific clinical and public health practice. There are no details about how the principles have been applied to questions of resource allocation, clinical obligations, restrictions on freedom of movement, medical application of unproven interventions, and so on, in order to generate action guiding advice. Unsurprisingly, the guidance also fails to meet the justification standard for ethics. The specific guidelines may well be the result of the application of some sort of procedure, but it is impossible to discern whether that is the case given that the experts charged with development of these guidelines do not make explicit its metaethical underpinnings. In important ways, then, the guidance is no more than an *ex cathedra* announcement by the experts appointed by the WHO.

These issues are compounded when we abstract the principles and their specifications away from the specific recommendations regarding resource allocation, triage, risk management, and so on, and employ them as an "ethical framework" or as "ethical considerations" to guide clinical and public health decision making during a pandemic. Take, for example, the "Public Health Ethics Framework" developed by the Government of Canada's Public Health Agency ("PHAC") in response to the COVID-19 pandemic.[43] The developers of this framework state that it is based on guidance and frameworks produced in Canada and internationally, including the aforementioned WHO ethical guidance. It has also significantly influenced more domain specific guidelines, including the "Preliminary Guidance on Key Populations for Early COVID-19 Immunization", issued by the Government of Canada's National Health Advisory Committee on Immunization (NACI), the issues with which we have already addressed elsewhere.[44] Like those chosen by the WHO, the PHAC's experts recognize that adequate ethical responses to pandemic-related clinical and public health issues require decision makers to "identify competing values and interests, weigh relevant considerations, identify options and make well-considered and justifiable decisions".[45] The framework begins with a list of ethical principles: trust, justice, respect for persons, communities and human rights, promoting well-being, minimizing harm and working together. It also contains a list of "procedural" principles, which are meant to facilitate "a solid, shared understanding of what values, principles and considerations are important", and thereby to guide and justify ethical decision making. These are: accountability, openness and transparency, inclusiveness, responsiveness and intersectionality. These principles are followed by the "Ethical Framework", a five-step procedural method that aims to: (1) identify the issue and gather the relevant facts; (2) identify and analyze ethical considerations and prioritize the values and principles that will be upheld; (3) identify and assess options in light of the values and principles; (4) select the best course of action; (5) evaluate.

Beginning with action justification, although the application of the five-step "Ethical Framework" should, according to the document, be guided by the aforementioned "procedural" principles, there is no discussion of how, for instance, stakeholder engagement relates to the other "relevant facts" the users are meant to identify and consider as part of step one of the framework. For instance, no detail is given about how different stakeholder views and concerns relate to "the relevant facts, scientific evidence and other contextual factors". This generates a problem when we reach step three of the framework, which demands that users "prioritize values and principles" and assess "the pros and cons of each option". Relatedly, if a user or set of users have assessed the options as part of step three, then what should be done if, as possible in step four, stakeholders are found to be "uncomfortable" with the "best course of action"? The point is that without a stated basis or associated procedure for working through such procedural conflicts, justification ultimately becomes a matter for the individual user or set of users, which, by prioritizing the vague principle of "accountability", can, in principle, merely be derived from the prioritization of their own principles and values.

The "Public Health Ethics Framework" attempts to get around these issues by stating that the principles of effectiveness, proportionality, reciprocity and precaution should be considered when weighing options. But without some sort of explicit procedure, theoretical foundation or set of criteria that helps the user understand how these four principles relate to one another and how they should be applied in specific instances, the justificatory burden is still borne by the individual user or set of users. For instance, what should a user do if scientific evidence suggests that the most "effective" intervention generates more harm than a less effective approach? Equally, what should a user do if an intervention stands to yield overwhelming benefits for the majority of the population but, at the same time, risks substantive burdens for a fraction of the most vulnerable? Indeed, the Canadian document acknowledges that action justification can only be supplied by decision makers when the procedural principles conflict: "given that it may not be possible in some circumstances to uphold all values and principles equally, it will be important for decision makers to explain how they prioritized them, and to justify the trade-offs made in each situation".[46]

As we have already seen, conflicts can arise not just between procedural principles, but also between stated ethical principles. In this instance, step two of the "Public Health Ethics Framework" asks users to determine the ethical values, principles and considerations involved in the issue, the values and principles that are in conflict and the values or principles that are most important. Once again, these requirements are question begging because there is no explanation of how the competing moral obligations of disparate ethical principles or values should be balanced with one another nor how potential conflicts between the principles should be resolved. For instance, should respect for communities be prioritized over individual freedoms? Alternatively, should respect for persons be prioritized over the greater good of society? Or should justice be prioritized over life-years preserved? The issue is that any priority is ultimately possible within a principlist framework. Although the

PHAC experts provide neither, there are at least two ways to resolve conflicts; (1) ordering the principles hierarchically or lexically; or (2) by introducing an organizing principle. The issue is that if pandemic ethical guidance does not resolve conflicts between principles, one has to draw on other sources, such as intuition or judgment, which, as we have seen, means that action justification procedures or criteria cannot be provided by the guidance itself. Instead, actions and interventions are justified by the implicit values and motivations of individual users.[47]

Let us turn now to the second question of this chapter: can COVID-19 ethical guidance documents, in principle, generate guidance that meets the needs of patients, practitioners and the public?

In a policy brief developed by the WHO's Health Ethics & Governance team concerned with the ethical dimensions of COVID-19 mandatory vaccination, the guidelines for ethical processes of decision-making state that "legitimate public health authorities that are contemplating mandatory vaccination policies should use transparent, deliberative procedures to consider the ethical issues outlined in this document in an explicit ethical analysis".[48] Such statements are legitimate and vital, and reflect those we have already encountered in the WHO and Canadian government's respective ethical guidance documents. However, as we have seen, on the one hand, COVID-19 ethical guidelines developed in the light of bioethical principlism have failed to make explicit the necessary metaethical basis for their ethical recommendations nor do they offer health practitioners any means of justifying decisions resulting from the application of the stated principles. On the other hand, by not providing users with procedures or criteria for specifying principles (and the relationships between them) or for resolving inevitable conflicts, the burden of applying principles to specific pandemic-related issues will be shouldered by individual providers, teams or specific individuals. Thus, despite what appears to be a consensus between the developers of COVID-19 ethical guidance documents for the need for *consistent* application of ethical guidelines and *publicly transparent* processes of justification, extant ethical guidelines derived from bioethical principlism do not give stakeholders a reason to believe that they will be applied consistently. Furthermore, the lack of adequate action justification criteria compromises the ability of stakeholders—the public writ large in particular—to determine the normative legitimacy of any clinical or public health decisions that result from the application of these guidelines.

8.4 Procedural Considerations for the Development of "Good" Ethical Guidance

It is not our intention to suggest anything other than honorable motives on part of those involved in the production of principlist approaches to pandemic ethical guidance. As individuals, they typically volunteered their time, and expert committees, panels, commissions and the like had difficult—if not impossible-to-meet—expectations to fulfil. However, even prior to the COVID-19 pandemic, questions were raised about the very legitimacy of these types of committees, panels and commissions.[49] On the one hand, answers to difficult normative questions were required, answers that oftentimes meant, if policy makers decided to act on them, that some people's lives would be prioritized over others', be it during triage decision making in ICUs or during the initial phases of the roll-out of vaccines. On the other hand, ethics committees, panels and commissions were operating in liberal democracies with their own foundational values (enshrined in constitutions and the like) and with a citizenry that held a wide range of diverse values. Of course, offering a straightforward consequentialist, deontological or virtue ethical analysis and guidance would not serve any practical purpose because each of these varieties of ethics frameworks would not speak to those citizens who hold other values. These frameworks may also have been in conflict with a given society's foundational values. It is not surprising, then, that principlism became popular, because it could have been seen to accommodate a more diverse set of values than other theory-driven frameworks.

As we have noted, "good" bioethics and, by extension, (bio)ethical guidance requires transparent decision-making processes, specifically, explicit, public discussion of the reasons and reasoning upon which public health and pandemic-related clinical decisions are made.[50] In liberal democracies, those who govern depend on the consent of the majority of those who are governed. Given that, during pandemics, policy options are considered that oftentimes infringe on individual freedoms, it matters a great deal that the governed are provided with considered, well-reasoned justifications, particularly as the "success" of such infringements is dependent on public cooperation. People whose liberty rights are infringed upon deserve a transparent justification that explains how a particular policy came about and why the objective it aims to support or achieve is deemed to be of sufficient importance that it justifies the infringement. This does not mean that people whose rights are infringed will necessarily agree with those justifications, but they are owed an explanation of the normative considerations, values and motivations on which such policies are based. What is unsatisfactory is "bullet-point ethics" like that endorsed in, for instance, the ethics guidance of PHAC's experts. The reason for this is that such ethical guidance documents also serve, importantly "as an ethical backstop in times of, for instance public health emergencies [...] It seems [then] unacceptable that they can be used to justify any action or none at all".[51]

Most of COVID-19 ethical guidance documents were authored by groups of (bio)ethicists (as well as, oftentimes, others with no particular ethics expertise). These groups needed to come up with some sort of consensus about specific guidelines for ICU triage, immunization priorities, the management of risk for health professionals and so on, and about specific ethical frameworks to guide public health and clinical decision making in general. If members of these groups were chosen to ensure diversity across different demographic groups, then it is reasonable to assume that they would have been unlikely to reach a consensus on any single value that should drive specific interventions or decision making in general. In relation to triage, for example, utilitarians may have agreed that lives preserved, or life-years preserved ought to be maximized, but that would not cut any ice with ethicists or others determined to prioritize equity. If advocates of utility and advocates of equity meet in a group, then it is conceptually impossible to end up with a coherent consensus document. When agreement regarding a single "organizing" principle or value cannot be reached, principlism becomes *pro tanto* "useful" as a normative framework: it allows all and sundry to contribute their values in the form of an ethical principle to the laundry list of values "that matter" or "to be considered" thereby postponing negotiations over particular policy recommendations until another day. This arguably explains the material content of the ethical guidance documents we discussed in this chapter: they mirror the values of those appointed to author these documents. They also explain the absence of any serious effort aimed at justifying why particular controversial principles were taken to trump other competing controversial principles (e.g., why equity should be prioritized over life-years preserved, or vice versa).

Jonathan Moreno hit upon the fundamental problem with attempting to develop the sorts of pandemic ethical guidance documents that we have considered here when he commented that "empirically, moral truth is in fact less likely to be achieved by groups, which are vulnerable to corruptions of political processes and interpersonal dynamics, than by well informed and reflective individuals".[52] However, as noted in the context of Beauchamp and Childress' "integrated" approach, there is also no reason to believe that a well-informed and reflective individual will deliver conclusions and decisions that all, or even a majority of, members of pluralistic societies will take to be morally legitimate. These related concerns lead us to suggest that ethical guidance documents, rather than attempting to merely provide "substantive" ethical content in terms of explicit principles and values, must primarily focus on making transparent the "procedural" conditions that have been fulfilled in generating and thereby justifying specific advice, and developing procedures that deliver transparent and consistent decision making. What considerations should inform the development of procedurally oriented pandemic ethical guidance?

The first consideration in the development of procedurally oriented ethical guidance ought to be transparency about how expert members have been appointed, by whom and with what mandate. There should be a transparent process that explains to the public, patients and practitioners how and why, say, a consequentialist was chosen as an expert on a committee while the equally available contractualist was not chosen, or vice versa. After all, the values expressed by specific ethical advice do not fall from heaven, and, as we have seen, they are almost always contested. Secondly, and relatedly, those chosen to develop such ethical guidelines ought to reasonably reflect the diversity of normative views prevalent in a given population.

Whoever gets appointed to serve as an ethics expert for a group, panel or committee will have their own ethical commitments. Given that the guidance documents to which they contribute will, to some extent, reflect those commitments, appointment procedures matter. Minou Friele reports that in Germany the first appointees to the country's national ethics council were criticized as being too close to, and handpicked by, the then Chancellor.[53] Caribbean-based bioethicist Cheryl Cox-MacPherson has flagged the failure of international guideline-producing bodies to consult stakeholders in the global south.[54] In the absence of genuine stakeholder consultation and participation, "the wider public might well begin to see a given national bioethics commission no longer as a group of professionals discharging their professional obligations in an unbiased manner, but instead as a group selected by the power of the day to conveniently serve an already pre-determined ideological agenda".[55]

The WHO has recognized the importance of transparency. It has produced a manual that governs the structures and processes of expert advisory panels and committees.[56] While the manual is far from perfect—note, for instance, the document's pervasive sexism—it highlights that the organization is cognizant that appointments to these sorts of panels and committees are never an exclusively expertise-based decision; they are also always significantly political decisions that require the ability of the appointer to explain why and how someone was appointed. The WHO's track record in terms of appointing uncontroversially the most knowledgeable global experts remains sketchy at best, despite its manual.[57]

Focusing on the procedural content of ethical guidelines, Norman Daniels and James Sabin have proposed and defended criteria that aim to establish a fair procedure for developing criteria for how scarce health care resources ought to be distributed.[58] Firstly, they stipulate that the criteria chosen must be made public and they must be justified. In other words, it is insufficient for the expert authors of such guidance documents to merely state, for instance, that equity or utility require XYZ or, worse, to preface advice with a list of ethical principles and then fail to connect recommendations for a specific intervention with those principles. Instead, when delivering specific advice or advocating for a specific intervention, they must explain the reasons for that advice or intervention and why, for instance, it necessitates prioritizing equity over utility (or vice versa). Secondly, Daniels and Sabin suggest that justifiable criteria are constituted by reasons, evidence and principles that a reasonable, well-informed person working toward a societally justifiable *modus operandi* could accept. Importantly, they also suggest that there ought to be in-built review and dispute resolution mechanisms. Those who disagree must be able to have their day in court, as it were.

This all seems probably quite obvious to the fair-minded observer, but authorities in many jurisdictions have kept these guidelines and criteria a secret, no doubt to avoid a public debate (and potential panic).[59] Equally, their ethics experts were almost always handpicked by government officials. There were no transparent public appointment procedures.

Two lessons can be drawn from these observations when it comes to developing pandemic ethical guidance focused on procedural conditions. First, and as we have discussed throughout, it is vital to get the buy-in from stakeholders who will be governed by the ethical guidance document regarding the transparency of the justifications provided by the hand-picked experts. There must also be a public consultation and a clear and transparent explanation of the ways in which the feedback received will be considered and incorporated into the final guidance. As Alex Friedman notes, "without greater opportunities for public participation…it is unclear how the process can hope to confer legitimacy on the decisions that it produces, or why it would be fair or reasonable to expect people not to object and fight back with any means necessary, including litigation, whenever they are disadvantaged for reasons that they do not understand or do not agree with".[60] Second, ethical guidance documents must be published widely. They cannot remain the policy makers' "dirty secret" as has all too often been the case during the COVID-19 pandemic. This kind of conduct is incompatible with the proper functioning of life in a liberal democratic society.

8.5 Conclusion

The COVID-19 ethical guidance documents that have proliferated during the pandemic highlight fundamental issues with approaches that focus predominantly on the substantive ethical content of such documents in terms of principles. Given that these documents rely on a narrow application of bioethical principlism, they cannot deliver either adequate action guidance or action justification (usually both), let alone the guidance and justifications necessary to meet the needs of patients, practitioners and the public. Taking into consideration the competing values that citizens within a pluralistic society will hold means that attempts to overcome the problems with principlism cannot fall back on single principle theories (e.g., utilitarianism) or inflexible, atemporal moral norms (e.g., deontology) without adequate, publicly transparent justifications for the decisions and interventions that are derived from those theories. Indeed, the same applies to principle-based approaches: substantive ethical recommendations derived from a set of *prima facie* and unranked principles require reasons and reasoning that those affected can perceive as legitimate even if they do not endorse the recommendations themselves. Shifting focus away from substantive ethical content to the procedural dimensions of action guidance and action justification allows those that develop pandemic-related ethical guidelines the flexibility to shape legitimate responses to ethical challenges in light of their own commitments and values (to the extent that such responses also—in a publicly transparent way—respond to the commitments and values representative of the public, patients and stakeholders). At the same time, however, it places the onus on guideline-developing organizations to ensure diversity in terms of the experts they choose to appoint to their committees and panels, and it demands that these committees and panels take (very) seriously the requirements for publicly transparent justifications as well as explicit procedures for transparent and consistent decision making.

Notes

1. Royal College of Physicians (2021); British Medical Association (2021).
2. Mannelli (2020).
3. McMillan (2018).
4. DeGrazia (2003).
5. Scottish Government (2020); Department of Health (2020), Royal College of Physicians, "Ethical Dimensions of COVID-19 for Frontline Staff;" BMA, "COVID-19 – Ethical Issues."
6. Beauchamp and Childress (2013).
7. Beauchamp (2010).
8. Schöne-Seifert (2006); Gert et al. (1997).

9. Gert et al. (2006).
10. Gert et al. (2006, p. 75).
11. Ibid., 87.
12. Ibid.
13. Beauchamp and Childress, Principles of Biomedical Ethics, p. 17.
14. Beauchamp (2011).
15. Gert et al. (2006, p. 89).
16. Ibid.
17. Beauchamp and Childress, Principles of Biomedical Ethics, p. 19.
18. Gert et al. (2006, p. 88).
19. Schöne-Seifert (2006), "Danger and Merits of Principlism."
20. Beauchamp and Childress, Principles of Biomedical Ethics, 3, 404, 408.
21. Ibid., 409.
22. Paulo (2016).
23. Beauchamp (2010, p. 159).
24. Paulo (2016, p. 114).
25. Beauchamp and Childress, Principles of Biomedical Ethics, p. 408.
26. For issues concerning Beauchamp and Childress' most recent approach to balancing and specifying principles, see, for example, Tom Tomlinson (2012), Paulo (2016). For issues concerning their approach to the common morality, see, for example, DeGrazia (2003), Turner (2003), Paulo (2016). For the limits and limitations of Beauchamp and Childress' appropriation of reflective equilibrium as a means of action guidance and action justification, see, for example, Arras (2009), Tomlinson (2012). And for broader issues concerning reflective equilibrium as a method for ethical inquiry, see, for example, Kelly and McGrath (2010), Scanlon (2014), McPherson (2015), Cath (2016), de Maagt (2017).
27. Earp et al. (2021).
28. McMillan, The Methods of Bioethics, p. 36.
29. BMA (2021, p. 8).
30. Ibid.
31. Archard (2020), Coggon and Regmi (2020), Fritz et al. (2020), Huxtable (2020), Wilkinson (2020).
32. Gert et al. (2006, p. 72).
33. Ibid., 75.
34. Gert, Culver and Clouser, Bioethics: A Systematic Approach, 2nd ed., p. 101.
35. WHO (2016).
36. Ibid., 8.
37. Ibid., 22.
38. Ibid., 10.
39. Ibid.
40. Ibid., 9.
41. Ibid.
42. Ibid., 21.
43. Government of Canada (2021).

44. Lewis and Schuklenk (2021).
45. Government of Canada (2021).
46. Ibid.
47. Paulo (2016, p. 156).
48. WHO (2021).
49. Friele (2003).
50. BMA (2021, p. 8).
51. Schuklenk (2013).
52. Moreno (1994).
53. Friele (2003).
54. Macpherson (2004).
55. Schuklenk (2004).
56. WHO (2007).
57. Schuklenk (2015).
58. Daniels and Sabin (2002).
59. Schuklenk (2020).
60. Friedman (2008).

References

Archard, David. 2020. Hard Choices at the Frontline, *Nuffield Council on Bioethics*, published March 27, 2020, Accessed July 23, 2021, https://www.nuffieldbioethics.org/blog/hard-choices-at-the-frontline

Arras, John. 2009. The Way We Reason Now: Reflective Equilibrium in Bioethics, In *The Oxford Handbook of Bioethics*, edited by Bonnie Steinbock, 46–71. Oxford: Oxford University Press.

Beauchamp, Tom L. 2010. *Standing on Principles: Collected Essays*. Oxford: Oxford University Press.

Beauchamp, Tom L. 2011. Making Principlism Practical: A Commentary on Gordon, Rauprich and Vollman. *Bioethics* 25 (6): 301-303. https://doi.org/10.1111/j.1467-8519.2011.01908.x.

Beauchamp, Tom L., and James F. Childress. 2013. *Principles of Biomedical Ethics*, 7th ed. Oxford: Oxford University Press.

British Medical Association. 2021. COVID-19—Ethical Issues. A Guidance Note, Accessed July 20, 2021, https://www.bma.org.uk/media/2226/bma-covid-19-ethics-guidance.pdf

Cath, Yuri. 2016. Reflective Equilibrium, In *The Oxford Handbook of Philosophical Methodology*, edited by Herman Cappelen and Tamar Szabó, 213–230. Oxford: Oxford University Press.

Coggon, John, and Sadie Regmi. 2020. Covid-19: Government Guidance on Emergency Rationing of Critical Care is Needed to Support Professional Decision Making, *BMJ Opinion*, published April 24, 2020, Accessed July 23, 2021, https://blogs.bmj.com/bmj/2020/04/24/covid-19-government-guidance-on-emergency-rationing-of-critical-care-is-needed-to-support-professional-decision-making/

DeGrazia, David. 2003. Common Morality, Coherence, and the Principles of Biomedical Ethics. *Kennedy Institute of Ethics journal* 13 (3): 219–230. https://doi.org/10.1353/ken.2003.0020

Daniels, Norman, and James Sabin. 2002. *Setting Limits Fairly—Can We Learn to Share Medical Resources?* Oxford: Oxford University Press.

de Maagt, Sem. 2017. Reflective Equilibrium and Moral Objectivity. *Inquiry* 60 (5): 443–465. https://doi.org/10.1080/0020174X.2016.1175377.

Department of Health. 2020. COVID-19 Guidance: Ethical Advice and Support Framework, last modified September 21, 2020, Accessed July 20, 2021, https://www.health-ni.gov.uk/sites/default/files/publications/health/COVID-19-Guidance-Ethical-Advice-and-Support%20Framework.pdf

Earp, Brian D., Jonathan Lewis, Vilius Dranseika, and Ivar R. Hannikainen. 2021. Experimental Philosophical Bioethics and Normative Inference. *Theoretical Medicine and Bioethics* 42 (3–4): 91–111. https://doi.org/10.1007/s11017-021-09546-z

Friedman, Alex. 2008. Beyond Accountability for Reasonableness. *Bioethics* 22 (2): 101–112. https://doi.org/10.1111/j.1467-8519.2007.00605.x.

Friele, Minou Bernadette. 2003. Do Committees Ru(i)n the Bio-Political Culture? On the Democratic Legitimacy of Bioethics Committees. *Bioethics* 17 (4): 301–318. https://doi.org/10.1111/1467-8519.00347

Fritz, Zoe, Richard Huxtable, Jonathan Ives, Alexis Paton, Anne Marie Slowther, and Dominic Wilkinson. 2020. Ethical Road Map Through the Covid-19 Pandemic. *BMJ* 369: m2033.

Gert, Bernard, Charles M. Culver and K. Danner Clouser. 1997. *Bioethics: A Return to Fundamentals*. Oxford: Oxford University Press.

Gert, Bernard, Charles M. Culver and K. Danner Clouser. 2006. *Bioethics: A Systematic Approach*, 2nd ed. Oxford: Oxford University Press.

Government of Canada. 2021. Public Health Ethics Framework: A Guide for Use in Response to the COVID-19 Pandemic in Canada, last modified February 16, 2021, Accessed July 28, 2021, https://www.canada.ca/en/public-health/services/diseases/2019-novel-coronavirus-infection/canadas-reponse/ethics-framework-guide-use-response-covid-19-pandemic.html

Huxtable, Richard. 2020. COVID-19: Where is the National Ethical Guidance? *BMC Medical Ethics* 21 (32). https://doi.org/10.1186/s12910-020-00478-2

Kelly, Thomas, and Sarah McGrath. 2010. Is Reflective Equilibrium Enough? *Philosophical Perspectives* 24 (1): 325–359. https://doi.org/10.1111/j.1520-8583.2010.00195.x

Lewis, Jonathan, and Udo Schuklenk. 2021. Bioethics Met its COVID-19 Waterloo: The Doctor Knows Best Again. *Bioethics* 35 (1): 3–5. https://doi.org/10.1111/bioe.12840.

Macpherson, Cheryl Cox. 2004. To Strengthen Consensus, Consult the Stakeholders. *Bioethics* 18 (3): 283–292. https://doi.org/10.1111/j.1467-8519.2004.00395.x

Mannelli, Chiara. 2020. Whose Life to Save? Scarce Resources Allocation in the COVID-19 Outbreak. *Journal of Medical Ethics* 46: 364–366. https://doi.org/10.1136/medethics-2020-106227.

McPherson, Tristram. 2015. The Methodological Irrelevance of Reflective Equilibrium, In *Palgrave Handbook of Philosophical Methods*, edited by Chris Daley 652–674. London: Palgrave Macmillan.

McMillan, John. 2018. *The Methods of Bioethics: An Essay in Meta-bioethics*. Oxford: Oxford University Press.

Moreno, Jonathan. 1994. Consensus by Committee: Philosophical and Social Aspects of Ethics Committees, In *The Concept of Moral Consensus*, edited by Kurt Bayertz, 157. Dordrecht: Springer.

Paulo, Norbert. 2016. *The Confluence of Philosophy and Law in Applied Ethics*. London: Palgrave Macmillan.

Royal College of Physicians. 2021. Ethical Dimensions of COVID-19 for Frontline Staff; last modified February 5, 2021, Accessed July 20, 2021, https://www.rcplondon.ac.uk/news/ethical-guidance-published-frontline-staff-dealing-pandemic

Schöne-Seifert, Bettina. 2006. Danger and Merits of Principlism: Meta-theoretical Reflections on the Beauchamp/Childress-Approach to Biomedical Ethics, In *Bioethics in Cultural Contexts*, edited by Christoph Rehmann-Sutter, Marcus Düwell and Dietmar Mieth, 111. Dordrecht: Springer.

Scanlon, T.M. 2014. *Being Realistic about Reasons*. Oxford: Oxford University Press.

Schuklenk, Udo, and Jason Lott. 2004. Bioethics and (Public) Policy Advice, In *Bioethics in a Small World*, edited by Felix Thiele and Richard E, 129–138. Ashcroft Berlin: Springer.

Schuklenk, Udo. 2015. Are International Ethical Guidance Documents and Statements Lacking Legitimacy? *Developing World Bioethics* 15 (2): ii–iii. https://doi.org/10.1111/dewb.12086.

Schuklenk, Udo. 2020. COVID19: Why Justice and Transparency in Hospital Triage Policies are Paramount. *Bioethics* 34 (4): 325–327. https://doi.org/10.1111/bioe.12744.

Schuklenk, Udo. 2013. Bullet Point Ethics as Policy Advice? *Bioethics* 27 (5): ii. https://doi.org/10.1111/bioe.12036.

Scottish Government. 2020. Coronavirus (COVID-19): Ethical Advice and Support Framework, last modified July 29, 2020, Accessed July 20, 2021, https://www.gov.scot/publications/coronavirus-covid-19-ethical-advice-and-support-framework/

Tomlinson, Tom. 2012. *Methods in Medical Ethics: Critical Perspectives.* Oxford: Oxford University Press.

Turner, Leigh. 2003. Zones of Consensus and Zones of Conflict: Questioning the 'Common Morality' Presumption in Bioethics. *Kennedy Institute of Ethics Journal* 13 (3): 193–218. https://doi.org/10.1353/ken.2003.0023.

WHO. 2021. COVID-19 and Mandatory Vaccination: Ethical Considerations and Caveats, last modified April 13, 2021, Accessed July 28, 2021, https://www.who.int/publications/i/item/WHO-2019-nCoV-Policy-brief-Mandatory-vaccination-2021.1.

WHO. 2007. *Regulations for Expert Advisory Panels and Committees* (Geneva: WHO, 2007), last modified June 14, 2007, Accessed July 27, 2021, https://www.who.int/ihr/procedures/en_ihr_roe_advisory_panel_regulations.pdf?ua=1.

Wilkinson, Dominic. 2020. ICU Triage in an Impending Crisis: Uncertainty, Pre-emption and Preparation. *Journal of Medical Ethics* 46: 287–288.

World Health Organization. 2016. *Guidance for Managing Ethical Issues in Infectious Disease Outbreaks* (Geneva: WHO, 2016), Accessed July 28, 2021, https://apps.who.int/iris/handle/10665/250580.

Chapter 9
Public Tasks During Contagious Disease Pandemics: A Rights-Based Perspective

Klaus Steigleder and Johannes Graf Keyserlingk

Abstract During a contagious disease pandemic the primary duty of a state is to protect the rights of its inhabitants without endangering its longer-term protective capacities. The effective and efficient mitigation of an epidemic requires a temporary rule of the plan. Besides, trust must be built up and sustained. The protection of life and health must not be confined to the protection from the contagious disease but must be balanced against other important (societal) aims. In addition, a state has duties to join efforts to combat the pandemic internationally and to support, if possible, other countries in containing the disease.

Keywords External perspective · Internal perspective · Rights · Rule of the plan · Public trust · National responsibility · International burden sharing

Acute contagious disease epidemics or pandemics involve urgent, difficult, and conflicting public tasks of sustaining a functioning economy and the functions of society, of providing for those infected, of limiting and pushing back the infection, and of protecting the (still) non-infected people, especially those at high-risk. These are tasks which are not confined to the national level. For states and societies and their economies are embedded in international or global relations, pandemics are cross-border events of global dimensions and, as is often said, contagious diseases do not naturally stop at borders, and many countries will only prevail with outside help. Thus, it is not only debated how the different obligations and tasks involved in contagious disease epidemics must be weighed against each other but also who must primarily fulfill these tasks.[1]

The original version of this chapter was revised: The author's name (Johannes Graf Keyserlingk) has been updated. The correction to this chapter is available at https://doi.org/10.1007/978-3-030-99692-5_14

K. Steigleder (✉) · J. Graf Keyserlingk
Ruhr-Universität Bochum, Bochum, Germany
e-mail: Klaus.steigleder@ruhr-uni-bochum.de

J. Graf Keyserlingk
e-mail: Johannes.GrafKeyserlingk@ruhr-uni-bochum.de

© The Author(s), under exclusive license to Springer Nature Switzerland AG 2022,
corrected publication 2022
M. Boylan (ed.), *Ethical Public Health Policy Within Pandemics*, The International Library of Bioethics 95, https://doi.org/10.1007/978-3-030-99692-5_8

In this article we will try to answer these questions at least in brief and will argue that rights-based moral theories are especially well-equipped to provide convincing answers. We will particularly argue that, first, states are the primary bearers of the different obligations and tasks concerning contagious disease epidemics or pandemics and that international or global duties of states must be approached from the internal perspective of involved parties whose primary obligation is the protection of the citizens or inhabitants of their respective countries. Second, while the protection of life and health is doubtlessly important, we argue against a one-sided focus on life- and health-protection during contagious disease epidemics which tends to prioritize life and health against other important tasks. For instance, the short-term, medium- and long-term-effects of protective measures must be balanced if such balancing is sensible. The details will, of course, depend on the perilousness of a disease and on how easy or difficult it is to contain it. It would be unjustified to treat, say, Covid-19 on par with Pest or Ebola, on the one hand, and with a cold, on the other hand. Third, and closely connected, not only the medical conditions but also the social conditions for increased vulnerability to contagious disease must be taken into account. Fourth, to avoid certain dilemmas in acute contagious disease epidemics or pandemics preventive measures are of the utmost importance. Modern societies may be better equipped to fight certain contagious disease epidemics, but, e.g. due to globalization, environmental degradation, and climate change they are also faced with considerable risks for pandemics.

9.1 Basic Assumptions of Rights-Based Ethics

We will assume that people have equal rights to the necessary conditions of being able to lead their lives, like freedom, life, physical and psychological integrity, and property.[2] Something like this is a widely acknowledged assumption in different human rights declarations and in the catalogues of fundamental rights of modern constitutions. It is also spelled out in varying details and emphases in different theories of rights-based ethics.[3] In the context of contagious disease pandemics various normatively important goals conflict with each other and different rights of different persons compete with each other. In order to deal with such complexities it will turn out to be of the utmost importance to focus from the very start on certain basic justificatory structures of the rights of people. Unfortunately, in the confines of this essay it is only possible to give a rough outline of these structures.

First of all, and as also pointed out, people have equal rights to the necessary conditions to lead their lives. Thus, the different rights or objects of rights are *related* to the ability (or, more precisely, to certain indispensable components of the ability) to lead one's life. The respective rights do not stand alone and may not be dealt with independently but are justified and related to each other by this fundamental relation. This is why the rights are not all on the same level but form a hierarchy among each other according to differences in their respective indispensability for being able to lead one's life. While all of the rights in question are overall or in the long run indispensable, many, if not most, of them can to different degrees be situationally dispensed with. So, while one's life is absolutely indispensable for continuing and, in this sense, leading one's life[4] certain kinds of non-essential property, for instance, may be situationally dispensable.

Second, the moral rights of people are basically approached (and justified) from within the viewpoint or the internal perspective of the bearer of the rights. A person holds and must hold that she is entitled to being able to lead her life and to the conditions necessary to do so. Thus, she forms certain normative expectations on or claims to the behavior of (the) other people. Within her standpoint, these expectations and claims are justified both in her sense of being of worth, so that in relation to (all) others she deserves to be able to lead her life, and in her dependence on the behavior of others, on whether these others will allow her to sustain or regain this capability. At the same time, she must acknowledge that (all) other persons are sufficiently similar to her and that they therefore possess the same worth, that they have basically the same dependence on the behavior or actions of others and that they therefore have the same justified normative expectations or claims on others regarding the conditions necessary to lead their lives.[5] This equality of the fundamental right to the basic abilities to lead one's life is in line with differences in the situational importance of particular rights of different people. Thus, the right to life of one person may situationally take precedence over, say, non-essential property of another person. Therefore, if there are three people, *A*, *B*, and *C*, and *A* is starving, *B* has food in abundance, and *C* has just enough food for herself, *A* and *C* may on *A*'s behalf take food from *B*.

Third, the picture sometimes painted that rights-based theories are *atomistic*[6] may be applicable to certain (implausible) libertarian theories, but it would gravely misunderstand a theory like the one outlined here. For the theory is based on the mutual acknowledgement of the equal worth and dependency or vulnerability of persons. Thus, the equal rights of people to the conditions necessary for being able to lead their lives require of us to acknowledge that we constitute both strict limits and important tasks for each other. We must be willing to restrict the pursuit of our actions and life plans out of respect for the potentially affected others and out of the acknowledgement of their own dependence on the necessary conditions of their ability to lead their lives. And we must be concerned about others when they need help.

Far from being atomistic the theory outlined is a theory of the normative necessity of mutual, albeit limited, concern. That we are vulnerable and may harm each other but also have the possibility to protect and support each other is not limited to infectious disease dynamics in which patients are both "victim and vector"[7] but is essential to the human condition and its normative relevance. This is, of course, highly relevant for infectious or contagious disease dynamics, but it is important to integrate this relevance into the broader picture of normative tasks. In fact, our vulnerability and the potential harm we can do to each other requires the state to foster and maintain those crucial but fragile forms of social cooperation on which any effective pandemic response depends. The barriers for such coordinated action are versatile though, like political polarization, poor leadership and, most fundamentally, low levels of public (or social) trust.[8] At any rate, the question of how to promote (or maintain) social cooperation and thus to make it more likely that people are willing to accept individual costs for the benefit of other people is a decisive one, not only for an effective and efficient pandemic response.[9] When answering that question, one should take cultural factors into account. There is evidence that cultural patterns, and particularly the commitment of citizens to the political collective, are important variables that inform a country's policy choices and determine its performance during a health crisis. As Bavel et al. point out, "[w]hile medical policies are different across societies, some differences in the response to the pandemic may be better described as cultural [...]."[10] To the extent that, as compared with the more individualist Western cultures, the stronger commitment to social norms in some Asian societies like South Korea allows for more effective responses to at least some of the public health (and broader societal) threats during a pandemic, the concern with culture, trust, and social cooperation should inform normative theorizing on the public tasks during a pandemic.[11]

The normative relevance of cooperation and thus of people's readiness to bear an individual cost in order to benefit a third party or, more generally, to promote the collective (societal) interest of public health, comes into full view when considering the fourth structural feature of the rights of people, namely that the moral rights of people are not only negative, i.e., rights to the forbearance of others, but also positive, i.e., rights to the assistance of others if certain conditions are fulfilled. Due to the equality of rights, rights to assistance are always situationally conditioned. One has a right to the assistance of others if one is not able to help oneself and another person is able to help "at no comparable cost".[12] One can see that this presupposes a hierarchy of rights. A theory for which all rights are on a par or on the same level cannot acknowledge positive rights, for positive rights would then of necessity be inconsistent with the equality of the rights between people. If A's right to X is endangered and B would be required to help A by endangering or setting back her own rights each of which is situationally of equal importance as X, then A's rights would be more important than B's rights. If, independent of any contractual obligations, Betty was required to save Amy's life by risking her own life, Amy's life would be more important than Betty's. Thus, if people possess equal moral rights against each other, there can situationally only be a moral right to be helped by another person if this does not affect rights of equal importance on the part of the potential helper, or if, in the formulation of Gewirth, the potential helper can help "at no comparable cost".

The other requirement that a person can only have a right to be helped if she is not able to help herself is also based on the equality of the rights between persons. If A had to help B even if B could help herself, B('s rights) would be more important than A('s rights).

Positive rights and the corresponding duties to help exemplify that the rights of people are originally approached from within the perspective of the bearers of the rights. The right to life of a person who is drowning in dangerous water and the equal right to life of a potential helper are basically not evaluated by an impartial observer who approaches the equality of rights from the outside but from within the perspective of the potential helper. From within this perspective the equal right to life of the potential helper may speak against trying to save the person by entering the water, because the potential helper has no duty to endanger her life in order to save the life of another person. This is even the case if several persons are drowning. The internal perspective is not maximizing. From within the internal perspective of one's own right to life the lives of, say, three other persons do not outweigh one's own life.[13]

Things are quite different when one is required to take an external perspective or the perspective of an outsider or impartial observer.[14] Suppose you are an uninvolved party and you could either save, without endangering your own life and with equal prospects of success, the two children drowning on your right side or the one child drowning on your left side, but you are unfortunately not able to save all three children. In such a case a maximizing perspective, trying to save as many children as possible, will probably take best account of the equal worth and equal rights of the affected children.

Thus, depending on whether an internal or an external perspective on the equal rights between persons may or must be taken, different rights or duties of agents will be pertinent. The neglect of the important question of when taking an internal or external perspective is justified is responsible for much confusion in contemporary political philosophy. For the determination of the public tasks in contagious disease epidemics or pandemics it will turn out to be of central importance.

The positive rights of persons normally lead to situationally pertinent duties of individual persons to help in cases of an acute emergency. Compared with this, in cases of chronic need constant or repeated help is required. Such a requirement may easily overburden the potential helper and negatively affect her ability to lead her life and thus her ability to help at no comparable cost. However, while persons may not be able to help in such cases individually, they may do so collectively and may institutionalize the required help. Concerning such cases, one's duties primarily consist in the support of the respective institutions.[15]

The effective protection of the rights of people by institutions is part of their rights. Thus, fifth, there must be the institutions of the state, including those of a welfare state, but also international and global institutions. Unfortunately, both theoretically and practically, the required international and global institutions are still underdeveloped, and in many places of the world the required state institutions are insufficient or seized by autocrats, dictators or an autocratic elite. Consequently, the rights of a huge number of people in the world are violated and unprotected. However, this does not speak against the relevance of states, and the relevance of existing states, for the protection of the rights of its citizens or inhabitants, nor does is speak against the relevance of defined borders and territories.[16] This is also the case for states whose constitutions and governments are, in view of the protection of the rights of their citizens, seriously defective. A limited rule of law may overall be better than no rule of law at all. And the abolishment of borders would in all probability bring down the protection of the rights of the former inhabitants and not create the desired protection of the new inhabitants.

A state, its officials and representatives must standardly take an external and impartial perspective on the rights of its citizens and inhabitants. And it must approach the rights of the inhabitants of other states from an internal perspective. That is because it must act as a custodian of the rights of its citizens and inhabitants whose effective protection is its primary responsibility. Thus, a state must not sacrifice the equal rights of its inhabitants in view of the endangered rights of other people. To give a topical example, suppose that during the pandemic of a life-threatening contagious disease a rich country possesses a considerable amount of vaccine doses but not enough to vaccinate all its inhabitants. Under such conditions, all else being equal, those responsible in the country are morally not allowed to take a considerable amount of the available vaccine doses and to donate them to a poor country which does not possess any of the required vaccine doses. By doing so, presupposing that the donated vaccines will actually be used to vaccinate the right people in the poor country, the donor country would accept the death of some of its inhabitants in order to save the life of inhabitants in the poor country. This would contradict the primary responsibility of a state for the protection of its own inhabitants.

It is important to note, however, that the priority treatment of its own inhabitants does not deny the universality of human rights, as the defenders of certain forms of cosmopolitanism would have it. Instead, the question is whether the universal moral rights may or must always be approached from an external or neutral perspective or whether and when they may or must be approached from within an internal perspective. It is also important to note that it does not follow from the importance of taking the internal perspective in certain problem situations that (the inhabitants of) rich states do not have urgent moral obligations in the face of the moral claims (of the inhabitants) of poor states. It is only to say that one should be aware of the dangers of misplaced moralizing given the complex and complicated state of the world.

Thus, to return to the vaccine example, while states have a primary obligation to fulfill the vaccination needs of their own citizens, they have at least in principle additional obligations to make considerable efforts to see to it that enough vaccines are produced for people living in countries which are not able to fulfill the respective needs of their population. This might be done both by arranging production capacities which exceed a country's own needs and by supporting the production and distribution of vaccines within the poor countries. However, the obligations in principle become concrete obligations only if ways of the effective distribution of vaccines in the poor countries are available.[17] Especially in the present context of fighting a pandemic, but also more generally in view of other global challenges like climate change, it is important to put this balancing between the individual state's core national and its wider international responsibilities into the broader perspective of the promises and limits of global cooperation. Although the story of human life on Earth may be characterized as "the story of increasingly complex cooperation",[18] it is the level of the nation state that to this day remains the most reliable system for the provision of those public goods that are required for the protection of rights. By itself, this may serve to confirm the normative principle that it is the primary responsibility of any individual state to concentrate on rights protection within the boundaries of its own jurisdiction. In this sense, any attempt to make progress toward international cooperation in our dealing with global health crises should start at the national level.[19] In the specific context of contagious disease pandemics, however, this focus on the responsibility to protect rights at home serves an additional, rather ambivalent function. On the one hand, the mutual assistance and coordinated efforts among states may send "strong signals of cooperation and shared values",[20] which could then foster deeper cooperation among peoples and states. On the other hand, the priority given to rights protection at the national level serves to anticipate a potential secondary threat that a pandemic situation poses to international cooperation. This threat lies in the experience of fear which the members of a political community (i.e. the in-group) tend to experience during a pandemic. Such fears are often associated with a growing sense of aversion, intolerance and outright hostility toward out-groups like people in other national communities.[21] The animosities faced by Asian Americans during the Corona pandemic are only one example of this phenomenon.[22] In view of the recent rise of populist, nationalist, and autocratic governments, a further rise in the levels of ethnocentrism and the associated increase in national isolationism would most certainly be a fatal development, morally and politically. Arguably, it is precisely in this context that for any individual state to fulfill its primary responsibility toward its own citizens and thus to prioritize the protection of their rights gains even further plausibility. For it is the effective protection of citizens' rights and the resulting sense of security that will minimize such fateful experience of threat and fear on the side of citizens, and that sense of security at home may then serve as the solid basis for seizing the beforementioned opportunities that a pandemic means for the prospects of deeper international cooperation. In sum, it is this ambivalence regarding the promises and limits of international cooperation during global pandemics that should inform the normative assessment of states' international obligations.

9.2 The State as the Primary Bearer of Tasks in Contagious Disease Pandemics

Epidemics or pandemics of potentially deadly contagious diseases threaten the fundamental rights of people and the functioning of the economy and of societies. Pandemics may have large global impacts, may affect the relations between countries, and may affect different countries differently. Even if a pandemic is not confined to a country, it is the state who is the primary bearer of the tasks of protecting its citizens or inhabitants, both those already infected and those threatened by an infection, and of sustaining, as far as possible, a functioning economy and the functions of society due to their strategic importance for the protection of the rights of the citizens.

In addition to the above-mentioned set of cooperation-related (pragmatic) reasons why it is reasonable for states to give priority to the protection of its citizens' rights, there is a more systematic rationale why the state should be the primary bearer of the indicated protective tasks: First, as a basic realization, such tasks are truly public ones which simply cannot be solved by individuals or on an individual level. Second, in principle the state is best positioned to make sure that the rights of its citizens or inhabitants are effectively protected by the required institutions and background conditions reaching from the enablement and protection of the civil liberties, the framework conditions of a functioning economy, the construction and maintenance of the necessary infrastructure, the build-up and preservation of a functioning health care system, the preservation and improvement of public health, the maintenance of a functional educational system to many other responsibilities. So, as an acute contagious disease pandemic threatens the effective protection of the rights of the citizens, this is a special case of the general responsibility of the state. At the same time a well-functioning state will have the means to fulfill the required tasks and must see to it that it will not lose its ability to effectively protect the rights of its citizens. Third, even if a single state cannot effectively fight the acute pandemic alone and must cooperate internationally, regionally and globally, as long as a state is able to take effective measures to fulfill its tasks, it must take these measures and must not delegate its tasks. For these tasks constitute genuine responsibilities of the state. A state must take an internal perspective to and a special advocacy of the rights of its citizens. And it must not seek help of others as long as it is able to help itself. Things are, of course, different if a state is overwhelmed or otherwise unable to fulfill its tasks. In such a case it must seek help from other states, relief agencies or international institutions. Fourth, the citizens of a state have special rights against their state and the institutions of the state because they have supported the state and its institutions. Therefore, they may rightly lay claim to being the primary beneficiaries of the institutions and capacities of the state. Correspondingly, the state has special duties to its citizens. It must fulfill its duties by taking up the tasks of containing and fighting the acute contagious disease pandemic.

As in normal times, the primary task of the state in the face of an acute contagious disease epidemic is the effective protection of the rights of its citizens. The difficulty is, of course, to spell out what this amounts to. Thus, on the level of the state no public sphere is introduced which would follow a different normative principle than the equal rights of persons to the necessary conditions for being able to lead their lives.[23] On the level of the state, this principle is not supplanted by, say, a principle of the maximization of cumulative wealth, health or happiness. However, as we have seen, the state must approach the equal rights of its citizens differently than the citizens may approach each other in their rights. While individual agents may approach each other from an internal perspective, the state must standardly approach the rights of its citizens from an external perspective, i.e., as an uninvolved party.

A notorious problem at the start of an acute contagious disease pandemic is that the problem is usually acknowledged too late.[24] Especially when the disease is caused by a new or unknown agent, there is a typical mix of political and economic interests in avoiding the consequences of false alarm and an accompanying tendency to sit on the fence and to soothe. When it can no longer be denied that an acute contagious disease is expanding on an epidemic or even pandemic scale it is increasingly difficult to contain the disease without drastic measures. If it is a new disease, many important facts will not be sufficiently known in the beginning, e.g., how deadly and how dangerous the disease is, in which ways it is communicated, when and how long an infected person is contagious or whether certain groups are especially at risk, say for medical or social reasons like poor or cramped living or working conditions. Therefore, initially the measures to be taken can only be inexact and rough.

There are three primary tasks here. First, the spreading of the disease must be stopped and further infections must be avoided. For the disease will impact the infected in their basic rights and the spread of the disease will negatively affect the workings of society and its institutions as well as the protection of the rights offered by them. Thus, in this perspective the already infected constitute both a direct and indirect threat to those not yet infected. Things are complicated by the fact that it may not be clear who is already infected and thus a vector of the disease while not yet showing any symptoms. Under such circumstances many asymptomatic persons may constitute a potential threat to each other. Therefore, the tasks of containment and protection involve the isolation of those already infected, quarantining those potentially infected and the prohibition of all avoidable contacts. This will include the closing of borders and the stop of passenger flights.[25]

Second, while being a risk to others justifies clear restrictions of one's rights one is, of course, not losing one's rights. Thus, those who are ill have rights to treatment and care if treatment and care is possible. Besides, the isolation and quarantine of people must be organized in such a way that the basic needs of the affected people are taken care of as far as possible. This pertains to food and drinking, to the possibility to occupy oneself with interesting activities and to stay in contact with others, e.g., electronically, but also to sustain one's abilities to meet one's financial obligations and to receive an income.

Third, those who treat or take care of the infected and also those who care for the quarantined must receive the best possible protection. This includes the sufficient availability of protective wear, disinfectants and so on, which in turn presupposes that adequate preparation for the case of pandemics is taken. It is also the task of the community of states and pertinent international organizations that appropriate preparations are made for being able to help poor countries with the necessary materials in emergency situations. These preparations must be supported and financed by the rich countries. It must also meticulously be observed that the disease is not, as is often the case in contagious disease epidemics, particularly spread by the involved doctors and caregivers. This is an important individual obligation of the involved doctors and caregivers whose abidance must be officially overseen.

9.3 The Unavoidable Ambivalence of Protective Measures and Its Normative Relevance

The measures to contain and fight the contagious epidemic are unavoidably deeply ambivalent. They aim at the protection of rights of the (still) healthy people and at the preservation of the important institutions of the society and the state. At the same time, they massively infringe the rights of those (possibly) infected and of those to be protected, and they massively interfere with the normal functioning of the economy, the exercise of occupations and social life. This has several important normative implications.

First, the measures and the attempted shutdown of the social life must be effective and efficient. The infringement of the rights of people can only be justified if the measures have the probable effect of containing the epidemic and of bringing the occurrence of infections down. This must be done with the least invasive measures possible. In fact, measures can be unjustifiably harsh or too lenient. There can, of course, be disagreement whether an almost complete but relatively short shutdown should be attempted which will bring large parts of economic production to a halt or a less complete and longer shutdown which tries to protect certain parts of the economy. The right strategy will depend on how "short" and how effective the "complete" shutdown is and how sustainable its effects will be. Such questions involve many uncertainties and are therefore difficult to answer. However, what must be avoided by all means is a substantial but ineffective shutdown.

Second, while the effectiveness of the overall measures is relatively easy to evaluate, an evaluation of the efficiency of the package and of single measures is much more complicated. As said, the measures of fighting a new contagious disease epidemic will initially be inevitably rough and, after the right start was missed, possibly too harsh. There is an urgent obligation to find out whether this is the case and, if need be, to correct it as soon as possible. The aim must be to establish what the required minimum measures are, how a state of using only these measures can be achieved as fast as possible, and how it can be sustained. In the face of a new disease, it will not be possible to answer this once and for all but only in relation to the present state of knowledge and to the present state of available means (e.g., tests, vaccines, therapeutics). The question may have no single answer and may only be answered by weighing different risks. Given the available means, one must find out what the aim concerning the disease should be, e.g. strict containment and elimination of any further infections in a country in the face of a devastating disease like Ebola (Ebola Virus Disease, EVD) or living with a disease and its regular but limited recurrence like standard influenza epidemics and possibly Covid-19. As measures of a shutdown directly or indirectly severely infringe the rights of the affected people, those who are responsible have a strict obligation to find out *on day 1* of a shutdown how the shutdown can be ended as quickly as possible.

This requires, third, that during an acute contagious disease epidemic or pandemic all levels of government (national to local) must be focused on the task of containing and fighting the disease effectively and efficiently, infringing the rights of the affected people to the least possible extent. This calls for what might be called the *rule of the plan*. For a first orientation one may think of a war economy. There is a need to focus on one, albeit complex aim and to make sure that it is reached in a coordinated way as soon and as sustainably as possible. At least for the time being this cannot be achieved by the decentral operations of the market. This constitutes a huge problem. In a market economy, to simplify a bit, governments are used to having many things dealt with decentrally on markets and to seeing their task mainly in influencing the framework conditions under which the markets operate. Contrary to this, fighting an epidemic or pandemic both effectively and efficiently in the explained sense requires a huge effort of continued planning and organization.

Thus, tasks must be defined, and means for their solution must be determined and employed in a coordinated way. Especially in the beginning, doing this will be complicated by huge knowledge gaps concerning the properties and dynamics of the disease and its spread. These gaps, especially the most important gaps, must be defined and systematically closed by means of international cooperation. While researchers will find many relevant research questions and ideas of how to answer them, it is important to define the pertinent questions whose treatment cannot be left to the contingency of whether a research group will take them up or not. Particular attention is needed to finance or coordinate investigations and research projects which are time-consuming and expensive like systematic postmortem examinations, their appraisal and publication or the drawing of a representative sample in order to establish how different groups or parts of the population are affected by the occurrence of the infection.

One may take the current Covid-19 pandemics to exemplify further tasks. Test capacities must be built up and systematic testing must be established especially of those who have close contact with high-risk persons or cannot avoid to work, teach or learn indoors in close proximity with other people. At the same time the necessary capacities must be established to isolate but also to look after those with a positive test result and to track, quarantine and test those who had contact with the positively tested persons. If possible, digital means should be used for signaling and tracing potential contacts of infected persons. As this may be incompatible with relevant data protection laws, the relevant regulations must possibly be suspended during a defined emergency situation and the necessity of doing so in view of the protection of situationally more urgent rights must be explained. School teaching must be reorganized. For example, attending classes must be connected with systematic testing, lessons must perhaps be shortened and given repeatedly and consecutively to smaller groups. School related local public transport must be reorganized in such a way that the infection risks of the children approaching and leaving schools are sufficiently reduced. For this, busses of travel organizations could be used which are not able to continue their normal business during the pandemic.

Special attention and care must be given to those who are working under cramped or confined working or living conditions. Enterprises must be obliged to ensure that working conditions are adapted and their employees are sufficiently protected.

9.4 Dealing with the Impediments of Bureaucracy

The required rule of the plan will be impeded by the normal workings of bureaucracy. To stress this is not to compare with embitterment the baneful workings of bureaucracy with the beneficial workings of markets. Nor is it meant as part of a comprehensive critique of bureaucracy.[26] Rather, it is only to highlight that the required rule of the plan needs organizational structures which are normally inexistent and that it will come across organizational structures which will be unsupportive or outright obstructive. For the elaboration, implementation, and adaptation of the required plans on the different levels of government and societal institutions will make it inevitable to secure the services of staff that is on the whole inexperienced in those tasks and occupied with other tasks. Besides, it will require regulatory flexibility of a kind that is often outright prohibited by the existing legal regulations, public procurement law and data protection law included. Finally, it will require of the persons responsible in different institutions a degree of initiative that will constitute a degree of nonconformism which at least under normal circumstances might have a negative impact on one's career prospects and which accordingly might be considered too risky. Thus, the normal workings of bureaucracy are not conducive to the degree of initiative needed in emergency situations.

We can see from this that the rule of the plan must to a large part consist in the creation and coordination of the required organizational structures on the different levels (national to local) of government and the supporting (ministerial, county, municipal, institutional) bureaucracies. Task forces must be created within the normal bureaucratic and institutional structures and its competencies must be defined and aligned. Existing expertise must be identified and used, e.g., the procurement or production of needed material, or the improvement of the necessary digital infrastructure through pertinent industries or enterprises, or the build-up of the personnel of public health offices with qualified persons who, due to the epidemic, cannot work in their normal jobs. Certain rules must be relaxed under such emergency conditions. For instance, emergency biddings must be allowed in connection with certain tasks. Besides, the rule of the plan does not and should not exclude that in order to learn from best practices different strategies will be attempted and compared with each other on the level of federal states, cities or municipalities.

Ideally, the needed organizational requirements are part of emergency plans done in advance and regularly reviewed and discussed on the different organizational levels. This constitutes, of course, a further bureaucratic task. The chances of its efficient implementation should not be overrated, especially when the memories of the last severe crisis begin to fade. During an emergency the measures taken must be continuously evaluated for their effectiveness and efficiency related to the above mentioned tasks of combating the epidemics while allowing for the greatest level of normalcy possible or the least restrictions necessary.

9.5 The Importance and Limitations of the Protection of Life and Health

There is a substantial danger of a one-sided focus on *a certain kind* of the protection of life and health, namely on the life and health threatened directly by the contagious disease or the underlying pathogen. For combatting a contagious disease epidemic seems to amount exactly to this. There is a further danger to overrate the *immediate* protection of life and health out of theoretical reasons.

We have seen that in the hierarchy of rights life is fundamental. We need our life in order to be able to lead our lives. This may induce one to assume that the protection of life is always paramount or that the right to life is absolute. However, this would be a mistake. For, as pointed out above, the right to life must be seen in relation to the equal right of persons to lead their lives. Absolute rights, if there are any, are a limiting case. Alan Gewirth has argued that there is an absolute right of all innocent persons "not to be made the intended victims of a homicidal project".[27] Thus, an absolute right to life would be a right against others to refrain from certain premeditated actions. However, it is evident that certain measures of actively protecting the right to life of people may have the effect of unduly restricting the equal rights of people to lead their lives. In this connection a helpful orientation can be gained from the Kantian idea of equal maximum freedom.[28] According to this, the equal right of people may be violated when the rights are equally restricted. Equality is not an isolated or freestanding moral imperative. Instead, each person has a right to the maximum freedom to lead his or her live that is compatible with the equal maximum freedom of all other persons to lead their lives. This constitutes an important general normative orientation for the evaluation and necessary reevaluations of the public restrictions aimed at containing and fighting a contagious disease epidemic.

Therefore, one is forced to work with the inevitably vague concept of sufficient protection as distinguished from complete protection. To illustrate this point, imagine a government wanted to establish as far as possible a complete protection against any murder within the legal sphere of the state. It would justify this by the necessity to protect the most basic right of people, i.e., the right to life. This could only be done or attempted to be approached by massive restrictions of the rights of the people and by amassing dangerous and possibly life-threatening power in the hands of the state. At the same time the measures would probably also be counterproductive because they would undermine the economic and social thriving of society and thereby undermine the abilities of the state and its institutions to effectively protect the rights of its citizens.

As applied to dangerous, i.e., potentially life-threatening diseases and disease epidemics the task is to find out what, according to the respective state of knowledge, according to the character of the disease and according to the available means to prevent or treat it constitutes a sufficient protection of life of all potentially affected. As the equal right to life is part of the equal right to lead one's life basically the public protection of the right to life of one person or certain groups of persons must not involve the thwarting of the ability of other persons or groups of persons to lead their lives. Besides, one has to be aware that certain measures aimed at the protection of life may negatively affect the right to life of others. Not receiving necessary treatments, postponing important surgeries, losing one's job, not being able to put to use skills one has acquired over a long time at great effort and expense like playing an instrument, not being able to meet beloved others, not being able to have the chance of life-changing encounters with possible future friends or life partners, not being able to make sport, not being able to go to school and to learn, being confined to cramped living conditions, being exposed to the aggression of others under those conditions, resorting to an unhealthy diet, and so on, may have massive effects on one's life chances, one's physical and psychological health and one's life expectancy. Except for the potential health effects different from the infectious disease, other important rights are affected too. Furthermore, a prolonged shutdown, the closure of businesses, universities and schools as well as the debts incurred by supporting affected industries or enterprises and by helping those who have lost their income due the protective measures may threaten the economic and social wealth of the society and thereby undermine the ability of a state to effectively protect the rights of its citizens, their right to life included.

Thus, it is of the utmost importance to approach the public tasks concerning contagious disease epidemics ultimately with the whole range of the involved problems and rights in view and not only in view of the immediate health problems connected with the infectious disease. The detailed weighing of the different problems in different areas and of the different rights of different groups will require further research. For this an overcoming of the constraint to defined problem areas like bioethics or economic ethics is needed. A further task of research is the normative treatment of relevant risks, i.e., the normative evaluation of only possible consequences. Despite some progress in certain defined areas, like the ethics of clinical trials, and despite attempts to circumvent the missing risk ethics with more or less ingenious auxiliary constructions like different uses of a precautionary principle[29] normative ethics is still mostly guided by the evaluation of actions with definite consequences.[30] We know that we must not use a car in order to overrun and kill another person. However, possibly we will run over and kill a person by using a car and we are less sure about the normative relevance of this possibility or risk.[31]

Infections with contagious diseases normally may not be conceptualized as direct threats to life. Instead, they are occurrences that involve multiple risks or uncertainties, namely at least the risk of getting infected, the risk of being infected and the risk of infecting others. Often, there will be uncertainty of whether one is an infection risk to others and if so, how much of an infection risk one is. As mentioned above, a disease as infectious and dangerous as Ebola requires a different treatment than Covid-19. In the case of Ebola strict containment and local eradication of the disease is necessary, which can be achieved because the disease is, unfortunately, so deadly and is spread via bodily fluids and not by airborne spread.[32] In contrast, if we look at Covid-19 independently of the availability of vaccines there seem to exist clear differences in the health risks for different groups. Groups like the elderly and those with preexisting conditions have a high risk of developing a severe and possibly deadly course of the disease, while groups like the young have a low risk of being affected by important symptoms. As the young or younger persons may nevertheless be infectious, protective measures pertaining to them as possible vectors of the disease are aimed at the protection of the persons in the high-risk groups. Such protection is, of course, important but must be limited in view of the rights and life prospects of the younger persons.

Thus, to develop more fine-grained criteria of what constitutes necessary and sufficient protection, the risks of different contagious diseases, the reliability of different protective measures as well as the impact of the different measures on the rights of all affected must be taken into account. Perhaps, different diseases can be classified in groups with comparable challenges, which may provide orientation for dealing with the outbreak of new diseases.

The preceding reflections pertained mainly to well-functioning and (relatively) rich states which in principle are able to use all the available means. A further important step is to define what can and must be done under much more unfavorable conditions in poorer states or less functioning states and how these states or the people living in these states can be supported. As the discussions about the effectiveness and potential harmfulness of development aid demonstrate, adequately dealing with the problems of support is outstandingly difficult.[33] One must resist the temptation to close existing loopholes by trying to save the world from one's desk with utterly unworkable or even objectively harmful proposals. There is possibly no alternative to first carefully studying what worked and what went wrong in previous attempts to prevent and fight epidemics in poor countries and then to proceed by using a method of trial and error.

9.6 Instead of a Conclusion: The Importance of Prevention and Preparedness

This article dealt with the public tasks during contagious disease epidemics and pandemics. Arguably, an existing epidemic is often a visible proof that warning signs were ignored, downplayed or even concealed and that the necessary preventive or protective measures come too late. It is therefore an important task to try to learn from a missed opportunity like the prevention of the Corona pandemic—and from examples of successful prevention or containment—how epidemics and pandemics can possibly be prevented and to try to establish or improve on early-warning systems. Arguably, to provide the necessary financial resources for doing this is mainly the responsibility of the rich countries. However, despite such efforts epidemic disease dynamics will be overlooked or cannot be detected in time. Therefore, being prepared for the advent of epidemics or pandemics is utterly important. As already mentioned, part of the preparation is to have sufficient protective wear available for those who must care for the infected people. Besides, the development of workable emergency guides is needed. It is to be hoped that both the criteria proposed here and the fulfillment of the task to detail them further could make a helpful contribution.

Notes

1. See, e.g., Faden et al. (2020), Verweij and Dawson (2007), and Battin et al. (2008).
2. Cf. Gewirth (1978). Gewirth himself focuses on the necessary conditions of being able to act successfully.
3. See, e.g., the overview given in Steigleder (2016), see also Gewirth (1984, 1986), Caney (2010), and Shue (2020).
4. However, certain forms of the prolongation of one's life may be in conflict with the life one has led or wants to lead.
5. Cf. also Gewirth (1978), 104–106.

6. Taylor (1985); for a rejection see also Gewirth (1996), 32f. and 91.
7. Battin et al. (2009).
8. Van Bavel et al. (2020) and Morse and Tsai (2017).
9. Greene (2013).
10. Van Bavel et al. (2020), 463.
11. For an instructive account of the functional relationship between social trust, mutual regard among members of the political community, and social cooperation, see Collier (2013).
12. Gewirth (1978), 218.
13. This is correctly pointed out by John Taurek, albeit without much recourse to normative theory. See Taurek (1977).
14. Here Taurek and some of his defenders go wrong. See, e.g., Timmermann (2004) and Lübbe (2008).
15. See Steigleder (2014).
16. See Graf Keyserlingk (2018).
17. It is important to note that "we" often do not know how to improve on bad states of affairs. In view of such situations one can only try to find ways of identifying and overcoming such knowledge deficits step by step. Moral rebukes that a bad state of affairs was not overcome are then misplaced. For instance, Smith and Upshur write in connection with the recent Ebola epidemic in West Africa: "Renewed commitments to improve global outbreak response capacities must not come at the expense of abdicating our arguably prior responsibility to prevent these outbreaks and their tendency to decimate the health of vulnerable populations." They then criticize "the failure to build robust health systems, strengthen resiliency" etc. Do Smith and Upshur know how "we" could (have) built up robust health systems in Guinea, Libera and Sierra Leone? Smith and Upshur (2015).
18. Greene (2013), 59.
19. Collier (2013), 235.
20. Van Bavel et al. (2020), 462.
21. Ibid.
22. Petri and Slotnik (2021).
23. Patricia C. Henwood analyses the initial tension between the containment of the Ebola epidemic and the care of the infected as a "tension between isolation for the public good and the highest possible standard of clinical care for the individual patient". From the perspective of rights-based ethics this is misleading, for the isolation and the prevention of further infections also aims at the protection of the rights of individual persons. This is not to deny that there nonetheless exists a cruel tension and that one must try to overcome it as far as possible. See Henwood (2016), 20.
24. "Truth is another casualty of plague. Some of the most damaging and self-injourious responses to an epidemic are denial and lies" writes Christakis (2020), 151. See also Horton (2021), vii–ix and MacKenzie (2020), 1–36.
25. For the ambivalence of closing boarders see, e.g., Horton, *The COVID-19 Catastrophe*, 24f.

26. For a critical exposition of such an attitude see e.g. Graeber (2015).
27. Gewirth (1981), 16.
28. Cf. Kant (1996), 387.
29. See, e.g., Steel (2015) and Hartzell-Nichols (2017).
30. See Hayenhelm and Wolf (2012) and Hansson (2013).
31. For an attempt to develop a rights-based risk ethics see Steigleder (2016) and (2018).
32. Stephen Goldstein (2016), 10f.
33. See e.g. Easterly (2002), Easterly (2006), Moyo (2009), and Acemoglu and Robinson (2012). For an optimistic view see Sachs (2005). For a somewhat intermediate position see Banerjee and Duflo (2011).

References

Acemoglu, Daron, and James A. Robinson. 2012. *Why nations fail: The origins of power, prosperity and poverty*. London: Profile Books.
Banerjee, Abhijit V., and Esther Duflo. 2011. *Poor economics. A radical rethinking of the way to fight global poverty*. New York: Public Affairs.
Battin, Margaret P., Charles B. Smith, Leslie P. Francis, and Jay A. Jacobson. 2008. Toward control of infectious disease: Ethical challenges for a global effort. In *International public health policy and ethics*, ed. Michael Boylan, 191–214. Doetinchem: Springer Science and Business Media.
Battin, Margaret P., Leslie P. Francis, Jay A. Jacobson, and Charles B. Smith. 2009. *The patient as victim and vector: Ethics and infectious disease* (New York: Oxford University Press.
Caney, Simon. 2010. Climate change, human rights and moral thresholds. In *Human rights and climate change*, ed. Stephen Humphreys, 69–90. New York: Cambridge University Press.
Christakis, Nicholas A. 2020. *Apollo's arrow: The profound and enduring impact of Coronavirus on the way we live*. New York: Little, Brown Spark.
Collier, Paul. 2013. *Exodus: Immigration and multiculturalism in the 21st century*. London: Penguin.
Easterly, William. 2002. *The elusive quest for growth: Economists' adventures and misadventures in the tropics*. Cambridge, MA: MIT Press.
Easterly, William. 2006. *The White Man's burden: Why the West's efforts to aid the rest have done so much ill and so little good*. New York: Penguin Press.
Faden, Ruth, Justin Bernstein, and Sirine Shebaya . 2020. Public health ethics. In *Stanford encyclopedia of philosophy*.
Gewirth, Alan. 1978. *Reason and morality*. Chicago: Chicago University Press.
Gewirth, Alan. 1981. Are there any absolute rights? *Philosophical Quarterly* 31 (1): 1–16.
Gewirth, Alan. 1984. The epistemology of human rights. *Social Philosophy & Policy* 1 (2): 1–24.
Gewirth, Alan. 1986. Why rights are indispensable. *Mind* 95 (379): 329–344.
Gewirth, Alan. 1996. *The community of rights*. Chicago: Chicago University Press.
Goldstein, Stephen. 2016. What is Ebola? In *Ebola's message: Public health and medicine in the twenty-first century*, ed. Nicholas G. Evans, Tara C. Smith, and Maimuna S. Majumder, 3–14. Cambridge, MA: MIT Press.
Graeber, David. 2015. *The Utopia of rules: On technology, stupidity, and the secret joys of bureaucracy*. Brooklyn, NY: Melville House Publishing.
Graf Keyserlingk, Johannes. 2018. *Immigration control in a warming world: Realizing the moral challenges of climate migration*. Exeter: Imprint Academic.
Greene, Joshua. 2013. *Moral tribes: Emotion, reason, and the gap between us and them*. London: Penguin.

Hansson, Sven-Ove. 2013. *The ethics of risk: Ethical analysis in an uncertain world*. London: Palgrave Macmillan.

Hartzell-Nichols, Laura. 2017. *A climate of risk: Precuationary principles, catastrophes, and climate change*. New York: Routledge.

Hayenhelm, Madeleine, and Jonathan Wolf. 2012. The moral problem of risk impositions: A survey of the literature. *European Journal of Philosophy* 20 (S1): E26–E51.

Henwood, Patricia C. 2016. Ebola in West Africa: From the frontline. In *Ebola's message: Public health and medicine in the twenty-first century*, ed. Nicholas G. Evans, Tara C. Smith, and Maimuna S. Majumder, 15–29. Cambridge, MA: MIT Press.

Horton, Richard. 2021. *The COVID-19 catastrophe: What's gone wrong and how to stop it happening again*, 2nd ed. Cambridge: Polity Press.

Kant, Immanuel. 1996. *The metaphysics of moral*, in The Cambridge Edition of the Works of Immanuel Kant, *Practical philosophy*, ed. Mary J. Gregor, 365–603. New York: Cambridge University Press.

Lübbe, Weyma. 2008. Taurek's no worse claim. *Philosophy and Public Affairs* 36 (1): 69–85.

MacKenzie, Debora. 2020. *COVID-19: The pandemic that never should have happened and how to stop the next one*. London: The Bridge Street Press.

Morse, Benjamin S., and Lily L. Tsai. 2017. Public health and public trust: Survey evidence from the Ebola virus disease epidemic in Liberia. *Social Science Medicine* 172: 89–97.

Moyo, Dambisa, and Dead Aid. 2009. *Why aid makes things worse and how there is another way for Africa*. London: Penguin Books.

Petri, Alexandra E., and Daniel E. Slotnik. 2021. Attacks on Asian-Americans in New York stoke fear, anxiety and anger. *New York Times*, 26 February.

Sachs, Jeffrey D. 2005. *The end of poverty: Economic possibilities for our time*. New York: Penguin Books.

Shue, Henry. 2020. *Basic rights: Subsistence, affluence, and U.S. Foreign Policy*, 40th Anniversary Edition. Princeton: Princeton University Press.

Smith, Maxwell J., and Ross E.G. Upshur. 2015. Ebola and learning lessons from moral failures: Who cares about ethics? *Public Health Ethics* 8 (3): 305–318.

Steel, Daniel. 2015. *Philosophy and the precautionary principle: Science, evidence, and environmental policy*. Cambridge: Cambridge University Press.

Steigleder, Klaus. 2014. Human dignity and social welfare. In *The Cambridge handbook of human dignity: Interdisciplinary perspectives*, ed. Marcus Düwell, Jens Braarvig, Roger Brownsword, and Dietmar Mieth, 471–476. Cambridge: Cambridge University Press.

Steigleder, Klaus. 2016. Climate risks, climate economics, and the foundations of rights-based risk ethics. *Journal of Human Rights* 15 (2): 251–271.

Steigleder, Klaus. 2018. On the criteria of the rightful imposition of otherwise impermissible risks. *Ethical Perspectives* 25 (3): 471–495.

Taurek, John. 1977. Should the numbers count? *Philosophy and Public Affairs* 6 (4): 293–316.

Taylor, Charles. 1985. Atomism. In *Philosophy and the human sciences: Philosophical papers 2*, ed. Charles Taylor, 187–210. Cambridge: Cambridge University Press.

Timmermann, Jens. 2004. The individualist lottery: How people count, but not their numbers. *Analysis* 64 (2): 106–112.

Van Bavel, Jay J., Katherine Baicker, and Paulo S. Boggio et al. 2020. Using social and behavioural science to support COVID-19 pandemic response. *Nature Human Behavior* 4: 460–471.

Verweij, Marcel, and Angus Dawson. 2007. The meaning of 'public' in 'public health." In *Ethics, prevention, and public health*, ed. Angus Dawson and Marcel Verweij, 13–29. Oxford: Oxford University Press.

Chapter 10
Allocating and Prioritizing Health Care in Times of Scarcity and Abundance

Rita Manning

Abstract The early response to the coronavirus pandemic revealed the United States as a failed state where a cascade of failures to allocate essential goods was the cause of unnecessary deaths. There are a number of questions I address as we assess how best to principally allocate essential health goods in this pandemic. Section I addresses some of the basic concepts in allocation and justice. Section II discusses features of the essential goods that we must allocate fairly. Section III looks at who is responsible for allocating these goods and how these responsibilities are legally authorized. Section IV, the most detailed section, describes the principles of justice that can be used to govern a principled allocation and closes with a look at the Crisis Standards of Care that have become prominent in this current pandemic.

Keywords Goods allocation · Distributive justice · Essential goods · Crisis Standards of Care

SARS-CoV-2 (coronavirus), the cause of COVID-19 (coronavirus disease 2019), emerged in Wuhan, China in December 2019 and subsequently spread around the world. In Europe, Italy was struck with such ferocity that by March ventilators had become such scarce items that doctors were contemplating sending elderly patients home to die.[1] Indeed, a prominent physician group warned that an "age limit for the admission to the ICU may ultimately need to be set."[2] Later an alarming number of deaths in nursing homes in Belgium inspired Médecins Sans Frontières to dispatch a team of experts to treat its nursing home residents.[3] The first patient in the United States was diagnosed in Washington state on February 25th but the CDC later concluded that community transmission in the U.S. had begun in late January or early February.[4] By April, New York City had a surge of COVID-19 cases which it valiantly fought with extra beds, ventilators, testing and contact tracing. By July, as we watched many nations and several states, including New York, recover from COVID-19 by following a well-thought out and disciplined plan, Texas was

R. Manning (✉)
San Jose State University, San Jose, CA, USA
e-mail: manning@ix.netcom.com

© The Author(s), under exclusive license to Springer Nature Switzerland AG 2022
M. Boylan (ed.), *Ethical Public Health Policy Within Pandemics*, The International Library of Bioethics 95, https://doi.org/10.1007/978-3-030-99692-5_9

sending elderly COVID-19 patients home to die because it could not accommodate all COVID-19 patients in its hospitals.[5]

When Italy was running out of ventilators and COVID-19 deaths piled up, it seemed a tragic but natural disaster where moral principles could make the resulting triage almost noble. But when Texas was sending COVID-19 patients home to die because they lacked ventilators, it was clear that the U.S. was a failed state where a cascade of failures to allocate essential goods was the cause of unnecessary deaths.

As I write this, there are more than 28 million coronavirus cases around the world and over 900,000 deaths.[6] In the United States, close to 7 million are infected and over 200,000 have died with more deaths predicted.[7] As the numbers of infections and deaths from COVID-19 continue to rise, we must come to a principled and effective plan to control this pandemic and address the destruction in its wake. One crucial element of this plan is a set of principles to govern allocation of the essential goods that are part of this effort.

While we cannot roll back the clock and begin with a set of principles that would have steered us on a safer and morally defensible path, we must take account of the failures to justly allocate the essential goods that were squandered and hoarded up to this point. This accounting will allow us to manage this pandemic going forward and prepare for the pandemics that are sure to emerge in the future. My purpose in this paper is not to endorse one particular set of principles, but to lay out the most plausible models along with some strengths and weakness. In addition, I hope to show that we need a model for allocations of essential health goods in all times, not just in times of scarcity and emergency.

There are a number of questions we need to ask as we assess how best to principally allocate essential health goods in this pandemic. Section I addresses some of the basic concepts in allocation and justice. Section II discusses features of the essential goods that we must allocate fairly. Section III looks at who is responsible for allocating these goods and how these responsibilities are legally authorized. Section IV, the most detailed section, describes the principles of justice that can be used to govern a principled allocation and closes with a look at the Crisis Standards of Care that have become prominent in this current pandemic.

10.1 Introduction to Justice and Allocation

Before we turn to these questions, there are a number of key concepts to distinguish.[8] I will use "allocation" to refer to distributing essential goods by appeal to a principle of justice. "Rationing" refers to any resource allocation strategy employed when there is scarcity, whether or not the scarce resource is an essential good which should be allocated by appeal to a principle of justice. "Triage" traces its roots to the battlefield where patients were distinguished by the severity of their injuries and the likelihood that they would survive with or without medical care. Today it refers to the process of ranking the severity of injuries in order to prioritize medical care, and is now seldom used to ration this care.[9] "Prioritization" refers to the process of ranking the individuals or groups to whom essential goods will be distributed.

10.1.1 Contexts in Which Allocation Decisions Are Made

10.1.1.1 Micro or Macro

There are important distinctions between types of allocation. The first is the context in which allocation is taking place. Micro-allocation is most commonly at the bedside where physicians have the power to limit care to a particular patient. Macro-allocation decisions can be made nationally, for example the commitment the United States made to make kidney dialysis available for all.[10] The broadest macro-allocation is global and the COVID-19 vaccine is an example of an essential good which will be distributed globally.

10.1.1.2 Private and Mixed Systems or Public Health System

A second distinction is whether allocation decisions are being made in a private and mixed health care system like the United States, or countries with publicly funded health care. In a system like the United States, allocation decisions are not uniform and centralized. In a publicly funded system like the United Kingdom, many decisions are centralized, including decisions about how to fund health care. In a publicly funded health care system, the funding of health care is an example of a macro-allocation.

10.1.1.3 Scarce Entitlements

Another important distinction is between the allocation of a good that is considered an entitlement that should be distributed to all who need it and which can be provided to all, and goods that may ordinarily be considered entitlements but are currently scarce. For goods that are both an entitlement and can be provided to all, a prioritization plan could be developed. An example of this good in a pandemic is a vaccine. Other examples in the United States are health care to stabilize an individual who presents at the emergency department with a medical emergency (EMTALA)[11] and kidney dialysis. Other goods might be considered an entitlement but because of their scarcity they cannot be made available to all who need it. Ventilators are the paradigm good in this category.

10.1.1.4 Conventional and Crisis Care

The last distinction to note is that allocations can occur during ordinary (called "conventional" times in Crisis Standards Care (CSC) models) or during an emergency. During ordinary times, there is both time to decide and a process to procure the needed care. During an emergency, both time and availability are in short supply. An emergency can involve just one patient, or it can involve multitudes. During a mass casualty event, such as a natural disaster, pandemic or terrorism attack, the emergency can be on a very large scale.

10.2 Essential Goods

Allocation decisions do not always require appeals to principles of justice. For many scarce goods, the market is a defensible mechanism for distributing them. The factors that strongly suggest that a justification is needed include (1) a scarcity of essential goods, (2) vulnerable persons who need those goods, (3) others on whom a related burden is imposed, and (4) life and health seriously impacted when those essential goods are not made available.

During the current pandemic, COVID-19 directly impacts life and health when people are infected and it has an indirect impact when lives and health of the entire community are affected by strategies to avoid widespread infection. For example, the CDC categorized eviction as health related when caused by a job loss which was caused by the shutdown imposed during the pandemic.[12]

The essential goods involved in the COVID-19 pandemic include those items needed to diagnose, screen and surveil the pandemic: testing[13] and contact tracing. They are also essential in the treatment of patients: ventilators, ECMO (extracorporeal membrane oxygenation), drugs, hospitalization, staff, equipment (including personal protective equipment (PPE)). Family members who care for infected family members and essential workers of all kinds will also need PPE to limit the spread of the infection. Isolating persons requires other goods such as food and housing.

Many other goods must be provided to combat this pandemic. While schools and workplaces are closed to limit the contagion, the technology for distance learning and child care for children who are distance learning, as well as compensation for lost work, must be provided. Without these goods, people will not be able to follow the restrictions designed to reduce contagion.

The effects on the economy should also be considered, e.g. unemployment payments, and money for schools to reopen. These effects are a consequence of the pandemic since without a shutdown the virus spreads uncontrollably. Hunger is another direct effect of the shutdown and is a public health issue in its own right.[14]

As we think about justifying allocation systems, we should also ask who will need the essential goods that provide care for the illness and protection from the virus in this pandemic. Some categories of persons are particularly vulnerable. Children might not be especially vulnerable to this virus, but they are vulnerable for other reasons:

because as children they lack the autonomy that allows them to choose risk and because they cannot protect themselves. The elderly are vulnerable because they are more likely to die from COVID-19 than younger patients. Nursing home residents are especially vulnerable because they are living in congregate settings and have been the primary victims of the disease. Incarcerated persons are vulnerable because they too are forced to live in crowded congregate settings and have been disproportionately infected by and died of the disease.[15] People of color, especially Latino/as and African Americans, have been infected and dying in widely disproportionate numbers during this pandemic. When we look at the question from a global perspective, we should note the ways that poorer countries are especially challenged by COVID-19. One of the most compelling current questions is how to fairly distribute vaccines globally.

Finally, we should ask who, in addition to those who are especially vulnerable, is especially burdened by this disease. Health care workers (HCW) are burdened with fighting this disease. Other essential workers are also especially burdened as they face a larger risk than those who can isolate and socially distance and they provide the resources that allow the rest of the population to isolate and socially distance.

10.3 Who is Responsible for Allocating Essential Goods

The responsibility for allocating essential goods has been debated in the U.S. since the virus arrived on our shores. States have taken much of the responsibility, federal health care agencies like the CDC and the NIH have tried to play an active role, and all the while President Trump largely ignored the crisis.[16] Local governments have taken charge while healthcare organizations have planned for and managed surges. In the meantime, a scarcity of crucial medical items has hampered the treatment of patients and the control of the disease.

One of the failures of controlling the virus in the U.S. was to put much of the burden on hospitals, as the hospitals did what hospitals do: "Get hospitals ready and wait for sick people to show," as Sheila Davis, the CEO of the nonprofit Partners in Health, puts it. "Especially in the beginning, we catered our entire [COVID-19] response to the 20 percent of people who required hospitalization, rather than preventing transmission in the community."[17]

10.3.1 Legal Authority and Responsibility

One of the fundamental purposes of any legitimate government is to promote the general welfare. The United States has a federal system of government with two levels of government, state and federal, which both have a certain amount of autonomy to make and enforce the laws that promote this general welfare. Both the states and the federal government have a significant amount of power to respond to public health emergencies.

The 10th Amendment of the Constitution grants state governments all powers not specifically given to the federal government, including the primary authority to control the spread of dangerous diseases within their jurisdictions. Individual states legislate different ways to exercise this power. Two Supreme Court cases illustrate the extent of this state power. In *Gibbons v. Ogden*, 22 U.S. 1 (1824) Chief Justice John Marshall cited the 10th Amendment in saying that police powers, including the ability to impose isolation and quarantine, are largely reserved to states for activities within their borders. The second case is *Compagnie Francaise &c. v. Board of Health*, 186 U.S. 380 (1902) which upheld Louisiana's ability to enact and enforce quarantine laws unless Congress had decided to preempt them. This is still good law and numerous courts have cited it as authority for state quarantines as recently as the Ebola outbreak.

States can allocate essential goods across state lines during large scale emergencies using the Emergency Management Assistance Compact (EMAC). This compact was created by Congress in 1996 (Public Law 104-321) to authorize 50 states, the District of Columbia, Puerto Rico, Guam, U.S. Virgin Islands and the Northern Mariana Islands to become EMAC members who can assist each other during an emergency and send personnel, equipment, and commodities to assist with response and recovery efforts in other states.

On the federal level there are a number of laws which impose considerable responsibilities on the president and federal agencies and also authorize significant power during emergencies.[18] Some of the most significant laws include: the Defense Production Act of 1950, reauthorized in 2009 (50 U.S.C. App. 2166) which was originally designed to incentivize the production of wartime needs but has been expanded to include natural or man-caused disasters, and acts of terrorism in the U.S. It allows the president to direct private companies to prioritize orders for needed supplies, to allocate materials, services, and facilities, and to restrict hoarding. The president may incentivize companies who provide these supplies through loans or loan guarantees, make purchases, and allow these companies to coordinate with each other, which might otherwise be in violation of antitrust laws. The Homeland Security Act of 2002 (6 U.S.C. §§ 311–321m) allows the DHS to coordinate during natural and manmade crises emergency planning. The Robert T. Stafford Disaster Relief and Emergency Assistance Act of 1988 (42 U.S.C. §§ 5121–5207) authorizes the President to declare a "major disaster" or "emergency" and trigger access to federal assistance to state and local governments and directs FEMA to coordinate this disaster relief. The Sandy Recovery Improvement Act of 2013 (42 U.S.C. §§ 5170, 5191) empowers the chief executive of a tribal government to directly request a disaster or emergency declaration from the President, as a state governor can do. Section 319 of the Public Health Service Act: Public Health Emergencies (42 U.S.C. § 247d) authorizes HHS to determine that a public health emergency exists and "take such action as may be appropriate" and use funds from the Public Health Emergency Fund. Section 311 of the Public Health Service Act: General Grant of Authority for Cooperation (42 U.S.C. § 243) states that the Secretary of Health and Human Services (HHS) shall assist states and local authorities in the prevention and suppression of communicable diseases and to help state and local authorities enforce quarantine regulations.

Section 319F-2 of the Public Health Service Act: Strategic National Stockpile and Security (42 U.S.C. § 247d-6b; 42 U.S.C. § 300hh-10(c)(3)(b)) authorizes HHS, in collaboration with CDC, to maintain a stockpile (including drugs, vaccines, biological products, medical devices, and other supplies) and deploy this stockpile in a public health emergency. The Public Health Security and Bioterrorism Preparedness and Response Act of 2002 (Pub. L. No. 107-188) requires HHS to "develop and implement" a national preparedness plan to protect the country against bioterrorism and other public health emergencies. Section 1135 of the Social Security Act: Authority to Waive Requirements During National Emergencies (42 U.S.C. § 1320b-5 Section 1135) authorizes the Secretary of HHS to waive or modify certain requirements of Medicare, Medicaid, and the State Children's Health Insurance Program during certain emergencies. The Public Readiness and Emergency Preparedness Act of 2005 (42 U.S.C. §§ 247d-6d, 247d-6e) authorizes HHS to issue a declaration that provides immunity from tort liability for claims of loss (except willful misconduct) sustained during countermeasures to a public health emergency. It also authorizes a fund in the U.S. Treasury to provide compensation for injuries directly caused by these countermeasures. Section 564 of the Federal Food, Drug, and Cosmetic Act 7 21 U.S.C. § 360bbb-3 if 1) authorizes HHS, upon determining that there is a public health emergency, to declare an Emergency Use Authorization (EUA) for an unapproved drug, device, or biological product, or for an unapproved use of an approved drug, device, or biological product.

During this pandemic, states have had an uneven record in responding,[19] but by and large they have provided the bulk of the work involved in allocating essential goods during the coronavirus pandemic. We have seen the federal government exercise some of its powers; for example, it allocated $50 billion in general distributions to Medicare facilities and providers impacted by COVID-19 out of the $100 billion appropriate by Congress in the CARES Act.[20] But many of the failures to respond adequately to the coronavirus pandemic include not exercising federal powers to an appropriate extent. For example, Trump's delay to use the Defense Production Act led to a serious shortage of PPE for health care workers.[21] Jared Kushner notoriously claimed that states should use their own stockpiles first: "And the notion of the federal stockpile was it's supposed to be our stockpile. It's not supposed to be states' stockpiles that they then use."[22]

We have seen that both the states and the federal government have considerable responsibility along with the legal authority to allocate essential goods during this pandemic. At the global level, sixty-four higher-income countries have taken on a corresponding responsibility by signing on to COVAX, an international agreement sponsored by WHO.[23] Thirty-eight more are expected to join with the notable exception of Russia, China and the United States.

10.4 Justice and Allocation

10.4.1 Bioethics

Most theorists and policy makers argue that allocation decisions are rooted in larger moral systems and hence justifications for these decisions depend in large part on moral principles. Other theorists argue that rather than look to principles of justice to ground ethical allocation decisions, we should focus on procedures for democratically deciding what allocations are fair.[24] Here, I shall assume that fair procedures are essential, but these procedures must be embedded in a larger moral system. I begin then with a sketch of the three types of moral systems that are predominant in bioethics: consequence based (Utilitarianism); virtue ethics based, and principle based.

10.4.1.1 Utilitarianism

Utilitarianism builds on the simple intuition that doing the right thing involves thinking about all the possible consequences of our actions and picking the alternative that maximizes social utility, the overall balance of negative and positive utility, over the long term, for all concerned. Over the years, utilitarians have offered different definitions of utility. Jeremy Bentham,[25] the first systematic utilitarian, defined it as pleasure and the absence of pain. John Stuart Mill[26] advocated happiness as a measure of utility. Happiness involves feeling pleasure (and pain) but more importantly it involves making judgments about our pleasures in the context of our life plan. Well-being is another measure and the advantage of using this measure is that we can come up with more or less objective standards to measure well-being.

10.4.1.2 Virtue Based Models

Virtue based models focus on the character of the individuals and organizations that are engaged in health care. Many professional codes of ethics illustrate central virtues. The American Medical Association Code of Ethics cites respect for persons, competence, compassion and responsibility as core virtues for physicians. Edward Pellegrino expands this list to include fidelity, benevolence, effacement of self-interest, compassion and caring, intellectual honesty, justice, and prudence as core virtues for physicians.[27] The American Nursing Association code of ethics includes compassion, respect, accountability and responsibility as core virtues. [28] Care ethics can be viewed as a type of virtue ethic that focuses on moral attentiveness, sympathetic understanding, relationship awareness, accommodation and harmony.[29] A caring person and organization would be aware of the failures of empathy and focus on minimizing these failures.

10.4.1.3 Principle-Based Models

Principle-based models prioritize respect for persons and human rights. Hence, they assume that justification involves more than an accounting of the consequences that various decisions can create. Rather they depend on basic moral principles. For Kantians, the fundamental principle is treat persons as ends in themselves and never merely as means. In bioethics, autonomy is a primary value as it respects the right of persons to make their own health choices.

Another source of principles in bioethics is Rawls' difference principle, "Social and economic inequalities are to be arranged so that (a) they are to be of the greatest benefit to the least-advantaged members of society."[30] Here, the worse off should not be made any worse off by any distribution of primary goods and a distributive system must be acceptable to any rational person who would be aware that under this system she may find herself to be the least well off.

Libertarians, who prioritize choice, view the market as a defensible mechanism for distributing at least some health care: "My view of this approach is Churchillian: a socially guaranteed basic health care minimum topped up by private philanthropy and genuine markets is the worst health care delivery system except for all others that have been tried from time to time."[31] Other defenders of libertarianism argue that a basic minimum of care can be equitable and just on libertarian grounds.[32] While making health care available through the market is widespread in the U.S., no defenders of models of allocation during a pandemic endorse this during a pandemic.[33] A prominent failure of the market model during this pandemic is that it often failed to supply enough essential goods. For example, N-95 respirator masks, a life-saving essential tool for health care workers, are still scarce in the U.S. because Trump did not use the Defense Production Act to compel companies to produce enough of these masks.[34]

10.4.1.4 Combined Models

One of the historic sources of principles in bioethics in the U.S. is the Belmont Report of the U.S. National Commission for the Protection of Human Subjects of Biomedical and Behavioral Research (National Commission 1978). This Report lays out a "set of basic moral principles that would justify corresponding practical guidelines in U.S. federal regulations. The purpose of the Belmont Report was to ensure that basic principles would become embedded in the United States research oversight system so that meaningful protection was afforded to all research participants."[35] The Belmont principles are a combination of principle-based systems and utilitarianism and include the principles of respect of persons, beneficence and justice.

Principle-based and utilitarian models are also combined in a widely adopted model that is called Principlism.[36] The principles are not ranked in terms of priority and are grouped under four general categories: (1) respect for autonomy, (liberty (the absence of controlling influences) and agency (self-initiated intentional action)); (2) nonmaleficence (do no harm); (3) beneficence (act for another's benefit); and

(4) justice (modeled on egalitarian social justice). Respect for autonomy reflects the influence of principle-based models. Nonmaleficence and beneficence address utilitarian concerns. Areas of justice in bioethics include: rules for allocating health care, and protection and aid for vulnerable and disadvantaged parties in health care systems locally or globally.

10.4.1.5 The Universal Declaration on Bioethics and Human Rights (UDBHR)

Substantive global agreement on ethics in health care is reflected in the Universal Declaration on Bioethics and Human Rights (UDBHR). This declaration was adopted by acclamation at the UNESCO General Conference on October 19th 2005.[37] This acclamation can be seen as clear evidence "that all 191 member states endorsed the Declaration despite different religious and socio-cultural backgrounds, [and] that UNESCO had managed to find some common grounds between nations, in order to set minimum standards for bioethics that are universally acceptable."[38]

The UDBHR adopted most of the principles that are central to Bioethics: human dignity and human rights (Article 3) (including rights to privacy and confidentiality, Article 9)); autonomy (Article 5), with its focus on informed consent (Article 6); equality and justice which prominently features nondiscrimination as a principle (Articles 10 and 11). Respect for cultural diversity and pluralism are listed as values, but human rights trump the interests of cultural diversity and pluralism: "…such considerations are not to be invoked to infringe upon human dignity, human rights and fundamental freedoms, nor upon the principles set out in this Declaration, nor to limit their scope" (Article 12). Utilitarianism is referenced in the values of benefit and harm (Article 4). Articles 16 and 17 express a commitment to including future generations and the environment in calculating benefits and harms. Justice is included explicitly in Article 10 (where justice is directly invoked) and 15 (where the obligation to share benefits is cited). The virtue of social responsibility is noted in article 14.

10.4.2 Bioethics and Allocation

Recall that allocation decisions take place in various contexts: where allocation is micro or macro, in private and mixed or public health systems, when goods are deemed to be entitlements and either scarce or available to all. Principles of justice apply to allocation decisions differently depending on the context.

Micro-allocation can be at the bedside where physicians have the power to limit care to a particular patient. The treating physician is responsible for allocation decisions and has a moral obligation to make decisions in the best interest of the patient and with the informed consent of the patient. The values stressed in the bedside setting are respect for persons (autonomy, informed consent) and beneficence where benefit is understood as furthering the best interest of the patient. In the context of a pandemic, many physicians argue that the attending physician should not make allocation decisions for her patient because this violates the obligation of the treating physician.[39] This policy is reflected in many allocation systems which put triage teams, and not treating physicians, in control of allocation decisions. Others argue that rather than limiting their focus to their patients, physicians should refocus their concern on the public which is endangered in the pandemic. This view has been soundly rejected by many theorists.[40]

The global distribution of the COVID-19 vaccine is an example of macro allocation and there are two models that are currently being debated: the WHO model[41] and the Fair Priorities Model.[42] The WHO model includes the following principles: human well-being, equal respect, global equity, national equity, reciprocity and legitimacy.[43] Legitimacy is a procedural principle. Global and national equity appeal to the Rawlsian difference principle. Human well-being is a utilitarian principle and equal respect is principle-based. Reciprocity is partly utilitarian and partly virtue based, where gratitude is cited as the virtue that would support reciprocity. Under this model, the vaccine is first distributed to countries for the first 3% of its population. Under later phases, the principles above apply. The Fair Priorities Model appeals to three fundamental values: benefiting people and limiting harm, prioritizing the disadvantaged, and equal moral concern. [44] Again we see utilitarian, Rawlsian and principle based models combined here. While the WHO and Fair Priorities Model share a commitment to widely held values, they differ in the details of prioritizing countries to receive the vaccine. The WHO model distributes the vaccine in the first phase to countries based on their total populations, whether or not the countries are rich or poor. The Fair Priorities Model considers relative wealth in the first phase.

In a private and mixed health care system like the United States, allocation decisions are not uniform and centralized. Given that over 30 million Americans do not have health insurance, many people never present themselves to a physician or health care organization that allocates the health care goods needed. Due in part to the complexity of this system, no one principle of justice governs allocation decisions. Allocation decisions are only made on the federal level for the health care funded by the federal government such as Medicare, the Veterans Administration, Medicaid, and services that are dictated by law, such as the Affordable Care Act,[45] the Emergency Medical Treatment and Labor Act (EMTALA)[46] and kidney dialysis.[47] The bulk of the rest of the decisions are made by insurance companies and patients who self-insure.

The UK is an example of a publicly funded health care system that makes resource decisions on a macro-level.[48] Health coverage in England has been universal since the creation of the National Health Service (NHS) in 1948. The NHS is allocated an overall budget by the UK which makes a political decision about how much tax revenue should be allocated to health care. The NHS then sets national budgets across various funding streams. Some of it goes to core allocations and the rest goes to Clinical Commissioning Groups (CCG) who are groups of general practitioners and nurses who prioritize the spending of their local community health organization. Many of their decisions will be made on the micro level where they are expected to apply principlism (which they call "the four principles") in making decisions:

Respect for autonomy: respecting the decision-making capacities of autonomous persons; enabling individuals to make reasoned informed choices.

Beneficence: this considers the balancing of benefits of treatment against the risks and costs; the healthcare professional should act in a way that benefits the patient

Non maleficence: avoiding the causation of harm; the healthcare professional should not harm the patient. All treatment involves some harm, even if minimal, but the harm should not be disproportionate to the benefits of treatment.

Justice: distributing benefits, risks and costs fairly; the notion that patients in similar positions should be treated in a similar manner.[49]

The next distinction is whether goods are entitlements that can be provided to all, or a scarce entitlement. A prioritization plan can be developed for goods that are entitlements that can be made available for all who need them. An example of this good in a pandemic is a vaccine and in response to a request from the NIH and CDC, the National Academies produced a plan for equitable allocation of vaccines against COVID-19.[50]

Other goods might be considered entitlements but, because of their scarcity, are not available to all who need it. Ventilators are the paradigm good in this category. These items are often allocated using Crisis Standards Care (CSC)).

The last distinction to note is that allocations can occur during ordinary times or during an emergency. Many federal agencies, states and professional health care organizations chose to adopt a unique standard of care during the COVID-19 pandemic, Crisis Standards Care.

We have already seen various bioethics models two of which, principlism and UDBHR, include both utilitarian and principle-based models. We now turn to the application of utilitarianism and principle-based models to allocation during emergencies.

10.4.2.1 Utilitarianism and Allocation

Some health economists measure well-being as in terms of the capacity to benefit per resource unit expended. They argue that scarce health care resources ought to be allocated so as to: maximize aggregate health; equally exhaust each person's capacity to benefit (CTB); most closely equalize final health states; and equally restore health states to population norms.[51]

Some bioethicists have used survival as the measure of utility.[52] Survival is often defined as surviving to hospital discharge, but it could also be defined as longer term survival. There are two ways of measuring survival: years of life saved or total number of lives saved.[53] Another more precise way of measuring utility in terms of life is Quality Adjusted Life Years (QALY).[54] Rationing by QALYs involves first selecting outcome measures that adjust life-years for quality, and then allocating so as to maximize QALYs.[55]

The relative sickness of patients is a relevant criterion for triage, whether or not utilitarianism is the model being applied, because care for patients who are either likely to survive without medical care or not likely to survive in any case would be seen as a waste of resources in times of scarcity. A utilitarian model would not stop at an either/or assessment on survival. Patients can be prioritized on the likelihood of their survival which allows the most efficient use of resources. One way to measure the likelihood of a patient's surviving is minimum qualifications for survival (MQS), which, in most systems, utilizes the Sequential Organ Failure Assessment (SOFA) score. For children, the scoring system most commonly used is the Pediatric Logistic Organ Dysfunction (PELOD).

10.4.2.2 Principle-Based Models and Allocation

Recall that a Kantian principle-based model prioritizes respect for persons and human rights. The Kantian principle applied to allocation decisions is to treat people equally. There are various interpretations of what it is to treat persons equally. Since everyone has an equal right to a scarce essential good, one way to allocate is by using a lottery principle. First-come, first-served is a version of a lottery principle but it is generally not accepted as a just principle in an emergency because it does not in fact treat people equally. People who have better access to transportation, for example, will arrive at the hospital first. The Life Cycle Principle (also called the "fair innings" principle) is another version of a lottery principle. The idea here is to give each individual an equal opportunity to live through the various phases of life.[56] Young patients are prioritized under this model because they have not had the same opportunity to live through as many phases of life as older patients.

Rawls' difference principle would allocate essential goods by giving priority to the worst off. Treating the sickest first is an obvious way to apply this principle during a pandemic. Another option is to view the youngest as the worst off because if they die from this illness, they would not have experienced the same years of life as an older patient.

All of these models have their problems and they are often inconsistent with each other. For these reasons, most models involve a combination of these kinds of principles. Currently, most models designed for use during a public health emergency are combination models which share a common thread: they include a prominent place for utilitarian principles. These models are called Crisis Standards of Care.

10.4.3 Crisis Standards of Care

By 2008, Koenig and Backer coined the term "crisis standard of care" to define "a substantial change in usual healthcare operations and the level of care it is possible to deliver, which is made necessary by a pervasive (e.g., pandemic influenza) or catastrophic (e.g., earthquake, hurricane) disaster."[57] Inspired by H1N1, the Institute of Medicine (IOM) developed a CSC model in 2009[58] and expanded and amended it in

2012[59] and 2013.[60] During the current COVID-19 pandemic, many health care institutions, professional societies, states and other governmental bodies, and theorists rushed to dust off their CSC models and put them into play.

10.4.3.1 The IOM Procedural Model

The CSC model assumes that in ordinary times, whether at the micro or macro level, conventional management systems focus on individual patients and during emergencies the standards of care shift to a focus on public health. This move involves a turn away from rights based moral principles to one based on utilitarianism.

There are many CSCs but I begin with the Institute of Medicine (IOM) model for developing a CSC plan. The IOM does not provide substantive allocation principles but rather assumes that states and healthcare organizations will develop their own substantive principles based on their own values and deliberations. They do however make one crucial assumption: "substantial change in the usual health care operations and the level of care it is possible to deliver... [are necessary because] public health disasters justify temporarily adjusting practice standards and/or shifting the balance of ethical concerns to emphasize the needs of the community rather than the needs of individuals."[61]

The CSC model includes two key procedural considerations: fairness of its standards and equitable processes to ensure that decisions and implementation of standards are made equitably. Fair standards are standards that are widely recognized as: fair; evidence based; responsive to specific needs; and focused on duties of compassion and care to steward resources, along with a goal of maintaining trust.[62] An equitable process requires transparency in the design and operation of the standards; consistency in application regardless of an individual's and group's race, age, disability, ethnicity, ability to pay, socioeconomic status, preexisting health conditions, social worth, perceived obstacles to treatment, past use of resources, proportionality of the scale of the emergency and degree of scarce resources, accountability of those who decide and implement the standards, and the governments who ensure appropriate protections and allocation of available resources.[63]

CSC comes into play when a catastrophic disaster occurs and persists well after the beginning of the disaster. This type of emergency is deemed to exist when: "[1] most or all of the community's infrastructure is impacted…; [2] local officials are unable to perform their usual roles for a period of time extending well beyond the initial aftermath of the incident; [3] most or all routine community functions—at places of work, recreation, worship, and education—are immediately and simultaneously interrupted; and [4] surrounding communities are similarly affected, and thus there are no regional resources to come to the aid of the affected local communities."[64] CSC is triggered when there is a critical infrastructure disruption, resource-sparing strategies (of staffing availability and material resources) are overwhelmed; and patient care space is severely challenged.

To understand how CSC works, IOM distinguished patient care as existing along a continuum.[65] At one end of this continuum health care organizations provide conventional care, patient services that are routine. The next spot on the continuum is contingency care which looks like routine care but allows some flexibility in the provision of routine care. During both conventional and contingency care, the individual is the focus of the health care organization. During crisis care, very limited resources are available and the shift is away from individual patient-centered care to population-centered outcomes. Here, decisions are not made primarily for the best interest of a particular patient, but out of a concern for the larger population, e.g. other patients whose needs may not be met if the particular patient's needs are met.

10.4.3.2 The CDC Model

The CDC accepts principlism as its basic ethical model, and lists a number of specific ethical considerations concerning the allocation of ventilators during a pandemic.[66] While they do not endorse a more definitive list of principles, they describe a variety of principles and ultimately endorse a multi-principle allocation approach that would require broad public deliberation about how to prioritize the various principles.

The specific ethical considerations include maximizing net benefits defined as maximizing the number of people who survive to hospital discharge. This fundamentally utilitarian principle has the advantage of satisfying non-utilitarians because each life has an equal claim to being saved and because no one life would be discriminated against on the basis of factors such as race and socioeconomic status. Maximizing years of life saved counts the overall years of life saved rather than the number of persons whose lives are saved. Another option is maximizing adjusted years of life saved. The adjustment is usually made on the basis of quality-adjusted life years (QALYs), or disability-adjusted life years (DALYs). The CDC worries about these options because they require considerable clinical information, likely would not be feasible in a public health emergency, and depend on arbitrary judgments regarding quality of life.

Social Worth is the second ethical consideration they address. They note that there has been a widespread rejection of social worth as a criterion for allocation of essential health goods because it assumes that one individual is intrinsically more worthy than another. They do, however, consider a related criterion, instrumental value (also referred to as "narrow social utility" and "multiplier effect") which refers to an individual's ability to play an essential role during a public health crisis. This has the virtue of incentivizing health care workers, and other essential workers, to be available during the public health crisis.

The next principle is the Life Cycle Principle (also referred to as "fair innings" and "intergenerational equity"). This principle grants individuals an equal opportunity to live through the various phases of life, childhood, young adulthood, middle age, and old age. In practice, it gives priority to younger patients over older patients. We shall see that a prominent criticism is that this principle discriminates against the elderly.

The final principle is the Fair Chances Principle. This principle is in response to a criticism of any version of maximizing net benefits. If essential goods are provided only to those with the highest priority under any maximizing net benefits schema, those who are not considered are deprived of a chance of survival.

10.4.3.3 The Core Guidance Checklist

The Core Guidance Checklist is a substantive CSC model developed by the Rand Corporation. This checklist was developed by consensus discussions with bioethicists, health care professionals, patient advocates and community members to support allocation decision-making during the COVID-19 crisis.[67] Among its "Clear and Consistent Criteria and Goals" are the following moral principles: respect for autonomy, nonmaleficence, beneficence, and justice in accord with general biomedical ethical practice; responsible resource stewardship; achieving the most good at a population level, rather than the usual standard of addressing individual patient-level wellbeing; avoidance of bias in allocation decisions based on nonclinical patient characteristics, such as race/ethnicity, gender, age, presence or absence of disabilities and presumed health-related quality of life before or after resource allocation.[68] Notice that while this model incorporates principlism, utilitarianism is given a special place in this model in the express instruction to address achieving the most good at the population level rather than achieving individual patient-level wellbeing. It also follows the UDBHR in specifically including nondiscrimination as a principle.

10.4.3.4 The Emanuel et al Model

This is a combined model which includes the following principles: maximize the benefits produced by scarce resources by saving the most individual lives or the most life-years defined in terms of likelihood to survive longest after treatment; treat people equally by randomly selecting patients; promote and reward instrumental value by prioritizing those who can save others, or have saved others in the past; give priority to the worst off defined as the sickest or the youngest.[69]

10.4.3.5 State Models

As I write this, twenty-six states have publicly available ventilator guidelines. There is significant variation in guidelines regarding exclusion criteria and the use of controversial factors, such as age and disability defined in terms of limited life expectancy and chronic conditions, to rank patients.[70]

Some states have not been as attentive about discrimination in their health allocation policies as they could be. Disability rights advocacy groups and persons with disabilities have filed complaints with the HHS Office of Civil Rights (OCR) against Alabama, Kansas, New York, Pennsylvania, Tennessee, Utah, and Washington alleging that the allocation guidelines followed by these states discriminated against persons with disabilities.[71] Other groups have alleged discrimination against people with disabilities, older adults, and people of color.[72]

Texas as a state does not have a CSC policy, but North Texas does. This policy excludes patients from care during a public health emergency and when essential health goods are scarce. They offer the following "Basic premises":

- The overall goal is to save as many lives as possible.
- Non-discrimination: Each patient will receive respect, care, and compassion without regard to basis of race, ethnicity, color, national origin, religion, sex, disability, veteran status, age, genetic information, sexual orientation, gender identity, exercise of conscience or any other protected characteristic under applicable law. Medical treatment, including scarce resources will not be allocated based on the patient's ability to pay. However, this does not mean that all patients should or will receive critical care services in the time of resource scarcity.
- These Guidelines should not be viewed as a first step toward any type of resource rationing under normal circumstances. It should be used only in genuinely extraordinary situations in which the demand for intensive care services overwhelms the available services, such as in pandemic respiratory crisis.
- Graded guidelines should be used to control resources more tightly as the severity of a pandemic increases.
- Priority should be given to patients for whom treatment most likely would be lifesaving and who have the best chance of returning to their prior functional status whatever that may be with treatment. Such patients should be given priority over those who would likely die even with treatment and those who would likely survive without treatment.
- Physician judgment should be used in applying these Guidelines including: 1) with individualized assessments of each patient based on best available, relevant, and objective medical evidence; and 2) modification of this Guidelines and tools based on the individual patient, when necessary.[73]

Note that while discrimination against persons with disabilities is expressly prohibited, the sole criterion for allocation of scarce care is survival: "the lowest priority for admission is given to patients with the lowest chance of survival with or without treatment, and to patients with the highest chance of survival without treatment. Physician judgment should be used in applying these guidelines, with individualized assessments of patients based on best available, relevant, and objective medical evidence." We shall see that this is cited as evidence of discrimination.

10.4.4 Critiques of CSC

10.4.4.1 We Don't Need CSCs. Basic Bioethics is Enough

To begin, it is not exactly clear why we need CSCs. Defenders of CSCs simply assume that scarcity requires that we shift the standard of care to emphasizing the needs of the community, while providing a lower standard of care for individuals. But why should we assume that the needs of the community become central when large numbers of individuals present themselves during a pandemic or other catastrophe? We could simply conceptualize this situation as one in which our focus should expand to include more individuals, e.g. future patients that we should expect to see. On the other hand, the impetus for CSCs might simply be to protect HCW from legal liability so that they will treat patients they would otherwise not be inclined to treat because of a concern about liability. But this move does not affect liability because the legal standard does not change when we move to crisis mode; liability is incurred when the physician fails to do what a reasonably responsible physician would do in a similar situation.[74] What changes is the situation that the reasonably responsible physician is facing in a crisis.

I should note in passing that it is ironic that CSC describes a transition from conventional management care to crisis management care during catastrophic disasters because, in practice, the U.S. essentially has no uniform conventional management care. The Affordable Care Act provides care in a patchwork of coverage provided by employers, plans bought and sold in the health insurance marketplace, and Medicaid. Medicaid coverage is provided through states but to date only 39 states (including DC) have adopted the Medicaid expansion.[75] During the pandemic, millions of Americans are without health insurance. Many Americans do not have a private physician and get the bulk of their care, when they get any care at all, in hospital emergency departments. Thus, conventional management care, outside the hospital doors, is that some have insurance that will cover part of their care, some can buy whatever care they need, and some have no insurance at all. For those without health insurance, EMTALA only requires hospitals to provide care to stabilize critically ill patients, and only if these patients presented to the emergency department, assuming that the hospital has an emergency department.

Changing the standards in CSC plans is doubly concerning when we note that it effectively lowers the standards by assuming that utilitarianism takes precedence in a pandemic. Combined bioethics models include utilitarianism and its appeals to consequences, but they do not assume that utilitarianism trumps all the other principles.[76]

10.4.4.2 Discrimination

Disability Rights Texas (DRTx) submitted a complaint against the North Central Texas Trauma Regional Advisory Council alleging that their guidelines deprive some persons of non-discriminatory access to health care and

> jeopardize the lives of adults and children with disabilities, older adults, individuals from communities of color, prisoners, and others with co-morbid conditions during the COVID-19 pandemic in violation of the Americans with Disabilities Act ("ADA"), Section 504 of the Rehabilitation Act, Section 1557 of the Patient Protection and Affordable Care Act ("ACA"), and the Age Discrimination Act of 1975 ("Age Act"). COVID-19 pandemic in violation of Title II of the Americans with Disabilities Act ("ADA"), Section 504 of the Rehabilitation Act, Section 1557 of the Patient Protection and Affordable Care Act ("ACA"), and the Age Discrimination Act of 1975 ("Age Act").[77]

The complaint offers detailed argument in favor of each claim, but here I will focus on just two: the claim that the guideline discriminates against persons with disabilities, and the claim that the guidelines discriminate against persons of color.

The claim of discrimination against persons with disabilities points to three discriminatory impacts of the exclusion criteria.

> First, many, if not all, of the criteria explicitly target certain disabling, pre-existing, or co-morbid conditions that are facially discriminatory and violate federal law. For instance, persons with certain neuromuscular conditions, like ALS, are wholly excluded from access to life-saving care. Second, the scoring system for determining the severity of a disabling, pre-existing, or co-morbid condition is itself discriminatory, by negatively weighting (and thus de-prioritizing) certain conditions and their impacts on long-term functioning, Finally, none of the exclusionary criteria allow for accommodations for persons with disabilities and many, if not most, of the scoring systems are based on "survivability" that is unrelated to COVID-19.[78]

The argument that persons of color are discriminated against refers to the following guideline: "Priority should be given to patients for whom treatment most likely would be lifesaving and who have the best chance of returning to their prior functional status whatever that may be with treatment. Such patients should be given priority over those who would likely die even with treatment and those who would likely survive without treatment."[79] Disability Texas notes that a higher chance of being saved and returned to a prior functional status is affected by past discrimination in the delivery of health care:

> communities of color have also experienced discrimination and marginalization in the delivery of health care, issues that continue in various forms today. People of color are more likely to experience co-morbid medical conditions like asthma, diabetes, hypertension, and heart conditions as a result of structural racism, environmental factors, occupational safety and health, and lack of access to health care. These health conditions can directly or indirectly factor into the various scoring systems underpinning the Guidelines and result in their exclusion from care altogether or de-prioritization for hospitalization and receipt of intensive care under the Guidelines.[80]

10.4.4.3 CSCs Are not Appropriate When Scarcity is Avoidable

There is a third reason why we need to be skeptical about the move to crisis management. CSC is not relevant when scarcity is avoidable. Before we assume that we should adopt CSC principles, we need to ask if the current crisis is entirely beyond our control or whether it is caused by human decisions. If the crisis is caused by human action or inaction, the scarcity is avoidable. If it is avoidable, CSC does not apply.

In the U.S., a cascade of failures shows that the scarcity of many essential goods was and is avoidable. First, there was a failure on Trump's part to recognize that the federal government has an obligation to fairly allocate the goods that are essential to life and health. In fact, when asked whether he takes responsibility for the lag in making test kits available, Trump's reply was "I don't take responsibility at all."[81] When governors were begging for federal help to acquire medical supplies, Trump replied "The Federal government is not supposed to be out there buying vast amounts of items and then shipping. You know, we're not a shipping clerk."[82] In fact, the president had the responsibility and a unique power to acquire and distribute the medical supplies needed by the states in the Defense Production Act.[83]

Scarcity of testing was one of the central failures. The public health community was well aware of the importance of testing: "Without systematic testing, 'We might as well put duct tape over our eyes, cotton in our ears, and hide under the bed,' said Dr. Margaret Bourdeaux, research director for the Harvard Medical School Program in Global Public Policy."[84] In spite of the obvious need for testing, the Trump administration failed to provide adequate testing and, even worse, hampered public health agencies' efforts to encourage testing. For example, CDC's website was edited by the HHS to include an instruction that non-symptomatic persons exposed to the virus did not need to be tested.[85] Fortunately, an outraged scientific community provided enough counter political pressure to rescind this terrible advice.

Transparency and full information are central public health values that were flaunted during the U.S.'s initial response to this pandemic. The CDC was pressured by the Trump administration not to release a report about the spread of the virus in a Georgia summer camp.[86] Trump's refusal to advocate masks and social distancing in spite of knowing full well that these protections were essential was another major failure. But Trump certainly shared the blame:

> almost everything that went wrong with America's response to the pandemic was predictable and preventable. A sluggish response by a government denuded of expertise allowed the coronavirus to gain a foothold. Chronic underfunding of public health neutered the nation's ability to prevent the pathogen's spread. A bloated, inefficient health-care system left hospitals ill-prepared for the ensuing wave of sickness. Racist policies that have endured since the days of colonization and slavery left Indigenous and Black Americans especially vulnerable to COVID-19. The decades-long process of shredding the nation's social safety net forced millions of essential workers in low-paying jobs to risk their life for their livelihood. The same social-media platforms that sowed partisanship and misinformation during the 2014 Ebola outbreak in Africa and the 2016 U.S. election became vectors for conspiracy theories during the 2020 pandemic.[87]

One way to highlight the U.S.'s early failure to respond adequately to the pandemic is to compare the U.S. with other countries. As I write this, 1,988 persons per 100,000 have been infected in the U.S.[88] Only nine countries have a higher infection rate: Qatar, Bahrain, Aruba, Panama, Chile, Kuwait, Peru and Brazil. Our immediate neighbors fare considerably better than the U.S.: Canada 367 infected per 100,000 and Mexico 526. Some of the most successful countries include New Zealand with 27 infections per 100,000, South Korea 43, Japan 60. Europe, the first outbreak outside China, has higher per capita numbers of infections than many countries but considerably lower than the U.S.: Italy 474, Germany 313, France 542, U.K. 549. The U.S, with a death rate of 59 per 100,000 has a death rate from the virus at a per capita rate five times that of Germany with a rate of 11 per 100,000. The next-closest death toll from the coronavirus is in Brazil, where 131,210 people have died, a per capita rate of 63 per 100,000.

The scarcities that bedeviled the U.S.'s response to the pandemic were most often avoidable and most CSC plans include the requirement that scarcity be addressed before the CSC standards are imposed. When scarcity is avoidable, rather than lower the standards of care, we could provide resources to raise the standard of care. This is not unusual. For example, by August, Kern County California became one of the worst hotspots in the country. Rather than lowering the standards for allocating the goods to combat the pandemic, the state of California responded by sending in strike teams to improve enforcement and $52 million to improve testing, tracing and isolation protocols.[89]

10.5 Conclusion

My purpose in this paper was not to endorse one particular set of principles, but to lay out the most plausible models along with some strengths and weakness. Here I looked at a number of models, including Crisis Standards Care. The focus on CSC in the absence of widely adopted models for care during ordinary times suggests that we need a model for allocations of essential health goods in all times, not just in times of scarcity and emergency.

We have seen that the magnitude of devastation of the coronavirus in the U.S. was largely preventable and caused in part by the U.S.'s initial failure to allocate the essential goods that were needed to treat patients and control infection. Given this failure, we cannot justify moving to CSC in order to lower standards of care for patients. Unfortunately, we can expect future emergencies that will involve unavoidable scarcity so the time spent developing CSCs has not been wasted. At the same time, we should not be content with the flawed CSC plans that are currently being challenged as discriminating against the elderly, persons with disabilities, people of color, those who are poor and uninsured, and those living in congregate and overcrowded housing.

Going forward, we should be vigilant about not adopting CSC plans until we are convinced that we have done all we reasonably can to address scarcities of essential goods. At the same time, we should also be vigilant in developing plans for emergencies that do not necessarily involve a scarcity of essential goods. Bioethics provides a wealth of insight on how to structure just allocation of all the essential goods needed in all kinds of health emergencies and the time for reflection is never too soon.

Notes

1. Mounk (2020).
2. Vergano et al. (2020).
3. "Left behind in the times of COVID-19," *Médecins Sans Frontières*, July 2020. The death toll of nursing home residents in Belgium has now reached 5700. Stevis-Gridneff and Apuzzo (2020). https://www.nytimes.com/2020/08/08/world/europe/coronavirus-nursing-homes-elderly.html?action=click&module=Top%20Stories&pgtype=Homepage.
4. "When Did the Coronavirus Start Spreading in the U.S.? Likely in January, CDC Analysis Suggests," *Stat News*, May 29, 2020. https://www.statnews.com/2020/05/29/cdc-local-transmission-coronavirus-united-states/.
5. Shepherd (2020).
6. "Mapping the Worldwide Spread of the Coronavirus," *Washington Post*, September 12, 2020. https://www.washingtonpost.com/graphics/2020/world/mapping-spread-new-coronavirus/.
7. "Mapping the Worldwide Spread," https://www.washingtonpost.com/graphics/2020/national/coronavirus-us-cases-deaths.
8. These definitions are adapted from Christian and Farmer (2009).
9. Christian, "Disaster Triage and Allocation of Scarce Resources," 13-3.
10. Kidney dialysis was deemed an entitlement when Section 299I was included in H.R. 1, the Social Security Amendments of 1972 as Public Law 92-603.
11. 42 U.S. Code § 1395dd—Examination and Treatment for Emergency Medical Conditions and Women in Labor Act.
12. CDC, "Temporary halt in residential evictions to prevent the further spread of COVID-19," last updated September 2, 2020. https://www.cdc.gov/coronavirus/2019-ncov/covid-eviction-declaration.html.
13. Testing is done to diagnose the illness in sick patients, to screen to identify who might need to be isolated, and to surveil to understand prevalence in a community to inform workplace, local, or regional policies. Right now, screening testing is especially lacking. See Silcox et al. (2020).
14. Hunger was identified as a public health issue as early as 1997. Sidel (1997). A 2016 study conducted in Massachusetts shows that it is still a public health issue there. See John T. Cook, Ana Poblacion, "The Estimated Health Related Costs of Food Insecurity and Hunger in Massachusetts," http://macostofhunger.org/wp-content/uploads/2018/02/full-report.pdf.
15. Thompson (2020).
16. Trump's failure was so immense that *Scientific American*, which had never endorsed a presidential candidate in its 175-year history, endorsed Joe Biden:

"The evidence and the science show that Donald Trump has badly damaged the U.S. and its people—because he rejects evidence and science. The most devastating example is his dishonest and inept response to the COVID-19 pandemic, which cost more than 190,000 Americans their lives by the middle of September." The Editors, October 1, 2020. https://www.scientificamerican.com/article/scientific-american-endorses-joe-biden/?print=true.
17. Yong (2020).
18. All the federal laws cited here are discussed in *Selected Federal Legal Authorities Pertinent to Public Health Emergencies Prepared by the Public Health Law Program Centers for Disease Control and Prevention.* Updated August 2017.
19. The Kaiser Family Foundation has extensive database on how individual states have responding to the coronavirus pandemic. https://www.kff.org/coronavirus-COVID-19/issue-brief/state-data-and-policy-actions-to-address-coronavirus/.
20. American Medical Association (2020).
21. The Congressional Research Service concluded that "The Administration's DPA implementation pattern appears sporadic and relatively narrow." Congressional Research Service, "Defense Production Act (DPA): Recent Developments in Response to COVID-19," Updated July 28, 2020. For reporting on Trump's use of the DPA, see Alvarez and Devine (2020).
22. Dale (2020).
23. Rauhala (2020).
24. John Rawls described justified principles as those principles "free and equal persons concerned to further their own interests would accept in an initial position of equality". He argued that in this initial position of equality, an rational person would agree that justified social and economic inequalities would be both: "(a) to the greatest benefit of the least advantaged, consistent with the just savings principle, and (b) attached to offices and positions open to all under conditions of fair equality of opportunity." Rawls (1971).
25. Bentham (1988).
26. Mill (2002).
27. Pellegrino (1985).
28. American Nursing Association code of ethics, American Nurses Association. (2015). Accessed September 23, 2020. http://www.nursingworld.org/MainMenuCategories/EthicsStandards/CodeofEthicsforNurses/Code-ofEthics-For-Nurses.html.
29. Manning (2009).
30. Rawls, *A Theory of Justice*, 302.
31. Lomasky (2015).
32. Menzel (2012).
33. Emanuel et al. (2020).
34. For a discussion of the scarcity of N-95s see Contrera (2020). In addition to the N-95s "77 percent of the clinics, long-term care facilities and rural hospitals

requesting goods in August reported that they had run out of at least one essential item, up from 65 percent in June." Jacobs (2020).
35. https://www.hhs.gov/ohrp/regulations-and-policy/belmont-report/index.html.
36. Beauchamp and Childress (2012).
37. UNESCO, *Universal declaration on bioethics and human rights.* Last updated June 2006. http://unesdoc.unesco.org/images/0014/001461/146180E.pdf.
38. Magnus (2016).
39. Glover (2019). See also Tilburt and Sulmasy (2017).
40. Annas (2020) and Schultz and Annas (2012).
41. WHO (2020).
42. Wolff et al. (2020).
43. WHO, SAGE (2020).
44. Jonathan Wolff et al., "An Ethical Framework for Global Vaccine Allocation."
45. Patient Protection and Affordable Care Act of 2010, Pub. L. No. 111–148, 124 Stat. 119 (2010).
46. The Emergency Medical Treatment and Labor Act (EMTALA was enacted by Congress in 1986 as part of the Consolidated Omnibus Budget Reconciliation Act (COBRA) of 1985 (42 U.S.C. §1395dd).
47. The Social Security Amendments of 1972 (P.L. 92-603), of Section 299I authorized Medicare entitlement for individuals with a diagnosis of chronic renal failure who were fully or currently insured under social security.
48. NHS "Allocations infographics," www.england.nhs.uk/wp-content/uploads/2020/02/nhs-allocations-infographics-feb-2020.pdf.
49. UK Cen Clinical Ethics Network, "The Four Principles of Biomedical Ethics," http://www.ukcen.net/ethical_issues/confidentiality/the_four_principles_of_biomedical_ethics.
50. The National Academies of Science, Engineering, Medicine, "A Framework for Equitable Allocation of Vaccine for the Novel Coronavirus," https://www.nationalacademies.org/our-work/a-framework-for-equitable-allocation-of-vaccine-for-the-novel-coronavirus#sectionProjectScope.
51. Carter et al. (2016).
52. Laventhal et al. (2020).
53. White et al. (2020). Accessed September 23, 2020. https://ccm.pitt.edu/sites/default/files/UnivPittsburgh_ModelHospitalResourcePolicy_2020_04_15.pdf
54. Scheunemann and White (2011).
55. Leslie P. Scheunemann and Douglas B. White, "The Ethics and Reality of Rationing in Medicine."
56. White et al. (2009).
57. Koenig et al. (2011).
58. Institute of Medicine (2009).
59. Institute of Medicine (2012).
60. Institute of Medicine (2013).
61. Institute of Medicine (2009).
62. Institute of Medicine (2009).

63. Institute of Medicine (2009).
64. Institute of Medicine (2012).
65. Institute of Medicine (2013).
66. For allocation of ventilators, the CDC adopted listed specific ethical considerations in a document, "Ethical Considerations for Decision Making Regarding Allocation of Mechanical Ventilators during a Severe Influenza Pandemic or Other Public Health Emergency" approved by the Ethics Subcommittee on February 18, 2011 and by the Advisory Committee to the Director on April 28, 2011. Accessed on September 23, 2020. https://www.cdc.gov/about/advisory/pdf/VentDocument_Release.pdf.
67. Lori Frank, Thomas W. Concannon, Karishma Patel, "Health Care Resource Allocation Decision Making During a Pandemic, "Resource Report, RAND Corporation, Santa Monica, Calif. © Copyright 2020.
68. Lori Frank, "Health Care Resource Allocation Decision Making During a Pandemic," 20.
69. Emanuel et al. (2020).
70. Piscitello et al. (2020).
71. Mello et al. (2020).
72. For a wealth of information on discrimination claims during the coronavirus pandemic, see Center for Public Representation, Update: July 22, 2020. https://www.centerforpublicrep.org/COVID-19-medical-rationing/.
73. North Central Texas Trauma Regional Advisory Council, Mass Critical Guidelines Document for Hospital and ICU Triage Guidelines for ADULTS. Accessed September 23, 2020. https://www.dallas-cms.org/tmaimis/Default.aspx?WebsiteKey=5857f487-9f64-4281-b4b7-67e6a2224be2&hkey=9f1e00e9-17f8-47f1-a874-2c315f147674&=404;https:%2F%2Fwww.dallas-cms.org:443%2FDCMS%2FPublic_Health%2FMass_Critical_Care.
74. For a fuller discussion of legal liability in a pandemic, see Schultz and Annas (2012).
75. The Kaiser Family Foundation provides a great deal of current information about health policy. For data on states and Medicaid, see https://www.kff.org/medicaid/issue-brief/status-of-state-medicaid-expansion-decisions-interactive-map/#:~:text=To%20date%2C%2039%20states%20(including,available%20in%20a%20table%20format.
76. Annas (2020).
77. Disability Rights Texas, Complaint Regarding North Texas Mass Critical Care Guidelines for Adults and Children. https://www.centerforpublicrep.org/wp-content/uploads/HHS-OCR-Complaint-re-North-Texas-Mass-Critical-Care-Guidelines.pdf.
78. Disability Rights Texas, Complaint, 10.
79. North Central Texas Trauma Regional Advisory Council, Mass Critical Guidelines Document for Hospital and ICU Triage Guidelines for ADULTS, 1.
80. Disability Rights Texas, Complaint, 16.
81. Voytko (2020).

82. Quote of the Day, *New York Times*, March 20, 2020, Section A, Page 3.
83. 50 USC Ch. 55.
84. Eban (2020).
85. Mandavilli (2020).
86. Sun (2020).
87. Yong (2020).
88. These figures are from the "New York Times, COVID World Map: Tracking the Global Outbreak," September 13, 2020. https://www.nytimes.com/interactive/2020/world/coronavirus-maps.html.
89. Branson-Potts (2020).

References

Alvarez, Priscilla, and Curt Devine. 2020. Trump administration's delayed use of 1950s law leads to critical supplies shortages. *CNN*, July 14. https://www.cnn.com/2020/07/13/politics/delayed-use-defense-production-act-ppe-shortages/index.html.

American Medical Association. 2020. HHS Public Health and Social Services Emergency Fund, July 27. https://www.ama-assn.org/system/files/2020-08/hhs-emergency-funding.pdf.

Annas, George J. 2020. Rationing crisis: Bogus standards of care unmasked by COVID-19. *The American Journal of Bioethics* 20 (7): 167–169.

Beauchamp, Tom L., and James F. Childress. 2012. *Principles of biomedical ethics*. Oxford: Oxford University Press.

Bentham, Jeremy. 1988 *The principles of morals and legislation* (originally published in 1789). Amherst, NY: Prometheus Books.

Branson-Potts, Hailey. 2020. Political battles, confusion reign in Kern County, one of worst U.S. Coronavirus hot spots. *Los Angeles Times*, August 18. https://www.latimes.com/california/story/2020-08-17/kern-county-pained-by-confusing-covid-19-guidance.

Carter, Drew, and Jason Gordon, Amber M. Watt. 2016. Competing principles for allocating health care resources. *Journal of Medicine and Philosophy* 41: 558–583, 562.

Christian, Michael D., and J. Christopher Farmer. 2009. Disaster triage and allocation of scarce resources. *Fundamental Disaster Management, Society of Critical Care Medicine* (13-2)-(13–14).

Contrera, Jessica. 2020. The N95 shortage America can't seem to fix. *Washington Post*, September 21. https://www.washingtonpost.com/graphics/2020/local/news/n-95-shortage-covid/?itid=hp-top-table-main.

Dale, Daniel. 2020. Trump administration edits national stockpile website a day after it contradicted Jared Kushner. *CNN*, April 3. https://www.cnn.com/2020/04/03/politics/stockpile-website-edited-kushner-claim/index.html.

Eban, Katherine. 2020. How Jared Kushner's secret testing plan went 'poof into thin air'. *Vanity Fair*. July 20. https://www.vanityfair.com/news/2020/07/how-jared-kushners-secret-testing-plan-went-poof-into-thin-air.

Emanuel, Ezekiel J., et al. 2020. Fair allocation of scarce medical resources in the time of COVID-19. *New England Journal of Medicine* 382 (21) (May 21): 2049–2055, 2051.

Glover, Jacqueline. 2019. The role of physicians in the allocation of health care: Is some justice better than none? *Kennedy Institute of Ethics Journal* 29 (1): 1–32.

https://www.washingtonpost.com/health/california-officials-blasted-for-prison-coronavirus-outbreak/2020/07/01/5062a04a-bbd8-11ea-97c1-6cf116ffe26c_story.html.

Institute of Medicine. 2009. Guidance for establishing crisis standards of care for use in disaster situations: A letter report, 3. https://www.ncbi.nlm.nih.gov/books/NBK219953/.

Institute of Medicine. 2012. *Crisis standards of care: A systems framework for catastrophic disaster response: Volume 1: introduction and CSC framework*. Washington, DC: The National Academies Press. https://doi.org/10.17226/13351.
Institute of Medicine. 2013. *Crisis standards of care: A toolkit for indicators and triggers*. Washington, DC: The National Academies Press 2013. https://doi.org/10.17226/18338.
Jacobs, Andrew. 2020. Despite claims, Trump rarely uses wartime law in battle against covid. *New York Times*, September 22. https://www.nytimes.com/2020/09/22/health/Covid-Trump-Defense-Production-Act.html?action=click&module=Top%20Stories&pgtype=Homepage.
Koenig, Kristi L., et al. 2011. Crisis standard of care: Refocusing health care goals during catastrophic disasters and emergencies. *International Journal of Clinical and Experimental Medicine* 3 (4): 159–165, 160, 161.
Laventhal, Naomi et al. 2011. The ethics of creating a resource allocation strategy during the COVID-19 pandemic. *Pediatrics*. Prepublication release, downloaded from www.aappublications.org/news by guest on September 11. https://doi.org/10.1542/peds.2020-1243.
Lomasky, Loren. 2015. Markets and mortality. *Georgetown Journal of Law & Public Policy* 13: 299–319, 317.
Magnus, Richard. 2016. The universality of the UNESCO universal declaration on bioethics and human rights. In *Global bioethics: The impact of the UNESCO international bioethics committee*, ed. Alireza Bagheri, Jonathan D. Moreno, and Stefano Semplici, 29–42, 30–31. Switzerland: Springer.
Mandavilli, Apoorva. 2020. C.D.C. testing guidance was published against scientists' objections. *New York Times*, September 17. https://www.nytimes.com/2020/09/17/health/coronavirus-testing-cdc.html?action=click&module=Top%20Stories&pgtype=Homepage.
Manning, Rita. 2009. A care approach. In *A companion to bioethics*, ed. Helga Kuhse and Peter Singer, 105–116. Oxford: Blackwell Publishing Ltd.
Mello, Michelle M., Govind Persad, and Douglas B. White. 2020. Respecting disability rights—Toward improved crisis standards of care. *The New England Journal of Medicine* 383 (5) (July 30): e26(1)–e26(4).
Menzel, Paul T. 2012. Justice, liberty, and the choice of health-system structure. In *Medicine and social justice: Essays on the distribution of health care*, ed. Rosamond Rhodes, Margaret Battin, and Anita Silvers, 35–46. Oxford: Oxford University Press.
Mounk, Yascha. 2020. The extraordinary decisions facing Italian doctors. *The Atlantic*, March 11. https://www.theatlantic.com/ideas/archive/2020/03/who-gets-hospital-bed/607807/.
Pellegrino, Edward. 1985. The virtuous physician, and the ethics of medicine. *Philosophy and Medicine* 17: 237–255.
Piscitello, Gina M., et al. 2020. Variation in ventilator allocation guidelines by US states during the Coronavirus disease 2019 pandemic a systematic review. *JAMA Network Open* 3 (6).
Rauhala, Emily. 2020. World Health Organization unveils plan for distributing coronavirus vaccine, urges cooperation. *Washington Post*, September 22. https://www.washingtonpost.com/world/coronavirus-vaccine-covax-who/2020/09/21/d21c7b4a-f9d3-11ea-a510-f57d8ce76e11_story.html.
Rawls, John. 1971. *A theory of justice*, 302. Cambridge, MA: The Belknap Press of Harvard University Press.
Scheunemann, Leslie P., and Douglas B. White. (2011). The ethics and reality of rationing in medicine. *CHEST* 140 (6) (December): 1625–1632, 627.
Schultz, Carl H., and George J. Annas. March 2012. Altering the standard of care in disasters—Unnecessary and dangerous. *MPH Annals of Emergency Medicine* 5 (3): 191–195.
Shepherd, Katie. 2020. South Texas County may send the sickest patients home to die as cases soar. *Washington Post*, July 24. https://www.washingtonpost.com/nation/2020/07/24/coronavirus-COVID-live-updates-us/?hpid=hp_hp-banner-main_virus-luf-1214am%3Aprime-time%2Fpromo#link-7YVGQTPOXBEA5JK5WC74HSD63I.
Sidel, Victor W. 1997. The public health impact of hunger. *American Journal of Public Health* 87 (12) (December): 1921–1922.

Silcox, Christina et al. 2020. A national decision point: Effective testing and screening for Covid-19. Duke-Margolis Center for Health Policy.

Stevis-Gridneff, Matina, and Matt Apuzzo. 2020. When COVID-19 hit, many elderly were left to die. *New York Times*, August 8. https://www.nytimes.com/2020/08/08/world/europe/coronavirus-nursing-homes-elderly.html?action=click&module=Top%20Stories&pgtype=Homepage.

Stuart Mill, John. 2002. *Utilitarianism* (originally published in 1863), available in *The basic writings of John Stuart Mill: On liberty, the subjection of women, utilitarianism*, ed. J.B. Schneewind. New York: Modern Library.

Sun, Lena H. 2020. Trump officials seek greater control over CDC reports on Coronavirus. *Washington Post*, September 13. https://www.washingtonpost.com/health/2020/09/12/trump-control-over-cdc-reports/?hpid=hp_hp-banner-main_virusmmwr-740pm%3Ahomepage%2Fstory-ans.

Voytko Lisette. 2020. Trump: 'No, I don't take responsibility' for botched Coronavirus testing rollout. *Forbes*, March 13. https://www.forbes.com/sites/lisettevoytko/2020/03/13/trump-no-i-dont-take-responsibility-for-botched-coronavirus-testing-rollout/#10689c9046f0.

Thompson, Don. 2020. California officials blasted for prison coronavirus outbreak. *Washington Post*, July 1.

Tilburt, Jon C., and Daniel P. Sulmasy. 2017. Context and scale: Distinctions for improving debates about physician 'rationing.' *Philosophy, Ethics, and Humanities in Medicine* 12 (5): 1–32.

Vergano, Marco, et al. 2020. Clinical ethics recommendations for the allocation of intensive care treatments, in exceptional, resource-limited circumstances. Italian Society of Anesthesia, Analgesia, Resuscitation and Intensive Care (SIAARTI), March 16. http://www.siaarti.it/SiteAssets/News/COVID19%20-%20documenti%20SIAARTI/SIAARTI%20-%20Covid-19%20-%20Clinical%20Ethics%20Reccomendations.pdf.

White, Douglas B., et al. 2009. Who should receive life support during a public health emergency? Using ethical principles to improve allocation decisions. *Annals of Internal Medicine* 150 (2) (January 20): 132–138, 132.

White, Douglas B., et al. 2020. University of Pittsburg, Department of Critical Care Medicine, School of Medicine, "Allocation of Scarce Critical Care Resources During a Public Health Emergency" April 15. Accessed September 23, 2020. https://ccm.pitt.edu/sites/default/files/UnivPittsburgh_ModelHospitalResourcePolicy_2020_04_15.pdf.

WHO. 2020. Fair allocation mechanism for COVID-19 vaccines through the COVAX facility final working version, September 9. Accessed September 23, 2020, https://www.who.int/publications/m/item/fair-allocation-mechanism-for-covid-19-vaccines-through-the-covax-facility.

WHO, SAGE. 2020. Values framework for the allocation and prioritization of COVID-19 vaccination, September 14. Accessed September 23, 2020, https://apps.who.int/iris/bitstream/handle/10665/334299/WHO-2019-nCoV-SAGE_Framework-Allocation_and_prioritization-2020.1-eng.pdf.

Wolff, Jonathan et al. 2020. An ethical framework for global vaccine allocation. *Science* 369 (6509): 1309–1312, originally published online September 3. Accessed September 23, 2020. https://science.sciencemag.org/content/369/6509/1309.

Yong, Ed. 2020. Anatomy of an American failure. *The Atlantic*, 33–47, 40, September.

Chapter 11
Addressing Pandemic Disparities: Equity and Neutral Conceptions of Justice

Debra A. DeBruin

Abstract The chapter begins by characterizing the COVID-19 disparities affecting BIPOC populations and summarizing research putting these disparities in historical context. It then presents a model explaining why these disparities arise. This background information grounds a discussion of why these disparities constitute inequities, and what justice requires in these circumstances. The analysis focuses primarily on obligations during pandemic but acknowledges that obligations do not end when pandemic does. It considers alternative conceptions of justice, focusing on questions about whether it is permissible to take race and ethnicity into account in pandemic response initiatives.

Keywords Justice · Health equity · Racial and ethnic health disparities · Pandemic ethics · Fair process · Equal opportunity

The human toll associated with the COVID-19 pandemic is staggering. Over 33.5 million people in the United States tested positive for COVID-19 between the start of the pandemic in early 2020 and mid-July 2021.[1] The illness led to 2,335,058 hospitalizations in the US from August 1, 2020 (when consistent reporting began) through July 18, 2021.[2] And as of July 14, 2021, 605,905 people in the US had died from COVID-19.[3] Many individuals who survive their illness experience longer term, debilitating effects from the disease—a phenomenon now commonly known as "long COVID".[4] In addition to the direct health effects of COVID-19, the pandemic is associated with a multitude of additional costs—including the health impact of delaying care for other conditions while sheltering from the pandemic; job loss, and housing and food insecurity associated with the pandemic's economic downturn[5]; and the social and emotional effects of isolation,[6] to name a few.

The tragic consequences of this pandemic have been borne disproportionately by Black, Indigenous, and other people of color ("BIPOC" populations). A high-level overview of data paints a stark picture.

D. A. DeBruin (✉)
Center for Bioethics, University of Minnesota, Minneapolis, MN, USA
e-mail: debru004@umn.edu

© The Author(s), under exclusive license to Springer Nature Switzerland AG 2022
M. Boylan (ed.), *Ethical Public Health Policy Within Pandemics*, The International Library of Bioethics 95, https://doi.org/10.1007/978-3-030-99692-5_10

Table 11.1 Risk for COVID-19 infection, hospitalization, and death by race/ethnicity[7]

Rate ratios compared to White, Non-Hispanic persons	American Indian or Alaska Native, Non-Hispanic persons	Asian, Non-Hispanic persons	Black or African American, Non-Hispanic persons	Hispanic or Latino persons
Cases	1.6x	0.7x	1.1x	2.0x
Hospitalization	3.3x	1.0x	2.9x	2.8x
Death	2.4x	1.0x	2.0x	2.3x

A more detailed analysis of the data reflects that certain subgroups within these racial and ethnic populations have even higher levels of elevated risk than represented in Table 11.1. For example, American Indian or Alaska Native individuals aged 18–49 are 5.7 times as likely to be hospitalized as Non-Hispanic White individuals in that age group.[8] Further data will be provided below. The US Centers for Disease Control and Prevention (CDC) acknowledges that "Long-standing systemic health and social inequities have put many people from racial and ethnic minority groups at increased risk of severe illness from COVID-19."[9]

This chapter will focus on equity as it relates to race and ethnicity in the COVID-19 pandemic, but equity concerns are not limited to the impact of the pandemic on BIPOC populations. For example, individuals with disabilities have also disproportionately suffered harms from COVID-19.[10] Sexual and gender minorities may also experience disparities in severe COVID-19 outcomes, but failures to gather necessary data hampers understanding of the vulnerabilities in these populations.[11] A fuller analysis of equity would need to attend to diverse populations and the ways in which the intersectionality of social identities affect social (dis)advantages and pandemic outcomes. Moreover, this chapter will primarily focus on the direct health effects of COVID-19—infections, hospitalizations, and death—and not the other costs of the pandemic noted above, which raise equity issues of their own.[12] The full array of pandemic-related equity issues deserves serious consideration, even though the scope of this chapter does not permit that I take them up here.

The chapter will begin by providing more data to better characterize the COVID-19 disparities affecting BIPOC populations and summarizing research that puts these data in historical context. I will then present a model that explains why these disparities arise. This background information will ground a discussion of why these disparities constitute inequities, and what justice requires in these circumstances. The analysis will focus primarily on our obligations during pandemic, but acknowledges that our obligations do not end when the pandemic does. I will consider alternative conceptions of justice offered by contemporary authors writing specifically about equity in the pandemic, focusing on questions about whether it is morally permissible to explicitly take race and ethnicity into account in pandemic response initiatives. I ultimately support an approach to doing so that I believe is not only morally permissible, but morally obligatory.

11.1 Racial and Ethnic Health Disparities During the COVID-19 Pandemic

One reason that the disparities affecting BIPOC populations during the COVID-19 pandemic are so troubling is that they are profound. A more detailed look at data concerning disparities reveals that BIPOC populations have significantly higher rates of hospitalizations, and at younger ages, than Whites do.

Table 11.2 Hospitalization rates per 100,000 population by age and race and ethnicity—COVID-NET March 1, 2020—July 3, 2021[13]

Age Category	Non-Hispanic American Indian or Alaska Native Rate[1]	Rate Ratio[2,3]	Non-Hispanic Black Rate[1]	Rate Ratio[2,3]	Hispanic or Latino Rate[1]	Rate Ratio[2,3]	Non-Hispanic Asian or Pacific Islander Rate[1]	Rate Ratio[2,3]	Non-Hispanic White Rate[1]	Rate Ratio[2,3]
0—17 years	62.3	2.8	66.3	3.0	72.2	3.2	25.3	1.1	22.4	1.0
18—49 years	927.7	5.7	570.6	3.5	677.6	4.1	172.7	1.1	163.6	1.0
50—64 years	1954.1	3.9	1582.8	3.2	1593.4	3.2	519.9	1.0	496.5	1.0
65+ years	2990.8	2.3	2970.0	2.2	2665.4	2.0	1126.9	0.9	1320.2	1.0
Overall rate[4] (age-adjusted)	1249.3	3.4	1016.9	2.8	1015.1	2.8	347.0	1.0	364.6	1.0

Note Rate ratios compare the rate of hospitalization in each group to that for Whites in the same age group

Presenting the data concerning death rates grouped by age reveals similar patterns: BIPOC populations are much more likely to die, and at younger ages, than Whites. In Table 11.3, the bars that extend above 0 demonstrate that "a given race/ethnicity group is experiencing a disproportionately high percent of COVID-19 deaths relative to their percent of the population." The bars that extend below 0 show the opposite—that the percent of COVID-19 deaths is smaller than these groups' percent of the population.[14] When visualized this way, the racial and ethnic disparities in death rates are quite striking, and disturbing.

Table 11.3 Differences by race and Hispanic origin between the percent of COVID-19 deaths and the population distribution, grouped by age[15]

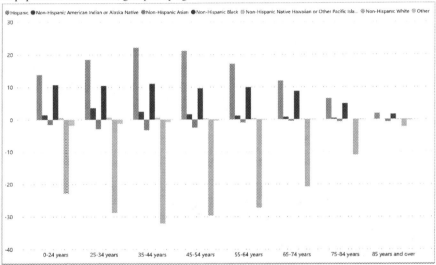

The more nuanced analysis of data presented in Tables 11.2 and 11.3 provides a much clearer understanding of the nature of COVID-19 disparities than the high-level overview provided by Table 11.1.

Situating these disparities in historical context is even more revealing. Wrigley-Field looks back to the effects of the 1918 pandemic—a severe influenza pandemic—and shows that "Whites' life expectancy in 1918 was far lower than in other twentieth century years—yet higher than Black life expectancy in all years but one between 1900 and 1918."[16] Based on this history, she asks whether the COVID-19 pandemic will result in "a spike in mortality for Whites that nevertheless remains lower than the mortality Blacks experience routinely, outside of any pandemic".[17] She analyzes demographic data and concludes:

> even in the COVID-19 pandemic, White mortality will remain lower than the lowest recorded Black mortality in the United States. If fewer than 400,000 excess White deaths occur in 2020, the COVID-19 pandemic for Whites will be less consequential to overall White mortality

than racial inequality is for Black mortality every year. And unless 2020 sees 700,000 to 1 million excess White deaths—a 31 to 46% mortality increase from recent years—life expectancy for Whites, even amid COVID-19, will remain higher than it has ever been for Blacks.[18]

Wrigley-Field notes that, given racial disparities in COVID-19 death rates, the pandemic will very likely exacerbate the racial gap in mortality.[19] Indeed, in July 2021, the CDC's National Center for Health Statistics released data showing that overall life expectancy in the US fell by 1.5 years during 2020, and racial and ethnic disparities in life expectancy grew during this time. Life expectancy declined by 1.2 years for Whites, by 2.9 years for Blacks, and by 3.0 years for Hispanic populations.[20] As we have seen, the racial and ethnic disparities in COVID-19 death rates are sobering. Wrigley-Field's analysis starkly captures how profound racial inequities in health status are, completely apart from the pandemic, and effectively clarifies why racism has been referred to as a public health emergency.[21]

11.2 Modelling Why Pandemic Disparities Arise

Historically, BIPOC and other socially disadvantaged populations have faced elevated risk of poor outcomes from infectious disease outbreaks. Blumenshine and colleagues offer a model to explain why such disparities arise. They point to differences among subpopulations in *exposure* to infectious disease, *susceptibility* to developing symptomatic illness—and especially severe disease—when exposed, and *access* to treatment when needed.[22] Differences in exposure are associated with factors such as housing density, reliance upon public transportation, and inability to work from home. Susceptibility issues relate to disparities in the incidence of underlying health conditions such as asthma and heart disease that increase risk from infectious diseases, as well as stress levels associated with social disadvantage. Access barriers can also affect susceptibility—for example, differential access to vaccines, once they become available, will affect susceptibility to illness or severe illness. Other access issues can also affect outcomes when individuals become ill—for example, financial barriers to seeking treatment including being uninsured or underinsured, lack of transportation to care, language barriers, and disparities in quality of care.[23] Additional research provides support for the model offered by Blumenshine et al.[24]

This analysis reveals another reason why the racial and ethnic disparities in the COVID-19 pandemic are so troubling: they were predictable. While no one could have predicted that this particular pandemic would occur at this particular time in history, experts have long acknowledged that pandemics will continue to occur, as they have historically.[25] Scientists studying coronaviruses noted in 2007 that "The possibility of the reemergence of SARS [Severe Acute Respiratory Syndrome] and other novel viruses from animals or laboratories and therefore the need for preparedness should not be ignored"—indeed, they described the risk as a "time bomb".[26] A duty to prepare is foundational.[27] Given the predictability of racial and ethnic disparities, preparedness ought to include measures to address them. Yet a systematic review of the preparedness ethics literature prior to the COVID-19 pandemic reveals little attention to equity issues.[28] There is serious danger in failing to admit the predictability of these inequities. As Valles states,

> [t]he more we treat the harm as unexpected—a fluke—the more we bolster the argument that no major structural changes need to be made.... [H]ealth inequities between populations are not biological destinies; they are the results of political choices, ones that we can ameliorate if we find the collective will to do so.[29]

Unfortunately, as Maness and colleagues note, "[t]he social and political will needed to correct these injustices has been, and continues to be, lacking."[30]

11.3 Health Disparities as Inequities

To clearly understand why health disparities such as those experienced by BIPOC populations during the COVID-19 pandemic constitute inequities, and to clarify social obligations to address these inequities, we need to get clear on what we mean by equity. The CDC characterizes health equity as follows:

> Health equity is achieved when every person has the opportunity to "attain his or her full health potential" and no one is "disadvantaged from achieving this potential because of social position or other socially determined circumstances." Health inequities are reflected in differences in length of life; quality of life; rates of disease, disability, and death; severity of disease; and access to treatment.[31]

Key to the CDC's characterization is the idea that "social position or other socially determined circumstances" ought not to disadvantage people regarding their health status. These social factors are referred to as the 'social determinants of health'.

The factors that increase BIPOC populations' *exposure* to COVID-19 and affect their *access* to vaccines and treatment are clearly social factors—jobs, housing, transportation, financial resources or appropriate insurance to secure treatment, and so on. The factors that increase these populations' *susceptibility* to poor outcomes when they become infected may appear to be biological rather than social, as these factors relate primarily to rates of underlying health conditions that increase COVID-19 risks. But these underlying conditions are also associated with social determinants of health. For example, given housing segregation, populations have differential access to healthy food and safe spaces to exercise, and are differentially exposed to environmental toxins that carry health risks. Inadequate access to healthcare may impede treatment for the chronic conditions such as heart and lung disease that increase COVID-19 risks. Persistent levels of stress associated with social disadvantage can also undermine health status.[32] Thus, social factors affect health status, and the underlying health conditions related to these social factors increase risk of progression to severe disease with COVID-19. Social position and other social factors do disadvantage BIPOC populations, both during pandemics and, in "normal"—interpandemic—times.

A closer examination of the nature of health disparities allows for a clearer understanding of our moral obligations to affected populations. Health disparities should be understood as

> systematic, plausibly avoidable health differences according to race/ethnicity, skin color, religion, or nationality; socioeconomic resources or position (reflected by, e.g., income, wealth, education, or occupation); gender, sexual orientation, gender identity; age, geography, disability, illness, political or other affiliation; or other characteristics associated with discrimination or marginalization.[33]

Saying that disparities are *systematic* does not imply that every member of the affected group will be disadvantaged to the same extent.[34] Rather, it means that they are connected to structural disadvantage—the "historical and contemporary policies, practices, and norms that create and maintain" social advantage and disadvantage for particular groups, e.g., based on race and ethnicity.[35] Thus, it is not simply that social factors happen to disadvantage people with respect to their health status; it is that those social factors are part of a network of social forces that *systematically produce* disadvantage. Given the detrimental impact of these disparities on populations, they also serve to *perpetuate* systematic disadvantage.[36] Thus, promoting health equity will require systematic change.

Saying that disparities should be understood to be *plausibly avoidable* does not mean that individuals in the affected groups can avoid them if they try—which would wrongly suggest that disparities are a matter of personal responsibility for those affected. Rather, it means that the disparities could be ameliorated through social change that alters the social determinants of health, assuming the knowledge and political will to enact change. Were the health differences unavoidable—due to natural genetic variation, for example—they might be tragic, but they would not be morally pernicious.[37] Were it impossible to alter the bases of these health differences, there would be no moral obligation to do so—'ought' implies 'can'. This analysis reveals a third reason why the racial and ethnic disparities in the COVID-19 pandemic are so troubling: there were avoidable.

Ameliorating routine (not pandemic-specific, but persistently long-term) disparities should help prevent—or at least diminish—disparities in pandemic outcomes. But that is not the primary reason to address routine disparities; they are serious inequities quite apart from their effects during public health emergencies. And it does not mean that the obligation to address routine disparities should fall primarily upon the public health and medical professionals responsible for pandemic preparedness and response. Routine disparities arise from systematic disadvantage and addressing them will involve systematic work—on residential and employment segregation, educational disparities, environmental injustice, barriers to accessing quality health care, and other social issues. Responsibilities should be broadly shared across our society. Much more must be said—and done—about this than can be addressed in a chapter on pandemic equity. But it is critical that this chapter acknowledges the role—and the depth and breadth—of these routine disparities in giving rise to racial and ethnic inequities in pandemics.

Given how profound these routine disparities are, we will likely not *achieve* health equity during a pandemic, when surging needs and strains on health and social systems demand that we focus resources and energy on the crisis at hand. That is, if we do not make substantial progress against routine disparities before the start of a pandemic, we are unlikely to be able to ensure that "every person has the opportunity to 'attain his or her full health potential' and no one is 'disadvantaged from achieving this potential because of social position or other socially determined circumstances'"[38] during the pandemic. This does not mean, however, that we cannot *make progress* toward equity during pandemic.

11.4 What Does Justice Require?

We should recognize that there is a diversity of views about what justice requires in pandemic response. A common theme relates to norms about the neutrality[39] of response efforts. There are variations on this theme. One approach is captured by a very influential account of pandemic ethics, which "recommend[s] an approach to justice that focuses on the procedures to be followed with the hope that good procedures will lead to fair outcomes."[40] The notion of *procedural justice* emphasizes "ensuring consistency in applying standards" and "identifying decision makers who are impartial and neutral."[41] These concerns about the nature of our duties of justice can be found not only in the published literature on emergency planning but also in public discussion. For example, in response to a commentary I published in the press on vaccine equity, some commenters objected that my message concerning equity inappropriately injected politics into vaccine allocation decision-making and conflicted with the view often expressed during the COVID-19 pandemic that science should drive pandemic response.[42] While science should inform discussions of ethical issues in pandemic response, it cannot, on its own, resolve them. Normative issues require normative analysis. However, the rejection of politics and valorization of science in this context communicates the embrace of an ideal that is neutral with respect to social context, race, and ethnicity.

Another variation on the theme about neutrality is expressed by Will, who articulates a view about the substantive commitments of justice, rather than focusing on procedural fairness. He explicitly applies this view to pandemic response efforts such as vaccine allocation but does not limit the scope of the view to pandemic ethics. For him, this view captures the nature of justice in general. He argues that pursuit of equity is "ignoble" because it abandons the "aspiration of colorblind equality" in favor of social interventions that focus on race and ethnicity to promote equity. Will contends that a focus on equity deviates from the foundational moral ideal of *equal opportunity* and so is intrinsically condemnable—that it "reveals the nation's moral regression".[43] He also suggests that pursuit of equity will yield problematic consequences. He contends that race- and ethnicity- conscious interventions may stigmatize BIPOC populations and make them dependent upon "government-dispensed special privileges."[44] Some legal scholars echo this substantive embrace of neutrality, and argue that explicitly taking race into account in decision-making may constitute racial discrimination and so be illegal.[45] These scholars raise the possibility that doing so may even "pit the races against each other or otherwise significantly exacerbate racial tensions."[46]

In the remainder of this chapter, I will consider the types of approaches that may promote equity during pandemic and discuss the concern that such approaches may be discriminatory and so actually violate justice. This is certainly not the only controversy about the initiatives that might be adopted to promote equity, but it does go to the heart of what kinds of interventions are ethically permissible.

11.5 Can Neutral Interventions Promote Equity?

It should be noted that some neutral interventions—i.e., interventions that do not explicitly consider race or ethnicity—may reduce racial and ethnic disparities during pandemic. For example, elevated COVID-19 risk in BIPOC populations is associated, in part, with patterns of employment.

> Workers originally deemed essential are disproportionately racial or ethnic minorities, are paid low wages, and do not have the option of working from home. The primary source of SARS-CoV-2 [the virus that causes COVID-19] exposure for many of these workers is their workplace, where workspace design precludes social distancing, personal protective equipment (PPE) is absent or limited, and sanitation and ventilation are inadequate.[47]

Indeed, Miller, Wherry and Mazumder found significantly higher death rates among "people working in occupations without work-from-home options."[48] Michaels and Wagner argue that the US Occupational Health and Safety Administration (OSHA) should issue an Emergency Temporary Standard to require that employers implement effective workplace safety measures to reduce transmission of the virus.[49] OSHA's intervention would do nothing to address underlying racial and ethnic patterns of employment—and so would not promote equity long-term—but implementing and enforcing pandemic-specific safety requirements could significantly reduce workplace transmission of the virus. Although this intervention does not specifically target BIPOC populations, given the demographics of the essential workforce, it could mitigate disparities in exposure during the pandemic.

Similarly, BIPOC populations constitute a disproportionate share of the population in prisons and jails. Not surprisingly, correctional facilities have been COVID-19 hotspots, given that people live and work in very close quarters, and those detained cannot control their movements through the facility or exercise control to protect themselves.[50] Miller, Wherry and Mazumder document "particularly large increases [in death rates] ... among those living in correctional facilities...."[51] These elevated risks facing populations in prisons and jails have fueled calls to "release unnecessarily incarcerated people and improve healthcare and conditions of confinement."[52] These interventions do nothing to address the underlying racial and ethnic disparities in incarceration, and they do not protect only BIPOC individuals, but they may mitigate COVID-19 exposure risks for these populations.

Interventions that address disparities in access also may not directly target race or ethnicity. For example, in January 2021, in response to the "exceptional circumstances caused by the ongoing COVID-19 pandemic," President Biden issued an Executive Order creating a special enrollment period for individuals to seek health insurance coverage under the Affordable Care Act.[53] The administration extended this enrollment opportunity to all regardless of race or ethnicity, but the Executive Order acknowledges racial and ethnic disparities in pandemic outcomes, and notes that BIPOC individuals are more likely to be uninsured.[54]

Thus, it may be possible in some cases to promote equity for BIPOC populations in pandemic using neutral interventions. The initiatives offered as examples here directly address exposure and access issues in a race- and ethnicity- neutral way, but may mitigate racial and ethnic disparities given the makeup of the populations affected by these risks. Indeed, given that discussions of these exposure and access issues sometimes note a worry with racial and ethnic disparities, it may well be that part of the intention behind adopting the initiatives is to mitigate these disparities. Contrary to Will's view, the pursuit of equity does not always abandon colorblind equality. And although they may promote equity for BIPOC populations, these interventions are not discriminatory, given their neutrality. As Persad argues, "Policies justified by race-neutral goals that involve no individual racial classifications are effectively insulated from equal protection concerns even if they also narrow racial disparities."[55]

11.6 Beyond Neutrality

However, neutral interventions sometimes perpetuate inequity; at times, group conscious initiatives are required to address disparities. Gostin provides a compelling example to illustrate this reasoning: during a natural disaster such as a hurricane, neutral recommendations to evacuate, for example, fail to protect disadvantaged populations that lack mobility or transportation to comply.[56] The impact of Hurricane Katrina illustrates the inequitable consequences that may follow from reliance on neutral approaches.[57]

The necessity of tailoring interventions to the needs of particular communities can also be seen in the context of pandemic planning and response. For example, participants in a pandemic planning community engagement process in Minnesota

> felt that many access barriers could be alleviated through outreach efforts in communities and partnership with community organizations that understand and are trusted by their communities. Participants strongly emphasized the need to bring educational campaigns into individual communities to better inform residents about influenza, pandemic planning, and available community health services. They proposed that educational campaigns be offered in multiple languages with a variety of teaching strategies rather than consist merely of distribution of written materials. They also advised that information be disseminated in multiple venues—such as neighborhood hubs—rather than simply be posted to the Internet. To improve trust, participants felt strongly that educators should be culturally competent and represent diverse groups found in the communities where the educational campaigns

would be offered. Participants stressed that to address issues concerning trust, transportation, mobility, and distance to care, resources should be brought into local communities, easily accessible sites or mobile units should be used for distribution of resources, and collaborations with trusted community organizations should be developed for providing care.[58]

Access depends upon more than insurance coverage. Unlike the previous examples, the basic strategy recommended here is to tailor interventions to the language, culture and needs of particular racial, ethnic, or other groups, in order to facilitate access.

However, this does not mean that the interventions proposed offer special privileges to some populations that are denied to others, or that they serve some populations while excluding others. Thus, while these approaches may not be designed to be neutral with respect to race and ethnicity (or other relevant aspects of social identity such as class or gender identity), they would not thereby be discriminatory or pit one group against another, so long as they fit into an overall response effort that does not attend only to the needs of select groups and ignore others. Rather, they recognize that, to achieve a common (neutral) goal of promoting fair access to care for all (equal opportunity), different group-specific strategies need to be employed to meet the needs of different communities. Thus, although all the interventions discussed above may promote equity, none should be seen as discriminatory.

11.7 Equity and Allocation of Resources

Discussions about equity tend to become most contentious when they relate to allocation of scarce resources. Plans may be needed for rationing resources during pandemic because widespread illness can create surges in demand for healthcare resources that may exceed available supplies. Even if other resources never become scarce, allocation plans are needed for vaccines and new therapies developed to treat pandemic illness. As we have experienced during the COVID-19 pandemic, once vaccines or therapies are developed for the specific pandemic disease threat, supplies will initially be limited until enough can be produced to meet the need. Allocation in contexts of scarcity involves significant ethical issues.

> Under normal circumstances, clinical ethics focuses directly on the needs and wishes of the individual patient; resources are to be allocated to patients largely based on commitments to promote patient well-being and respect patient autonomy. … In public health crises involving significant shortages of resources, public health and health care systems become overwhelmed and the norms guiding care must shift to focus on community benefit rather than individual well-being or autonomy. From a moral point of view, such a shift is profound.…[59]

Ethicists and public health emergency response professionals describe this shift as a move from conventional standards of care to crisis standards of care (CSC).[60]

How should we understand equity in allocation decision-making? To put this in the context of the model of pandemic disparities offered by Blumenshine et al., allocation particularly relates to disparities in susceptibility to severe disease.[61] As we have seen, these disparities are connected to racial and ethnic disparities in underlying health status. But there is little that can be done once the pandemic begins to alter underlying health status—rates of asthma, heart disease, diabetes, and so on. Therefore, to affect disparities in susceptibility to severe disease, we need to address allocation of resources. We may be able to avert poor outcomes if we use available public health and healthcare resources to try to prevent infections from progressing to severe disease or resulting in death. Measures to promote equitable access to resources are relevant here. But when there are insufficient resources to meet need, access is not the only issue. Ethical guidance about who should receive priority in allocation to limited resources also becomes central.

Allocation could take race and ethnicity into account at two different levels. First, ethics guidance for allocation across populations sometimes recommends allocating greater amounts of the supply of scarce resources to geographic areas where more at-risk populations are located.

> Once at-risk groups are identified, distribution of resources such as vaccines and antivirals to sites across the state should track target groups. In other words, more resources should be sent to communities with greater numbers of prioritized recipients, so that those at highest priority have best access to the resources. … In contrast, if vaccine [for example] is shipped throughout the state in amounts proportional to area population, priority groups may not be reached as needed.[62]

Given that BIPOC populations face extremely high risk of poor outcomes, race and ethnicity could be considered (along with other factors) in decisions about geographic allocation of scarce resources. The principle justifying this type of distribution is neutral: distribute resources to promote access for populations at greatest risk of poor outcomes. Which populations confront greatest risk is an empirical matter; data should ground decision-making about distribution. Race and ethnicity should be factors in decision-making to the extent to which they are associated with elevated risk. This approach does not involve decision-making about which individuals should be allocated resources; it involves no "racial preference" or "special privileges"[63] in allocation of resources to individuals. Thus, this approach to geographic distribution should not be considered discriminatory from a moral perspective. It is beyond the scope of this chapter to analyze whether this approach would be deemed discriminatory from a legal point of view. As noted above, however, Persad maintains that initiatives "justified by race-neutral goals that involve no individual racial classifications"[64] would not be legally objectionable.

What about allocation of resources to individuals? Might it be morally permissible to consider race and ethnicity in these decisions? Some scholars argue that explicitly taking race into account in allocation decision-making constitutes racial discrimination and is most likely illegal. Schmidt, Gostin and Williams note that "[t]here is no direct precedent in which courts have considered race in allocating scarce health care resources."[65] Persad agrees.[66] However, as he explains,

> Currently, policies that treat individuals differently on the basis of race, even in order to address disparities, must satisfy "strict scrutiny": they must be narrowly tailored to satisfy a compelling governmental interest. While some policies have satisfied this exacting test, the

steep barrier strict scrutiny presents led it famously to be described as "strict in theory, fatal in fact."[67]

Existing precedent, "while not about the allocation of scarce medical resources, suggests that allocating scarce medical interventions based on individual patients' race would not pass legal muster."[68]

I aim to focus here, not on the question of whether allocation decisions that consider an individual's race and ethnicity are legal, but whether they are ethical. Sometimes law and ethics diverge in their determinations of the acceptability of practices. There may be a compelling argument for the moral appropriateness of race- and ethnicity-conscious allocation decisions, even if they would be illegal. Of course, it is important to understand the legal implications for such practices, as legal action against allocation plans could disrupt pandemic response in ways that ultimately work to the detriment of many patients. The legal analysis matters, but it is worth analyzing if it differs from an ethics analysis. Of course, Will's analysis is a moral one. On his view, taking race into account in allocating resources such as vaccines constitutes a "racial preference", and gives "special privileges" to some individuals over others based on their race or ethnicity. Since he believes that equal opportunity requires color-blindness, he views such "preference" as immoral.[69]

One might reject the consideration of race and ethnicity in individual allocation decisions out of a concern with procedural justice rather than the more substantive ideal of justice embraced by Will. Hodge and colleagues ground their argument in the nature of the decisions being considered in allocation. They explain that

> allocations of life-saving and other treatment resources at the bedside should be based on "individualized assessments of each patient" using the best available medical evidence concerning likelihood of death prior to, or imminently after, hospital discharge for the patient's diagnosis. .... CSC systems advocating for considering specific social groups (e.g., ethnicity, [Area Deprivation Index, which measures social vulnerability]) or relative age (e.g., prioritizing younger patients) are not making medical decisions, but rather expressing social priorities that require advance community assent and legal support.[70]

Essentially, Hodge and colleagues focus on neutral decision-making processes. They express concern about disparities but believe that it is more appropriate to address them using approaches other than factoring race and ethnicity into allocation decisions.[71]

On the other hand, some ethicists argue that to be equitable, allocation decisions should explicitly consider the race and ethnicity of patients needing care. Schmidt, Roberts and Eneanya contend that an approach to allocation which considers only data about the patient's health status favors patients who have benefitted from social advantage during their lives, given the link between underlying health conditions and systemic social (dis)advantage. They state that a critical question about the use of allocation scoring systems "is about the extent to which such approaches should be sensitive to, or ignore, social justice implications."[72]

Sederstrom maintains that allocation decisions must incorporate social justice considerations. She worries that many CSC plans are guided by one goal: to save the most lives. She considers how such a plan would handle allocation decisions for Black patients with underlying health conditions that raise their risk of poor COVID-19 outcomes. She illustrates with the case of a middle-aged Black patient who presents to the emergency department "with shortness of breath and clearly in distress."[73] Given his underlying health conditions, the patient faces substantial risk of death even if he is allocated to receive mechanical ventilation, such that he is categorized into the group of patients with the poorest prognosis. Since, in this scenario, ventilators are scarce and other patients are likely to fare better with treatment, the CSC plan recommends withholding the available ventilator from him to allocate it to a patient who is more likely to benefit. The case is undeniably tragic; Sederstrom maintains that it is also inequitable. Given that racial and ethnic disparities in underlying health status are connected to systemic disadvantage, she recommends that the CSC plan give this patient extra "points" in the triage calculation to counteract that disadvantage. This racial correction to his triage score would mean that he would not be grouped with the patients with the poorest prognosis, thus increasing his chances of being allocated a ventilator.[74] She maintains that her proposal "creates an opportunity to level the playing field," and describes it as "a form of medical reparations...."[75]

11.8 An Alternative Approach

The controversy over the ethical appropriateness of considering race and ethnicity in individual allocation decisions thus gets cast as a debate between those who appeal to equal opportunity or procedural justice to maintain that allocation decisions should be based solely upon race- and ethnicity- neutral clinical considerations, and those who embrace the moral appropriateness of a social justice goal such as reparations for health inequities. I believe that there is a middle ground: factoring race and ethnicity into clinical calculations to better capture and mitigate disparities in risk, without broadening allocation decision-making to include concern with reparations. To be clear: this analysis will not take a position on the moral permissibility (or obligatoriness) of reparations for health (or other) inequities. Rather, I will defend an alternative proposal for including race and ethnicity into allocation decisions as a way of promoting equity, one that I will argue is not discriminatory and should be acceptable even to those who embrace neutrality as a requirement of justice. I will illustrate this approach by talking about the allocation of two resources: monoclonal antibody therapies, and vaccines.

The U.S. Food and Drug Administration (FDA) has authorized the use of monoclonal antibodies (mAbs) for high-risk patients with mild to moderate COVID-19 and for post-exposure prophylaxis in some patients facing high risk of poor outcomes if they became infected.[76] In May 2021, the FDA provided updated guidance about what types of risk factors make patients eligible for mAbs.[77] In addition to providing a list of medical conditions that may substantially increase risk of poor outcomes with COVID-19—including immunosuppressive disease, diabetes, and chronic lung disease, among others—the FDA notes:

Other medical conditions or factors (for example, race or ethnicity) may also place individual patients at high risk for progression to severe COVID-19 and authorization of [mAbs] under the [Emergency Use Authorization] is not limited to the medical conditions or factors listed above.[78]

This guidance raised many questions for health care providers, given that it appears to deviate from standard clinical decision-making that considers only medical factors, not social ones such as race and ethnicity. Not only does the guidance appear to suggest that a patient could be eligible for mAbs based on their race or ethnicity alone when there is sufficient capacity to meet the needs of all patients seeking mAbs treatment, it also prompted many to ask whether race and ethnicity could, or should, factor into allocation decisions even in conditions of scarcity requiring rationing.

I will argue that race and ethnicity should factor into these allocation decisions. Clinicians may not be accustomed to explicitly considering race and ethnicity in the risk assessments that inform allocation decisions. However, the FDA's inclusion of race and ethnicity as risk factors reflects a great deal of evidence—some of which we have reviewed in this chapter—that BIPOC populations experience profound disparities in COVID-19 risk. The goal of mAbs therapy is to prevent infection, or progression of infection to severe disease or death, in populations at high risk of poor outcomes from COVID-19. All factors that significantly elevate risk should be considered in allocation, whether they are strictly clinical or social factors. The consideration of race and ethnicity in this situation promotes a neutral public health goal of mitigating clinical risk. They may be social factors but including them in allocation decision-making does not by itself transform those decisions to pursue social goals such as securing reparations for long-term structural disadvantage.

One might nevertheless object that, if structural disadvantage is associated with higher rates of underlying health conditions that increase COVID-19 risks, we should focus solely on those underlying health conditions, and not race or ethnicity, when we allocate mAbs. The problem with this approach is that these risk-elevating underlying conditions are underdiagnosed in BIPOC populations, given disparities in access to care, and disparities in quality of care.[79] Thus, limiting consideration to underlying health conditions when assessing a patient's risk factors will predictably result in underestimation of the risks for BIPOC populations, with the result that they will continue to be under-protected from risk. Thus, insisting on an allocation schema that is blind to race and ethnicity will perpetuate disparities in severe illness and death for these populations. One might further object that considering both race/ethnicity and underlying health conditions to assess a patient's risks will double count risk factors and so unfairly advantage these populations in allocation. However, the allocation model need not be additive this way—one point for race, one for cardiovascular disease, and so on. Moreover, no one objects when we consider both age and underlying conditions when we assess risks for elderly patients, although part of the reason age elevates risk may be the frequency of underlying conditions in elderly patients.[80]

Having all the factors that affect one's risk of poor outcomes considered in allocation decisions is not a special privilege, even if one of those factors is one's race or ethnicity. It is not a special privilege to take a patient's cardiovascular disease or chronic lung disease into account when allocating mAbs. Similarly, it is not a special privilege to take inclusion in BIPOC populations into account, given evidence of risk. White individuals are not unfairly denied privileges if their race is not considered among their other risk factors (e.g., cardiovascular disease, diabetes), because white race has not been shown to elevate COVID-19 risks. And White race does not deprioritize or exclude individuals for mAbs allocation; it simply does not prioritize them, because it is not associated with heightened risk. Although critics of race- and ethnicity- conscious allocation tend to compare it to affirmative action in education, the analogy does not hold given the model of allocation being proposed here. This is not "reverse discrimination"—it is not discrimination at all, from a moral point of view. It is the consideration of all factors that elevate risk of poor outcomes when allocating health resources geared toward preventing poor outcomes.

Given this, the argument in favor of considering race and ethnicity extends to vaccine allocation as well. Wrigley-Field and colleagues analyzed the impact on mortality of different vaccine allocation approaches. Using data from two states (California and Minnesota), they determined the consequences of the age-based plan for vaccine allocation that was used in these states (as was common across the US) for death across populations. They

> found that sequential age-based prioritization [-- vaccination that starts with the oldest people and progressively extends eligibility for younger groups --] alone would result in substantial racial/ethnic disparities in deaths averted. For example, vaccinating all people aged 75+ would have prevented nearly two-thirds of white COVID-19 deaths (CA: 65%; MN: 65%). Yet, for California and Minnesota respectively, this age-based prioritization alone would have prevented only 40% and 33% of Black COVID-19 deaths, 35% and 27% of Latino COVID-19 deaths, and 61% and 32% of Asian and Asian-American COVID-19 deaths…. These stark differences reflect both that the white population is substantially older than most BIPOC populations and that COVID-19 mortality reaches high levels at substantially younger ages in BIPOC populations…. Age-based prioritization therefore reduces much more of the total risk in white populations compared to BIPOC populations.[81]

They then compared these results to other potential allocation models to identify the model that best reduced risk of death across populations. First, they considered a schema that included younger BIPOC populations facing comparable risk of mortality to the age groups prioritized in the actual allocation plan. So, for example, this hypothetical plan would allocate to BIPOC individuals aged 50–64 at the same time as allocating to individuals aged 65–69, because those younger BIPOC populations face comparable risk of death to the older population. They "found that prioritizing vaccination for race-age groups with the highest risk would better target vaccination to high-risk individuals…"[82] However, recognizing the opposition to explicitly factoring race and ethnicity into allocation plans, they went on to consider other options as well. These other options promoted equity to a greater extent than age-based allocation, but typically did not address risk as well as the allocation model that explicitly factored race and ethnicity into eligibility.[83]

While this research considered the impact of these various vaccine allocation plans for only two states, it does provide evidence demonstrating that race- and ethnicity- conscious allocation plans can best mitigate risk, at least in some contexts. Given that vaccine allocation is meant to prioritize the populations facing highest risk, this study shows that the best way to achieve that end may be to factor race and ethnicity into allocation models. As with mAbs allocation, considering race and ethnicity in this context does not bestow special privileges on some races that are denied to others, any more than considering age bestows special privileges on some age groups. Considering race and ethnicity does not in any way alter the fundamental goal of allocation plans. Rather, it improves the ability of vaccine allocation to meet its goal, because it extends protection from risk to all populations facing comparable risk.

Contrary to Will's assumptions, this discussion of mAbs and vaccine allocation shows that pursuing equity does not necessarily constitute an abandonment of the ideal of equal opportunity. In both cases, explicitly considering race and ethnicity in allocation promotes equal opportunity for protection from risk. And despite Hodge and his colleagues' worries that consideration of social groups in allocation would mean that we would no longer be "making medical decisions, but rather expressing social priorities,"[84] that would not be the case when the overall goal of decision-making remains the minimization of severe illness and death. While Sederstrom's proposal for reparations in ventilator allocation[85] does appear to alter the nature and goals of the allocation process, the proposals for allocation of mAbs and vaccine that I have discussed above do not. I have not taken a stand on the question of whether altering the goals of allocation may be permissible. I simply mean to defend the moral appropriateness—indeed, I would argue, the moral obligatoriness—of one type of approach to promote equity in individual allocation by directly considering race and ethnicity, at least for some resources in some contexts. When the purpose of allocation is to mitigate risk, insisting on turning a blind eye to racial and ethnic disparities in risk to maintain neutrality in allocation decision-making would be unjust, and may "significantly exacerbate racial tensions."[86]

A note about data: the argument I have provided here depends upon evidence concerning racial and ethnic disparities in risk, as well as evidence that allocation would less effectively mitigate risk in BIPOC populations if we did not consider race and ethnicity in allocation decisions. At this point in the pandemic, there should be no doubt that substantial evidence solidly establishes disparities in risk. As for the effectiveness of allocation: the analysis provided by Wrigley-Field et al. provides extremely strong evidence that vaccine allocation would best address risk if it took race and ethnicity into account. We do not have quite the same kind of evidence for mAbs—that is, we have not analyzed the effects on hospitalization and death of differing mAbs allocation plans. I do not think that we need this level of evidence to say, with confidence, that we need to consider race and ethnicity in allocation plans. As I mention above, we have good reason to believe that allocating solely based on underlying conditions would under-protect BIPOC populations, given underdiagnosis of chronic conditions in those populations. Insisting that we not incorporate race and ethnicity into mAbs allocation decisions until we have even stronger evidence will likely result in unnecessary hospitalizations and deaths in these populations. We ought not to tolerate that outcome.

11.9 Conclusion

Ameliorating racial and ethnic inequities during pandemic will require addressing the disparities in exposure, susceptibility and access outlined by Blumenshine and colleagues. As we have seen, it is commonly held that justice requires the interventions we adopt to be neutral with respect to race and ethnicity, either to preserve fair decision-making processes, or to meet substantive requirements for equal opportunity. Given the dominance of these views of justice in our culture, it is important to determine their implications for the pursuit of equity.

Some interventions that are neutral with respect to race and ethnicity may nevertheless promote equity for BIPOC populations during pandemic. However, we will predictably fail to address pandemic disparities—and so will perpetuate them—if we insist on avoiding all explicit consideration of race and ethnicity.

I have argued that this neutral view of justice does not require this avoidance. It is a mistake to think that explicit consideration of race and ethnicity necessarily undermines what is fundamentally valued in this view of justice: fair, neutral processes or a commitment to equal opportunity. Color-blindness is not the central commitment of this view of justice; it is assumed to be necessary to promote fair process or equal opportunity. But that assumption is incorrect, at least in some circumstances. Indeed, for at least some interventions, preserving fair process and ensuring equal opportunity may *require* that we explicitly factor race and ethnicity into our decision-making. Unfortunately, this mistaken understanding of the requirements of justice misdirects our pursuit of equity—and undermines protection of health and life in BIPOC populations. Justice requires that we correct course—both during pandemic and in "normal" times.

Notes

1. US Centers for Disease Control and Prevention (CDC), "COVID Data Tracker Weekly Review, Interpretive Summary for July 16, 2021," https://www.cdc.gov/coronavirus/2019-ncov/covid-data/covidview/index.html.
2. CDC, "COVID Data Tracker United States at a Glance," last updated July 20, 2021, https://covid.cdc.gov/covid-data-tracker/#new-hospital-admissions.
3. CDC, "COVID Data Tracker Weekly Review July 16, 2021," https://www.cdc.gov/coronavirus/2019-ncov/covid-data/covidview/index.html.
4. Nalbandian et al. (2021).
5. Center on Budget and Policy Priorities, "Tracking the COVID-19 Recession's Effects on Food, Housing, and Employment Hardships," updated July 20, 2021, https://www.cbpp.org/research/poverty-and-inequality/tracking-the-covid-19-recessions-effects-on-food-housing-and.
6. Holt-Lunstad (2020).
7. CDC, "Risk for COVID-19 Infection, Hospitalization, and Death By Race/Ethnicity," updated June 17, 2021, https://www.cdc.gov/coronavirus/2019-ncov/covid-data/investigations-discovery/hospitalization-death-by-race-ethnicity.html#print.

8. CDC, "Disparities in COVID-19-Associated Hospitalizations: Racial and Ethnic Health Disparities," updated July 9, 2021, https://www.cdc.gov/coronavirus/2019-ncov/community/health-equity/racial-ethnic-disparities/disparities-hospitalization.html.
9. CDC, "Disparities in COVID-19-Associated Hospitalizations," https://www.cdc.gov/coronavirus/2019-ncov/community/health-equity/racial-ethnic-disparities/disparities-hospitalization.html.
10. CDC, "COVID-19: People with Certain Medical Conditions," updated May 13, 2021, https://www.cdc.gov/coronavirus/2019-ncov/need-extra-precautions/people-with-medical-conditions.html
11. Heslin and Hall (2021, 149–154).
12. Brown (2020).
13. CDC, "Disparities in COVID-19-Associated Hospitalizations: Racial and Ethnic Health Disparities," updated July 9, 2021, https://www.cdc.gov/coronavirus/2019-ncov/community/health-equity/racial-ethnic-disparities/disparities-hospitalization.html#print.
14. CDC, "Disparities in Deaths from COVID-19: Racial and Ethnic Health Disparities," updated December 10, 2020, https://www.cdc.gov/coronavirus/2019-ncov/community/health-equity/racial-ethnic-disparities/disparities-deaths.html#print.
15. CDC, "Disparities in Deaths from COVID-19: Racial and Ethnic Health Disparities," https://www.cdc.gov/coronavirus/2019-ncov/community/health-equity/racial-ethnic-disparities/disparities-deaths.html#print.
16. Wrigley-Field (2020, 21854).
17. Wrigley-Field (2020, 21854).
18. Wrigley-Field (2020, 21854–21855).
19. Wrigley-Field (2020, 21855).
20. Arias et al. (2020).
21. American Public Health Association, "Racism Is a Public Health Crisis," accessed July 21, 2021 at https://www.apha.org/topics-and-issues/health-equity/racism-and-health/racism-declarations.
22. Blumenshine et al. (2008, 709–715).
23. Blumenshine et al. (2008, 710–712).
24. See, for example, Quinn et al. (2011). See also Hutchins et al., on behalf of the Racial and Ethnic Minority Populations Subgroup of the Centers for Disease Control and Prevention's Pandemic Influenza Working Group on Vulnerable Populations (2009). Hutchins et al. do not explicitly discuss Blumenshine et al.'s model, but their findings about the factors that elevate risk overlap significantly with the model provided by Blumenshine et al.
25. Taubenberger et al. (2007, 2025).
26. Cheng et al. (2007, 683).
27. Kinlaw et al. (2009, S185–S192). Cf. Minnesota Department of Health (MDH), "Minnesota Crisis Standards of Care Framework: Ethical Guidance," updated: 01/10/2020, https://www.health.state.mn.us/communities/ep/surge/crisis/framework.pdf: 8–9.

28. Leider et al. (2017, e1–e9).
29. Valles (2020, 192, 208).
30. Maness et al. (2021, 18).
31. CDC National Center for Chronic Disease Prevention and Health Promotion, "Health Equity," page last reviewed March 11, 2020, https://www.cdc.gov/chronicdisease/healthequity/index.htm
32. US Department of Health and Human Services Office of Disease Prevention and Health Promotion, "Social Determinants of Health," accessed July 21, 2021 at https://www.healthypeople.gov/2020/topics-objectives/topic/social-determinants-of-health. See also Braveman (2012, 665–667). See also Singu et al. (2020).
33. Braveman et al. (2011, S150).
34. Braveman et al. (2011, S151).
35. Urban Institute, "Structural Racism in America," accessed July 21 2021 at https://www.urban.org/features/structural-racism-america
36. Braveman et al. (2011, S150).
37. Braveman et al. (2011, S151–S152).
38. CDC National Center for Chronic Disease Prevention and Health Promotion, "Health Equity."
39. Bruce and Tallman (2021, 209).
40. Kinlaw et al. (2009, S188).
41. Kinlaw et al. (2009, S188).
42. See comments to DeBruin (2021).
43. Will (2021).
44. Will (2021).
45. Persad (2021); cf. Schmidt et al. (2020).
46. Persad (2021, 1103).
47. Michaels and Wagner (2020, 1389).
48. Miller et al. (2021, 5).
49. Michaels and Wagner (2020, 1389–1390).
50. Franco-Paredes et al. (2021, e12).
51. Miller et al. (2021, 5).
52. Brennan Center for Justice, "Reducing Jail and Prison Populations During the Covid-19 Pandemic," last updated July 14, 2021, https://www.brennancenter.org/our-work/research-reports/reducing-jail-and-prison-populations-during-covid-19-pandemic. Cf. Franco-Paredes et al. (2021, e10–e15).
53. Biden Jr. (2021).
54. Biden Jr. (2021).
55. Persad (2021, 1112).
56. Gostin (2007, 3).
57. Van Spall et al. (2020, 3390–3393).
58. DeBruin et al. (2012, 589).
59. DeBruin and Leider (2020, 306).
60. DeBruin and Leider (2020, 307). Cf. Institute of Medicine (2012).

61. Considerations other than susceptibility may be relevant, however. For example, in some circumstances, workers who provide services in high-risk settings should be prioritized for access to resources given their exposure risks. We owe them protection because they take on risk to serve the community.
62. DeBruin et al. (2010, 38).
63. Will (2021).
64. Persad (2021, 1112).
65. Schmidt et al. (2020, 2023).
66. Persad (2021, 1101).
67. Persad (2021, 1101). Cf. Schmidt et al. (2020, 2024).
68. Persad (2021, 1103). Cf. Schmidt et al. (2020, 2024).
69. Will (2021).
70. Hodge Jr. et al. (2021, 3).
71. Hodge Jr. et al. (2021, 2).
72. Schmidt et al. (2020, 4).
73. Nneka Sederstrom, "The 'Give Back': Is There Room for It?" posted July 16, 2020, https://www.bioethics.net/2020/07/the-give-back-is-there-room-for-it/.
74. Nneka Sederstrom, "The 'Give Back': Is There Room for It?" posted July 16, 2020, https://www.bioethics.net/2020/07/the-give-back-is-there-room-for-it/.
75. Sederstrom and Wiggleton-Little (2021, 30).
76. U.S. Food and Drug Administration (FDA), Letter to Yunji Kim, PharmD, Regeneron Pharmaceuticals, Inc. (July 30, 2021), https://www.fda.gov/media/145610/download. See also FDA, Letter to Christine Phillips, PhD, RAC, Eli Lilly and Company (February 9, 2021), www.fda.gov/media/145801/download.
77. FDA, "Fact Sheet for Health Care Providers Emergency Use Authorization (EUA) of Bamlanivimab and Etesevimab" (May 2021), www.fda.gov/media/145802/download. See also FDA, "Fact Sheet for Health Care Providers Emergency Use Authorization (EUA) of Regen-Covtm (casirivimab and imdevimab)" (June 2021), www.fda.gov/media/145611/download.
78. FDA, "Fact Sheet for Health Care Providers Emergency Use Authorization (EUA) of Bamlanivimab and Etesevimab." See also FDA, "Fact Sheet for Health Care Providers Emergency Use Authorization (EUA) of Regen-Covtm (casirivimab and imdevimab)."
79. Singu et al. (2020, 3–4). See also Agency for Healthcare Research and Quality (2020, D2).
80. Mueller et al. (2020).
81. Wrigley-Field et al. (2021, 2–3).
82. Wrigley-Field et al. (2021, 3).
83. Wrigley-Field et al. (2021, 2–3).
84. Hodge Jr. et al. (2021, 3).
85. Nneka Sederstrom, "The 'Give Back': Is There Room for It?" posted July 16, 2020, https://www.bioethics.net/2020/07/the-give-back-is-there-room-for-it/. See also Sederstrom and Wiggleton-Little (2021).
86. Persad (2021, 1103).

Acknowledgment I would like to thank the members of the Minnesota COVID Ethics Collaborative for rich discussions of equity matters in COVID-19 response over the course of this pandemic. I would like to especially acknowledge JP Leider, PhD, for conversations about these issues (and many others in the ethics of disaster response) over the course of several years. While I certainly benefitted from their thoughtful engagement, my views in this chapter are my own. These colleagues have not reviewed or endorsed the analysis I provide in this chapter, and all of the errors herein are mine.

References

Agency for Healthcare Research and Quality. 2020. 2019 National Healthcare Quality and Disparities Report, December.

Arias, Elizabeth, Betzaida Tejada-Vera, Farida Ahmad, and Kenneth D. Kochanek. 2021. Provisional Life Expectancy Estimates for 2020. Vital Statistics Rapid Release report no. 015. https://www.cdc.gov/nchs/data/vsrr/vsrr015-508.pdf.

Biden, Joseph R., Jr. 2021. Executive Order on Strengthening Medicaid and the Affordable Care Act. January 28. https://www.whitehouse.gov/briefing-room/presidential-actions/2021/01/28/executive-order-on-strengthening-medicaid-and-the-affordable-care-act/.

Blumenshine, Philip, Arthur Reingold, Susan Egerter, Robin Mockenhaupt, Paula Braveman, and James Marks. 2008. Pandemic Influenza Planning in the United States from a Health Disparities Perspective. *Emerging Infectious Diseases* 14 (5): 709–715.

Braveman, Paula A. 2012. Health Inequalities by Class and Race in the US: What Can We Learn from the Patterns? *Social Science and Medicine* 54 (5): 665–667.

Braveman, Paula A., Shiriki Kumanyika, Jonathan Fielding, Thomas LaVeist, Luisa N. Borrell, Ron Manderscheid, and Adewale Troutman. 2011. Health Disparities and Health Equity: The Issue is Justice. *American Journal of Public Health* 101 (Suppl. 1): S150.

Brown, Steven. 2020. The COVID-19 Crisis Continues to Have Uneven Economic Impact by Race and Ethnicity. Urban Wire: The Blog of the Urban Institute, July 1. https://www.urban.org/urban-wire/covid-19-crisis-continues-have-uneven-economic-impact-race-and-ethnicity.

Bruce, Lori, and Ruth Tallman. 2021. Promoting Racial Equity in COVID-19 Resource Allocation. *Journal of Medical Ethics* 47: 208–212.

Cheng, Vincent C.C., Susanna K.P. Lau, Patrick C.Y. Woo, and Kwok Yung Yuen. 2007. Severe Acute Respiratory Syndrome Coronavirus as an Agent of Emerging and Reemerging Infection. *Clinical Microbiology Reviews* 20 (4): 683.

DeBruin, Debra A. 2021. Speed Should Not Overrun Ethics in Vaccine Rollout. *Star Tribune*, January 29. https://www.startribune.com/editorial-counterpoint-speed-should-not-overrun-ethics-in-vaccine-rollout/600016774/?refresh=true.

DeBruin, Debra A., and Jonathon P. Leider. 2020. COVID-19: The Shift from Clinical to Public Health Ethics. *Journal of Public Health Management and Practice* 26 (4): 306.

DeBruin, Debra A., Mary Faith Marshall, Elizabeth Parilla, Joan Liaschenko, J.P. Leider, Donald J. Brunnquell, J. Eline Garrett, and Dorothy E. Vawter. 2010. Implementing Ethical Frameworks for Rationing Scarce Health Resources in Minnesota During Severe Influenza Pandemic, 38. https://www.health.state.mn.us/communities/ep/surge/crisis/implement.pdf.

DeBruin, Debra A., Joan Liaschenko, and Mary Faith Marshall. 2012. Social Justice in Pandemic Preparedness. *American Journal of Public Health* 102: 586–591.

Franco-Paredes, Carlos, Nazgol Ghandnoosh, Hassan Latif, Martin Krsak, Andres F. Henao-Martinez, Megan Robins, Lilian Vargas Barahona, and Eric M. Poeschla. 2021. Decarceration and Community Re-entry in the COVID-19 Era. *The Lancet Infectious Diseases* 21: e12.

Gostin, Lawrence O. 2007. Why Should We Care About Social Justice? *Hastings Center Report* 37 (4): 3.

Heslin, Kevin C., and Jeffrey E. Hall. 2021. Sexual Orientation Disparities in Risk Factors for Adverse COVID-19-Related Outcomes, by Race/Ethnicity—Behavioral Risk Factor Surveillance System, United States, 2017–2019. *Morbidity and Mortality Weekly Report (MMWR)* 70 (5) (February 5): 149–154. https://www.cdc.gov/mmwr/volumes/70/wr/mm7005a1.htm.

Hodge, James G., Jr., Dan Hanfling, John L. Hick, and Jennifer L. Piatt. 2021. Diminishing Disparities in U.S. Crisis Standards of Care: Medical and Legal Challenges. *EClinicalMedicine—The Lancet* 34: 3.

Holt-Lunstad, Julianne, 2020. The Double Pandemic of Social Isolation And COVID-19: Cross-Sector Policy Must Address Both. Health Affairs Blog, June 22. https://www.healthaffairs.org/do/10.1377/hblog20200609.53823#:~:text=Immediate%20effects%20of%20social%20isolation,emotional%20or%20overeating%2C%20may%20increase.

Hutchins, Sonja S., Kevin Fiscella, Robert S. Levine, Danielle C. Ompad, and Marian McDonald. 2009. Protection of Racial/Ethnic Minority Populations During an Influenza Pandemic. *American Journal of Public Health* 99 (S2): S261–S270.

Institute of Medicine. 2012. *Crisis Standards of Care: A Systems Framework for Catastrophic Disaster Response*, vol. 1. Washington, DC: The National Academies Press.

Kinlaw, Kathy, Drue H. Barrett and Robert J. Levine. 2009. Ethical Guidelines in Pandemic Influenza: Recommendations of the Ethics Subcommittee of the Advisory Committee of the Director, Centers for Disease Control and Prevention. *Disaster Medicine and Public Health Preparedness* 3 (Suppl. 2): S185–S192.

Leider, J.P., Debra DeBruin, Nicole Reynolds, Angelica Koch, and Judy Seaburg. 2017. Ethical Guidance for Disaster Response, Specifically Around Crisis Standards of Care: A Systematic Review. *American Journal of Public Health* 107 (9): e1–e9.

Maness, Sarah B., Laura Merrell, Erika L. Thompson, Stacey B. Griner, Nolan Kline, and Christopher Wheldon. 2021. Social Determinants of Health and Health Disparities: COVID-19 Exposures and Mortality Among African American People in the United States. *Public Health Reports* 136 (1): 18.

Michaels, David, and Gregory R. Wagner. 2020. Occupational Safety and Health Administration (OSHA) and Worker Safety During the COVID-19 Pandemic. *Journal of the American Medical Association* 324 (14): 1389–1390.

Miller, Sarah, Laura R. Wherry, and Bhashkar Mazumder. 2021. Estimated Mortality Increases During the COVID-19 Pandemic by Socioeconomic Status, Race and Ethnicity. *Health Affairs* 40 (8): 5.

Mueller, Amber L., Maeve S. McNamara, and David A. Sinclair. 2020. Why Does COVID-19 Disproportionately Affect Older People? *Aging* 12 (10): 9959–9981.

Nalbandian, Ani, Kartik Sehgal, Aakriti Gupta, et al. 2021. Post-acute COVID-19 Syndrome. *Nature Medicine* 27: 601–615.

Persad, Govind. 2021. Allocating Medicine Fairly in an Unfair Pandemic. *University of Illinois Law Review* 2021 (3): 1085–1134.

Quinn, Sandra Crouse, Supriya Kumar, Vicki S. Freimuth, Donald Musa, Nestor Casteneda-Angarita, and Kelley Kidwell. 2011. Racial Disparities in Exposure, Susceptibility, and Access to Health Care in the US H1N1 Influenza Pandemic. *American Journal of Public Health* 101 (2): 285–293.

Schmidt, Harald, Lawrence O. Gostin, and Michelle A Williams. 2020. Is It Lawful and Ethical to Prioritize Racial Minorities for COVID-19 Vaccines? *Journal of the American Medical Association* 324 (20): 2023–2024.

Schmidt, Harald, Dorothy E. Roberts, and Nwamaka D. Eneanya. 2021. Rationing, Racism and Justice: Advancing the Debate Around 'Colourblind' COVID-19 Ventilator Allocation. *Journal of Medical Ethics* 48 (21): 126–130.

Sederstrom, Nneka, and Jada Wiggleton-Little. 2021. Acknowledging the Burdens of 'Blackness'. *HEC Forum* 33: 19–33.

Singu, Sravani, Arpan Acharya, Kishore Challagundla, and Siddappa N. Byrareddy. 2020. Impact of Social Determinants of Health on the Emerging COVID-19 Pandemic in the United States. *Frontiers in Public Health* 8: article 406.

Taubenberger, Jeffery K., David M. Morens, and Anthony S. Fauci. 2007. The Next Influenza Pandemic: Can It Be Predicted? *Journal of the American Medical Association* 297 (18): 2025.

Valles, Sean A. 2020. The Predictable Inequities of COVID-19 in the US: Fundamental Causes and Broken Institutions. *Kennedy Institute of Ethics Journal* 30 (3–4): 191–214.

Van Spall, Harriette G.C., Clyde W. Yancy, and Keith C. Ferdinand. COVID-19 and Katrina: Recalcitrant Racial Disparities. *European Heart Journal* 41 (36) (September 21): 3390–3393.

Will, George. 2021. Pursuing Equity Over Equality Reveals the Nation's Moral Regression. *The Washington Post*, July 30. https://www.washingtonpost.com/opinions/2021/07/30/pursuing-equity-over-equalityreveals-nations-moral-regression/.

Wrigley-Field. Elizabeth. 2020. US Racial Inequality May Be as Deadly as COVID-19. *PNAS (Proceedings of the National Academy of Sciences of the United States of America)* 117 (36): 21854–21856.

Wrigley-Field, Elizabeth, Mathew V. Kiang, Alicia R. Riley, Magali Barbieri, Yea-Hung Chen, Kate A. Duchowny, Ellicott C. Matthay, David Van Riper, Kirrthana Jegathesan, Kirsten Bibbins-Domingo, and Jonathon P. Leider. 2021. Geographically-Targeted COVID-19 Vaccination Is More Equitable and Averts More Deaths Than Age-based Thresholds Alone. *Science Advances* 7 (40): eabj2099. https://doi.org/10.1126/sciadv.abj2099.

Chapter 12
COVID-19 in Skilled Nursing Homes and Other Long-Term Care Facilities (LTCFs): Could Stronger Public-Health Measures Have Made a Difference?

Rosemarie Tong

Abstract As a result of co-chairing the North Carolina Institute of Medicine/Department of Public Health Task Force on Ethics and Pandemic Influenza Planning in 2007, I had the opportunity to learn a great deal about how a major pandemic would be ethically challenging. For the most part, the NC Ethics Task Force provided good ethical guidelines for determining health care workers' and "critical-industry" employees' responsibilities to work during a life-threatening pandemic. It also produced good ethical advice for balancing the protection of individuals' rights against the maintenance of society's welfare in a pandemic, and for prioritizing the use of limited health care resources in a pandemic. However, the NC Ethics Task Force failed to consider in any detail how residents in long-term care facilities (LTCFs) might be disproportionately impacted by a virus like the avian flu, let alone by a virus like COVID-19. Had LTCFs received and followed clearer public health guidelines, recommendations, and mandatory rules from the inception of COVID-19, they might have better served their vulnerable population. But "politics" was pitted against "science" with respect to even the most basic public health measures—wearing a mask, practicing social distancing, hand washing, and avoiding large group activities.

Keywords COVID-19 · 2007 North Carolina Ethics Task Force on public health measures during a pandemic · Health care workers' responsibilities in a pandemic · Critical industry workers' responsibilities in a pandemic · Individual rights versus social welfare in a pandemic · Prioritizing limited health care resources in a pandemic · Long-term care facilities (LTCFs) · Long-term care industry · Ethical ideals versus political pressures · Ethics of justice · Ethics of care

In 2007 I had the privilege to co-chair with Leah Devlin[1] the North Carolina Institute of Medicine, Department of Public Health Task Force on Ethics and Pandemic

---

R. Tong (✉)
Department of Philosophy and Healthcare Ethics, Center for Professional and Applied Ethics, Charlotte, USA
e-mail: rotong@uncc.edu

© The Author(s), under exclusive license to Springer Nature Switzerland AG 2022
M. Boylan (ed.), *Ethical Public Health Policy Within Pandemics*, The International Library of Bioethics 95, https://doi.org/10.1007/978-3-030-99692-5_11

Influenza Planning.[2] At that time, I was both the Distinguished Professor of Healthcare Ethics at the University of North Carolina, Charlotte (UNCC) and the Director of its Center for Professional and Applied Ethics (CPAE).[3] The NC Ethics Task Force was convened to address concerns that the H1N1/HFN1 virus, colloquially known as the avian flu, might morph into a full-scale pandemic. Several years before the avian flu threatened the United States, Canada had direct experience with the SARS (Severe Acute Respiratory Syndrome) pandemic, a virus it was able to control within a relatively short amount of time.[4] Wanting to be maximally prepared for a virus, potentially more contagious and deadly than SARS, NC public health officials and clinicians discussed with their Canadian counterparts their SARS' successes and failures. Noteworthy about the NC Task Force was its desire to stockpile *ethical* guidelines in advance of a possible pandemic at least as bad as SARS if not worse. Not wanting to wait until the last minute before a severe influenza pandemic hit, the NC Ethics Task Force aimed to develop objective ethical criteria for handling the kind of emotional questions typically raised during a pandemic, especially the question of who shall live when not all can live.

Members of the NC Ethics Task Force included faith community leaders, physicians, nurses, epidemiologists, social workers, ethicists, maternal and childhood development experts, food supply administrators, transportation officials, advocates for persons with disabilities, energy executives, community preparedness and disaster managers, school superintendents, public health authorities, an administrator of a rehabilitation and healthcare facility, and a representative from the American Association of Retired Persons (AARP). No doubt, this list of experts is impressive and inclusive, but looking back at it through the lens of the COVID-19 pandemic, I think the NC Task Force lacked an adequate number of representatives from skilled nursing homes, assisted living facilities, correctional institutions, and other congregate living centers. Had we had more representation from these groups, we may have produced a more complete set of ethical guidelines not only for the avian flu but also for the COVID-19 influenza pandemic that hit North Carolina, the United States, and the world.

In this chapter, I will share the NC Ethics Task Force's ethical considerations on four matters: (1) healthcare workers' responsibility to provide care during an influenza pandemic; (2) responsibility of workers in critical industries to work during an influenza pandemic; (3) balancing the rights of the individual and the need to protect the public; and (4) prioritization and use of limited resources during an influenza pandemic. For the most part, the NC Ethics Task Force provided good ethical guidelines for managing these four matters, but its "crystal ball" failed to see that residents in long-term care facilities (LTCFs), and other congregate living facilities like prisons and homeless shelters would be disproportionality impacted by COVID-19. Thus, any future NC Ethics Task Force would need to look longer and harder at the members of these vulnerable populations, especially the 75 + population in LTCF's. The residents of these establishments are getting older, sicker, and more cognitively impaired. Moreover, they are growing in number. By 2060 the number of Americans age 65 and older is projected to double from 52 to 95 million, meaning that this age group will constitute 23% of the US population.[5] At present, there are approximately 15,505 nursing homes in the United States.[6] In addition, there are approximately 28,900 assisted living residences.[7] Because more and more US people are living to 80, 90, or even 100, the supply of LTCFs will have to increase substantially to meet the projected demand for them.

12.1 Introduction

Stockpiling Solutions: North Carolina's Ethical Guidelines for an Influenza Pandemic[8] was written in the event that the H1N1/H5N1 strain of avian flu would hit the state of North Carolina dramatically. The virus didn't do this, but fear of it gave North Carolina the opportunity to ask many what-if questions about the avian flu. According to the *Stockpiling Solutions* authors, "there are typically three influenza pandemics every century."[9] The twentieth century saw the Spanish Flu (H1N1 virus) between 1918 and 1919; the Asian Influenza (H2N2 virus) between 1957 and 1958; and the Hong Kong Influenza (H3N2 virus) between 1968 and 1969.[10] The first of these pandemics led to 675,000 fatalities in the United States; the second to 7000 fatalities; and the third to 34,000 fatalities.[11]

The editor of this anthology, Michael Boylan, Ph.D., refers to the Spanish Flu (but neither to the Asian influenza nor to the Hong Kong Influenza) as a twentieth century pandemic in his very helpful chapter on the ethics of public health. As a matter of conjecture, Boylan may have glossed over the Asian and Hong Kong influenzas because they resulted in relatively few US fatalities. Interestingly and rightly, Boylan counts HIV-AIDS, from 1981 to 2021 and beyond as a twentieth/twenty-first century pandemic.[12] He notes that between 1981 and 2006, 500,000 Americans died from HIV-AIDS, making it a close runner-up to the Spanish flu in terms of fatalities.[13] As he sees it, HIV-AIDS in the United States would have been far less deadly had it not been associated with "sex, homosexuality, and intravenous drug use."[14] Boylan also includes Ebola in 1975, 2014, and 2019 as a twentieth/twenty-first century pandemic.[15] This especially deadly and contagious disease was not considered by the NC Ethics Task Force probably because Ebola has been confined mostly to West Africa where there have been approximately 12,000 to 15,000 fatalities.[16] Both Boylan and the NC Ethics Task Force counted Severe Acute Respiratory Syndrome (SARS) in 2003 as a twenty-first century pandemic. Although 192 cases of SARS and no fatalities were documented in the United States,[17] 438 cases of SARS and 44 fatalities were documented in Canada.[18] The NC Ethics Task Force was particularly interested in Canada's response to SARS, viewing it as an opportunity to prepare North Carolina *ethically* as well as *epidemiologally* for an outbreak of the avian flu.[19] As it turned out, the avian flu had very little impact on either the United States or North Carolina.[20] But the same cannot be said for the COVID-19 pandemic of 2020 to 2021.

Before COVID-19 arrived in the United States via a Washington state passenger on a plane headed back home from Wuhan China, the WHO estimated that "a new influenza pandemic in the United States would lead to approximately 45 million outpatient visits, 865,000 to 9,900,000 hospitalizations, and 209,000 to 1, 903,000 deaths."[21] By January 31, 2021, the WHO's forecast was alarmingly on target. There have been 110 million cases of COVID-19 worldwide and 2.4 million deaths since February 2020.[22] During the same period of time, there were 25.7 million cases of COVID-19 and 431,882 deaths in the United States.[23] In the state of North Carolina alone, there were 759,955 cases of COVID-19, resulting in 9381 deaths.[24] At the national level, 120,000 of all COVID-19 deaths occurred in LTCFs[25]; and at the state level, 40% of all COVID-19 deaths occurred in the same.[26] Although there are now several vaccines available for COVID-19 with as much as 95% efficacy, the roll out of these life-saving pharmaceuticals has been slower than originally anticipated.[27] Still there is good reason to believe that these vaccines will be able to control the spread of COVID-19 in the world, the United States, and North Carolina, but not before millions more people are infected with the virus and thousands more die from it. Until enough Americans are vaccinated to achieve herd immunify, US public health officials advise people to wear masks, practice social distancing, and sanitize their hands frequently. Moreover, because it is still not known whether vaccinated individuals can be carriers of COVID-19,[28] vigilance seems to be the order of the day as new strains of COVID-19 are reported around the world.[29] At this point in the pandemic, it is anyone's guess whether the vaccines already developed for COVID-19 can also protect people from COVID-19 variants.[30]

12.2 Healthcare Workers' Responsibility to Provide Care During an Influenza Pandemic

Examining the guidelines of the 2007 NC Ethics Task Force for healthcare workers' responsibility to provide care during an influenza pandemic, it is clear that most of them applied to *licensed* healthcare personnel like physicians, nurses, and psychologists. Some mention was made of nurse aides,[31] most likely Certified Nurse Assistants (CNAs) who do not have licenses. As the North Carolina Ethics Task Force saw it, all healthcare personnel (licensed or non-licensed) have an ethical responsibility to perform their regular employment duties during a pandemic and to help out with work they ordinarily do not do should a need arise.[32] But surveys available in 2007 indicated that not all licensed healthcare personnel would agree with this observation. A 2003 survey of US physicians "found that 80% of physicians "were willing to continue to care for patients in the event of a potentially deadline outbreak.""[33] Less (55%) thought "there was a duty to treat patients when endangering one's own health; fewer still (40%) were willing to put themselves at risk of contracting a deadly illness to save other lives."[34] Like physicians, nurses were ambivalent about working during a pandemic, and this despite the fact that refusing to care for COVID-19 patients could result in disciplinary measures unless, for example, nurses weren't given N95 masks to protect themselves, their patients, and their loved ones from COVID-19.[35] In order to ameliorate safety fears among physicians and nurses, the NC Ethics Task Force promised them that in return for their willingness to do hazardous work, they would be given priority status for personal protective equipment (PPE), COVID-19 tests, anti-virals, ventilators, ICU beds, ventilators, and vaccines. As the NC Ethics Task Force saw it, this quid pro quo arrangement was fair[36]; and, as it turned out, this arrangement kept a very high percentage of NC physicians and nurses at their posts during the current COVID-19 pandemic.[37]

Although the NC Ethics Task Force spoke in considerable detail about physicians' and nurses' duties in hospitals, it did not say much, if anything, about the unlicensed healthcare workers that staff nursing homes and other LTCFs. Typically, most of the direct care work done in these establishments is done by certified nurse assistants (CNAs), supervised by relatively few registered nurses (RNs) and a physician who may only be available on call. CNAs get anywhere from 75 h to three-months training, but in a crisis, "nurse aides" with as little as eight hours of training may care for residents.[38] The median wage of these workers is $13.48 an hour.[39] Most of them are women and many of them are members of US racial and ethnic minorities.[40] In a growing number of cases, however, many direct caregivers are immigrants who may or may not be able to speak fluent English.[41]

Because the pay is so low (an average of $28,980)[42] and the work so physically taxing and emotionally stressful, a significant number of nursing home staff leave as soon as they are able to get a higher paying, less demanding job, often in retail stores or even fast-food restaurants.[43] However, other direct caregivers in nursing homes can't imagine doing anything other than eldercare. They love the work, but cannot get enough hours at any one LTCF to earn a living wage. It is not unusual for such workers to clock in for a morning shift at a nursing home, drive to an assisted living facility for an afternoon shift, and then drive again to deliver several hours of home healthcare.[44] Such a schedule is grueling for direct caregivers, especially if they have small children or elderly relatives back at home with special care needs. Moreover, it is anxiety-producing for them, if they have concerns about jeopardizing not only their own health but that of their loved ones. A registered nurse in a LTCF may also have the same worries, but she will not be doing jobs like diapering, showering, and feeding residents. Moreover, she will also be earning much more than the CNAs or other less credentialed caregivers she manages. The median salary for RNs in the United States is $35.17 per hour[45] and that of physicians is $100.00 per hour.[46]

Because the primary focus of the NC Ethics Task Force was on hospitals, it did not offer enough specific ethical guidelines for LTCFs, and this despite the fact that, even in a non-pandemic situation, many elderly and disabled people see-saw between a LTCF and one or more hospitals routinely. This back-and-forth motion is rooted in a perverse relationship between Medicare and Medicaid funding.

According to the AARP, the bills of three-fifths of a typical nursing home's population are paid by Medicaid, the US federal-state healthcare insurance program for poor people. This program gives the nursing home about $200 dollars a day per Medicaid resident, not nearly enough to cover his or her care, yet alone keep the nursing home financially afloat.[47] Where the typical nursing home makes its money is from the other two-fifths of its population. Medicare, the US healthcare insurance program for elderly and disabled people, provides an average of $535 dollars per resident for up to 100 days after a hospital stay. If a Medicare resident at a nursing home gets ill after these 100 days, they can be transferred back to the hospital. If they get well enough, they can then be transferred back to the nursing home for rehabilitation up to another 100 days and so on. Because $535 per Medicare resident covers their care and then some, says Harris Meyer, "nursing homes rely on a relatively small number of well-paying residents to make up for the money they say they lose on the rest."[48] During the COVID-19 pandemic, elective surgeries were postponed and hospitals admitted only the worst cases of COVID-19, thereby shrinking nursing homes' supply of Medicare-funded residents, a situation which weakened their ability to provide quality care to their Medicaid patients.[49]

Realizing that the see-sawing described above needed to be halted as the number of COVID-19 victims in nursing homes and hospitals swelled, public health officials issued guidelines for limiting the transfer of COVID-19 residents to hospitals and accepting COVID-19 patients from them.[50] Around the same time, they also realized that it was not so much the residents of nursing homes and assisted living facilities who were giving staff COVID-19 but vice versa.[51] Although the Centers for Medicare and Medicaid Services (CMS) and the Center for Disease Control (CDC) were slow in issuing guidelines for testing the residents and staff of nursing homes,[52] they eventually determined that testing, testing, and then some more testing was the best way to halt the spread of COVID-19 in nursing homes and other LTCFs. However, these two federal public healthcare agencies urged LTCFs to test their residents and staff with the slower and costlier Polymerase Chain Reaction (PCR) method as opposed to the quicker and less expensive antigen method. Supposedly, the former testing method is more accurate than the latter testing method. Although quick turnover tests made more sense to LTCF administrators than slow PCR tests, many states nonetheless required them to use the PCR method of testing and pay for a considerable percentage of its costs.[53] Similarly, both federal and state agencies were slow to send nursing homes adequate Personal Protective Equipment (PPE), masks for residents, and other supplies.[54] On the plus side, because many nursing homes and other LTCFs had experience with quarantining or isolating infectious residents, they were quick to designate whole wings of their establishments for COVID-19 positive residents, as well as those with severe symptoms of COVID-19. Unfortunately, about one-third of a typical nursing home's residents are cognitively impaired. Many of them can't understand the benefits of quarantine, isolation, or testing. Neither can they understand the value of mask-wearing, social-distancing, and hand-sanitizing. In worst case scenarios, pharmacological treatment may need to be used "when individuals living with dementia have severe symptoms or have the potential to harm themselves or others."[55] Physical restraints should be avoided altogether.[56]

Although staff-turnover rates are high in the best of times in nursing homes, they are even higher in the worst of times.[57] Still, CNAs will stay at their jobs if properly motivated. Higher wages and better work conditions are, of course, appreciated by those at the bottom of a LTCF's hierarchy, but so is a pervasive ethics of care. For example, at a 60-bed nursing home in Georgia, its administrators joined with a team of nurses, nurse-aids, and other employees, including a maintenance technician for an 11-week "lock in."[58] This group of 33 dedicated care workers moved into Pebblebrook at Park Springs nursing home in Stone Mountain, Georgia, sleeping in spare rooms, on air mattresses, or in tents in order to keep their establishment COVID-19 free and their families back at home safe. Blessed with the support of Pebblebrook's owners who fed the team, paid them overtime, and gave them a bonus, the nursing home remained COVID-19 free while administrators figured out ways to manage the establishment in a less restrictive manner.[59] The fact that the administrators joined with their staff in the "lock in" explains to a great degree why it worked. The team truly felt like a family whose members were equally valued for their unique contribution to the good of all, especially the residents of the nursing home. The nursing home administrators made it clear that they were no better than their staff, providing an example for all to emulate.

12.3 Responsibility of Workers in Critical Industries During an Influenza Pandemic

The NC Ethics Task Force referred to the US Department of Homeland Security's list of 17 critical industries in a disaster to determine which of them would be most essential in a pandemic. On the list of these critical industries was "public health and healthcare personnel.[60] Unlike public health and healthcare personnel, especially licensed ones, many other critical workers do not have a special obligation to risk their health and lives for the common good. But they may have a contractual obligation to keep on working under adverse conditions so that society does not collapse. One thinks here of food providers, energy suppliers, police officers, fire fighters and so forth. Such critical workers may lose their jobs if they fail to be on call during an influenza pandemic. The NC Ethics Task Force stressed that because of such possible penalties, "employers should be sensitive to the appearance of favoritism or inequity that could result if only lower-paid employees are required to work on-site while the higher-paid executives or managerial staff is allowed to work off-site."[61] In other words, "decisions about who must work on-site and who may work off-site should be guided solely by the responsibilities of the job and not by salaries, job titles, or any other aspects unrelated to job functions."[62]

In the abstract, this arrangement sounds fine, but, in reality, most white-collar jobs can be done off-site, while almost all blue-collar jobs have to be done on site. The NC Ethics Task Force considered the food industry in particular. Shelf stockers and cashiers have to work on-site and, for all practical purposes, so do managers (but not owners). In an effort to protect both customers and employees from COVID-19, groceries began to offer more in the way of contact-free home deliveries and curbside pick-ups. Some of them even adopted a credit-card only policy, thus avoiding potentially dangerous cash transactions. Still most people in North Carolina continued to walk the aisles of grocery stores which all stayed open during the 2020–2021 COVID-19 pandemic. There were no panicked assaults on groceries as the NC Ethics Task

Force imagined.[63] The worst thing that happened was an irrationally high purchase of toilet paper.

Because of federal and state public health requirements, restaurants were initially prohibited from any in-restaurant dining. Like the grocery stores described above, restaurants began to offer more in the way of pick-ups and deliveries. When NC restaurants were permitted to open their doors first at 25% capacity, then at 50%, and finally at 75% capacity, diners came, but the pick-ups and deliveries remained popular. Unfortunately, during the more restrictive stages of the COVID-19 lock down, many small restaurants were not able to survive on pickups and deliveries alone. They had to shut down, leaving their wait staff, cooks, and cleaners without jobs. As in the grocery industry, what most workers in the restaurant business seemed to fear was not so much contracting COVID-19 but being without employment.[64]

As we noted above, public health and healthcare personnel are regarded as critical workers and, as such, have at least a contractual obligation, if not also a professional obligation to keep on working despite risks to their health and, in extreme circumstances, to their lives. The residents of nursing homes are a particularly vulnerable group that cannot survive without caretakers. Many of them are over the age of 80 and unable to perform one or more Activities of Daily Living (ADL) like dressing, feeding, and toileting themselves. The more fortunate nursing home residents have loved ones who visit them regularly and help with their care, but in the 2020–2021 COVID-19 pandemic, visitations were curtailed or limited in one way or another.[65] Worse off are nursing home residents without any attentive family members or friends. They are especially dependent on nursing home staff for human interaction. I noted above, more often than not, nursing homes are understaffed. CNAs and other aides are stretched to the limit and the handful of RNs on staff have a hard time addressing the medical needs of the people entrusted to their care let alone their non-medical needs. Thus, according to the NC Ethics Task Force, it is especially important that every one working at a LTCF feels "as safe, compensated, and supported as possible."[66] This is a tall order, however, and not every NC nursing home was able to fill it during the early months of the COVID-19 pandemic, despite the fact that the federal government allocated $15 billion to the nursing home industry.[67] According to the AARP, in all too many cases, this money went to "administrative costs" or the pockets of owners of large, For-Profit (FP) LTCF-chains.[68] Relatively little of the government money went to increasing the salaries of the staff, especially the lowest-paid ones. Not every nursing home is like the Pebblebrooke Nursing Home described above. Sometimes negligence, greed or self-interest influence the way money is spent in a nursing home or other LTCF.

12.4 Balancing the Rights of the Individual and the Need to Protect the Public

According to the NC Ethics Task Force, in a crisis situation, public health officials along with government officials should "act to protect the overall health and well-being of the population."[69] To limit deaths and slow the progress of an influenza pandemic like COVID-19 public health officials may need to limit individuals' freedom by means of isolation, quarantining, or less restrictive social distancing measures like keeping six feet apart. Whereas isolation applies to those "who actively have a disease,"[70] quarantine applies to individuals who "may have had contact with an infected person and may be contagious to others."[71] Such persons may be required to stay at home or at a designated location.

Early on in a pandemic, isolation and quarantine is an effective way to control its spread. But as we noted above, without frequent testing of staff and residents, nursing-home administrators cannot really know who needs to be confined to quarters or banned from work for at least two weeks. A single asymptomatic resident or staff member can spread COVID-19 like wild fire. For example, at the Aston Park nursing home in Asheville, NC, the spread of COVID-19 began when one member of the staff came down with the disease in May 2020. Eleven days later, 55 staff members and residents tested positive for COVID-19. Of them, three residents and one staff member died.[72] Situations such as this one prompted federal, state, and local public health officials to issue very strict "no visitor" rules. In many instances, these rules prevented family members from helping out with their loved ones' physical and psychological needs. Well aware of inadequate staffing at many nursing homes, families often visit their parents or grandparents to make sure they are drinking and eating enough, given adequate palliative care, showered, and kept in clean diapers.[73] Although the majority of nursing homes deliver quality care to their residents, some do not. Mike Dark, staff attorney for California Advocates for Senior Care Reform, said that during the first-half of the COVID-19 pandemic, nursing home residents were "getting sicker and sicker behind closed doors,"[74] and he was constantly fielding phone calls from people worried sick about their loved ones.

Of all the tradeoffs between balancing the rights of the individual and the need to protect the general public or group, the "no-visitor" policy proved most onerous. Years ago my father had to go to a nursing home twice for extended periods of rehabilitation. I soon realized his liberty was being curtailed in all sorts of ways. He couldn't go to sleep and wake up as he pleased, get out of his pajamas or not depending on his mood, eat "unhealthy" meals every once in a while, and so forth. As understandable as these restrictions to my father's liberty were—afterall, a LTCF can't cater to everyone's idiosyncratic desires—, I couldn't stand seeing him growing depressed, and because I had the means, I found alternative care for him in his own home, his beloved "castle." Thus, my heart goes out to people who do not have the means to arrange adequate home care for their loved ones, as they watch them growing increasingly thin, unkempt, and unhappy through a window or plastic screen. Fortunately, many visitor restrictions in nursing homes and assisted living residences were relaxed in September 2020. The Centers for Medicare and Medicaid Services (CMS) clarified its "compassionate care" exception to the non-visitor rule. Provided adequate protective measures were taken, visitors could see a LTCF resident when he or she was dying, "struggling" to adjust to nursing home life, "grieving" after the recent death of a family member or friend, needing "help and encouragement with eating or drinking," or "seldom speaking, and crying frequently."[75]

Importantly, when public health officials emphasized that in order to curb the spread of COVID-19, all Americans should wear masks, practice social distancing, sanitize their hands avoid unnecessary trips, and shun large groups, "politics" caused significant numbers of Americans to ignore one, more, or all of these recommendations. In fact, many supporters of then President Donald Trump took it as a badge of honor to attend his very large re-election rallies unmasked and crowded together.[76] Moreover, whatever their political persuasion, Democrat or Republican, many Americans decided to travel considerable distances during the 2020 Thanksgiving and Christmas holidays.[77] Predictably, COVID-19 cases spiked after these holidays,[78] but apparently not highly enough for all segments of the US population to stay at home as much as possible.

As we shall see in the next section, worries about developing a priority system for anti-virals, COVID-19 tests, ventilators, ICU beds, and vaccines worried the NC Ethics Task Force. But what it did not expect was the number of healthcare workers who would refuse COVID-19 vaccinations. As of February 2021, 60% of nursing-home staff in Ohio said they had no plans to be vaccinated.[79] In Florida, at least two-thirds of the staff at one hospital refused the vaccine, prompting the hospital to "give away shots to the general public."[80] Dr. Anthony Fauci, President Biden's chief Medical Advisor for the COVID-19 pandemic, pleaded with front-like healthcare workers to get vaccinated. He said: "It's important to protect yourselves, to protect your family, but as important, symbolically, as healthcare providers, to show confidence in the vaccine so that other people in this country follow suit."[81] In addition, among the general public, minority groups, especially African-Americans, were hesitant about getting vaccinated. Well aware of tragic "treatment" programs for African-Americans like the 40-year long Tuskegee Syphilis Study, during which researchers continued to watch the "natural course" of syphilis in a group of Black men even after the discovery of penicillin which could have cured them, many Black people are waiting to see how the vaccine affects white people before they roll up their sleeves for "the shot."[82] This situation is particularly worrisome because COVID-19 has hit the African-American community and other racial and ethnic groups in a disproportional way.[83]

Although the CDC says the United States is on target to vaccinate enough people by the third quarter of 2021 for everyone to return to "regular" life,[84] its projections may be too optimistic. Indeed, there is evidence that among the general population, a sizable number of Americans don't want to be vaccinated.[85] Among these people are some healthcare workers in hospitals and nursing homes.[86] Even some patients in these establishments are hesitant to receive the COVID-19 vaccine. The question then becomes how to handle uncooperative staff members and residents of LTCFs. Should nursing home workers be fired or suspended if they refuse to be vaccinated? If so, who will replace them? Would a better approach be to frequently test staff for COVID-19 and make sure they all follow a strict hygienic regime? Chances are that LTCFs would opt for increased-testing programs over mandatory-vaccination programs. But what about the residents of LTCFs? Should they be forced to be vaccinated, or should they simply be persuaded that, in comparison to isolation, quarantining, daily COVID-19 tests, no-visitor rules, or dismissal from their "home," vaccination is the more attractive alternative? Seemingly, public health officials should follow the lead of the NC Ethics Task Force and develop guidelines to address these situations, especially if residents cannot give their informed consent to any of the options just mentioned. To be sure, family members may give consent to one or more of these options for their loved ones living with dementia, but such a strategy might further confuse some already confused residents.[87]

12.5 Prioritization and Use of Limited Resources During an Influenza Pandemic

During the early days of the COVID-19 outbreak in the United States there was a shortage of ventilators and ICU beds to treat serious cases of COVID-19. In addition to this, there was, as we noted above, a shortage of PPE, COVID-19 tests, anti-virals, and ICU beds. The ventilator crisis was eventually solved by states with few COVID-19 cases sending ventilators to states with many COVID-19 cases. The federal government also released ventilators from its stash of them, and the makers of ventilators doubled their efforts to manufacture as many ventilators as possible.[88] Soon, the ventilator crisis ended, as did the PPE, COVID-19 tests, anti-viral and ICU bed crises. And now, every effort is being made to manufacture and distribute vaccines as quickly as possible, especially to hospitals and LTCFs.[89] The general population as well as hospitals and LTCFs are breathing a sigh of relief. But the situation might have gone the other way. There could have been a shortage of all anti-COVID-19 tools. Back in 2007, the NC Ethics Task Force considered several ways to prioritize limited health care resources during the pandemic if this happened. They were as follows:

1. Priority should be given to assure the functioning of society; for example, workers in utilities, food distribution, communications, law enforcement, and so on.
2. Priority should be given to reduce the incidence or spread of the disease—for example, children, who, in an ordinary flu season, are generally the most likely to spread the disease, or those who are more likely to catch the disease or be at risk for influenza complications, or those subpopulations who have the best chance of surviving the disease, but only if they get the limited healthcare resources, as soon as possible.
3. Priority should be given to protect people with the most years of life ahead of them.

4. No groups should receive priority for the distribution of limited healthcare resources, in order to ensure that everyone has an equal chance of being protected. Individuals should be eligible for limited healthcare resources on a first-come, first-serve basis or through a lottery.
5. Priority should be given to those with the most *quality* of life years left (the life-cycle principle); that is, each person should have an opportunity to live through all stages of life, modified to give priority to 20-year-olds over 1-year-olds because the older individuals have more developed interests, hopes and plans but have not had the opportunity to realize them.[90]

Importantly, the NC Ethics Task Force stressed that decisions about the allocation of scarce healthcare resources should not be made on the basis of "race, color, religion, nationality, ethnicity, gender, age, disability, sexual orientation, geography, economic status, or insurance,"[91] a noble goal but one that is especially difficult to honor with respect to age. For example, when hospitals in some states learned that some nursing homes were using ventilators to keep 80-year-olds in a persistent vegetative state (PVS) or in a deep coma alive, they suggested that nursing home staff should remove these people from ventilator support and send the ventilators to hospitals able to use them for COVID-19 patients with a good chance of full recovery.[92] This suggestion was not welcomed by the families of nursing-home residents on ventilators, however. They viewed their loved ones' lives as worth preserving no matter what. Although many people would not want to go on "living" in a persistent vegetative state, some do.[93]

The NC Ethics Task Force emphasized that depending on the healthcare resource under consideration—PPE, tests, anti-virals, ventilators, ICU beds, vaccinations, and so forth—one or more of the prioritizations considered above would emerge as the one(s) to follow. Although the NC Ethics Task Force stated that, ideally, "allocation guidelines should be developed at the state level in advance of a pandemic,"[94] it is difficult to do this without knowing what population(s) a given influenza pandemic might choose as its main target(s).

12.6 Conclusion

Because it has been 13 years since I co-chaired the NC Ethics Task Force, my memory of its deliberations is probably faulty. But I do remember that the NC Ethics Task Force was strongly in favor of prioritizing front-line health care personnel and other critical workers for most if not all the healthcare resource allocations discussed above. There was also strong support for prioritizing the young over the old with the caveat that such prioritizing should be reconsidered if an influenza pandemic targeted the old as opposed to the young, which turned out to be the case in COVID-19. Still, I remember several members of the NC Ethics Task Force speaking passionately about their willingness to die so that their children and/or grandchildren could live. Moreover, I remember thinking how important public health measures are for securing and maintaining society's well being. Public health should not be viewed as the "step child" of the healthcare system. Because of dramatic achievements in curative medicine, it is easy enough to overlook the value of preventative medicine. But if the COVID-19 pandemic has taught us anything, it is the importance of a strong public health system in which federal, state, and local government officials work together. Far fewer COVID-19 cases and deaths would have occurred in the United States had clearer guidelines, recommendations, and mandatory rules been issued from the get go.[95] But as mentioned above, "politics" was pitted against "science" with respect to even the most basic public health measures—wearing a mask, practicing social distancing, hand washing, and avoiding large group activities, especially in poorly ventilated spaces. This mistake is one not to make again.

With respect to people's health worldwide, nationwide, and statewide, science, not politics is the best authority. But just as important is an ethics informed by both justice and care. Here I wish to quote from Leah Devlin's and my preface to *Stockpiling Solutions*.

> As important as an ethics of justice will be during an influenza pandemic, even more important will be an ethics of care. Under dire circumstances, the value of the common good must be weighed more heavily than the value of respecting individual rights and personal autonomy. During a pandemic, rationing can help us maintain the value of justice, provided it is done ethically –that is, by directing scarce resources to where they will do the most good for us all and by letting everyone know why it is we have chosen a particular distribution method. It is the ethics of caring that will see us through this crisis.
>
> In the end, we human beings are a very vulnerable lot. We are radically dependent on each other for survival, and we need to view ourselves as passengers in a lifeboat in the middle of the ocean with no visible sign to rescue. If there aren't enough supplies to go around until help arrives, we can do several things: we can ask for volunteers to jump off the boat; we can start drawing straws for who gets pushed off the boat; we can have a majority vote about which lives are most dispensable; or we can look in each other's eyes and see ourselves – fearful, hopeful, and in need of compassion – and then we can start paddling together to get to shore, knowing that although we might not all make it, we didn't turn on each other in our panic. What we most need to weather a pandemic is an ethics of trust, reciprocity, and solidarity. If we have that, we will have the most precious health care resource of all.[96]

These two paragraphs made sense to me in 2007 during the avian flu scare. Thirteen-years later, as we live through the COVID-19 pandemic, these same paragraphs make even more sense to me. Ethics, together with science, are our best defense against COVID-19 and any other pandemic that may follow it.

Notes

1. In 2007, Leah Devlin, DDS, MPH was the State Health Director, Division of Public Health, NC Department of Health and Human Services.
2. Henceforward referred to as the NC Ethics Task Force.
3. My department base was the Philosophy Department at UNCC.
4. University of Toronto, Joint Center for Bioethics, "Stand on Guard for Thee: Ethical Considerations for Pandemic Preparedness Planning," https://utoronto.ca.libroxy.lib.unc.edu/job/home/documents/pandemic.pdf.2005.
5. Population Reference Bureau (2019).

6. Meloa (2021).
7. Ameri Living, "Assisted Living Facts and Figures," www.ahcancal.org.Facts-and-Figures/2009.
8. North Carolina Institute of Medicine (2007).
9. Ibid.
10. Ibid.
11. Ibid.
12. Michael Boylan, "The Context and Foundations of Ethical Public Health Policy".
13. Ibid., 9.
14. Ibid., 11–12.
15. Ibid., 11–13.
16. Ibid.
17. Department of Health (2011).
18. Goldfinger (2020).
19. University of Toronto, Joint Center for Bioethics. "Stand on Guard for Thee".
20. Branswell (2019).
21. World Health Organization. "Current WHO Phase of Pandemic Alert," https://www.who.int.libproxy.lib.unc.edu/car/disease/avian_influenza/phase/en/index.html.
22. MNT News, "COVID-19 Live Updates: Total Number of Cases Pass 110 Million," *Medical News Today*, February 19, 2021, www.medicalnewstoday.com-articles-live-updates-c.
23. Center for Disease Control and Prevention (2021).
24. Ibid.
25. Kim (2021).
26. Harrar et al. (2021).
27. Blythe (2021).
28. Ibid.
29. CNBC.com staff (2021).
30. Ibid.
31. North Carolina Institute of Medicine (2007, 27).
32. Ibid., 33.
33. Cited in ibid.
34. Cited in ibid.
35. Paul P. Murphy, "They Were Placed on Leave for Refusing to Work Without N95 Masks. COVID-19 Unit Nurses Are Now Back to Work," *CNN*, April 23, 2020, www.cnn.com-california-coronavirus-nurses-return-trnd.
36. North Carolina Institute of Medicine (2007, 30).
37. McCausland (2020).
38. Harrar et al. (2021, 36).
39. Kinder (2020).
40. Ibid.
41. Zellman et al. (2019, 919–926).
42. Chen et al. (2021).

43. Ibid.
44. Kim (2021, 4).
45. Kinder (2020).
46. Ibid.
47. Meyer (2020, 28).
48. Ibid.
49. Ibid.
50. Ibid.
51. Chen et al. (2021).
52. Hoffman et al. (2020).
53. Rav et al. (2020).
54. Ibid.
55. Alzheimer's Association, "Coronavirus (COVID-19): Tips for Dementia Caregivers in Long-Term or Community-Based Settings," www.alz.org-professionals-professional-providers. Accessed February 14, 2021.
56. Ibid.
57. Schroeder (2020).
58. Ravitz (2021, 27).
59. Ibid.
60. North Carolina Institute of Medicine (2007, 35),
61. Ibid., 37.
62. Ibid.
63. Ibid.
64. Nunley (2021).
65. Kennerly (2020).
66. North Carolina Institute of Medicine (2007, 37).
67. Joseph G. Ouslander and David C. Grabowski, "COVID-19 in Nursing Homes: Calming the Perfect Storm," *Journal of the American Geriatrics Society* (July 31, 2020), https://doi.org/10.1111/jgs.16784.
68. Ibid.
69. North Carolina Institute of Medicine (2007, 37).
70. Ibid.
71. Ibid.
72. Kestin (2020).
73. MacLellan (2020).
74. Ibid.
75. Riechmann (2020).
76. Lush (2020).
77. Bose (2021).
78. Ibid.
79. Wernau (2021, A.7).
80. Ibid.
81. Cited in Ibid.
82. Kleindl (2021).
83. Center for Disease Control and Prevention (2021).

84. Lovelace and Diggins (2020).
85. Kaplan (2020).
86. Wernau (2021).
87. Ouslander (2020).
88. Ibid.
89. Staff writer, "Feds Unveil Plan to Get COVID-19 Shots to Nursing Homes" (2020).
90. North Carolina Institute of Medicine (2007, 49–50).
91. Ibid.
92. Faryon (2020).
93. Ibid.
94. North Carolina Institute of Medicine (2007, 51).
95. Jeneen Interlandi, "Why We're Losing the Battle with COVID-19," *The New York Times Magazine,* July 31, 2020, 30–39, 51, 53.
96. North Carolina Institute of Medicine (2007).

References

Alzheimer's Association. "Coronavirus (COVID-19): Tips for Dementia Care Professionals." www.alz.org-professionals-professional-provides. Accessed February 20, 2021.

American Health Care Association, National Center for Assisted Living. "Assisted Living—Facts and Figures." www.ahcancal.org.Facts-and-Figures/2009.

Blythe, Anne. 2021. "Even as Vaccine Distribution Begins, North Carolina's Top Public Health Official is the 'Most Wanted' She's Been Since the Start of the Pandemic." January 8, 2021. https://www.northcarolinahealthnews.org/2021/01/08/coronavirus-today_lizations-more-vaccine-plan-details-uncch-delays-in-person-olasses/.

Bose, Devna. 2021. "Holiday Travel Led to Worsening Coronavirus Caseload in Charlotte Here's What to Know. *The Charlotte Observer*, January 23, 2021. www.charlotteobserver.com-news-article-24843834.

Boylan, Michael. "The Context and Foundations of Ethical Public Health Policy."

Branswell, Helen. 2019, February 13. "What Happened to Bird Flu: How a Major Threat to Human Health Faded from View." *STAT* (February 13, 2019). www.statnews.com-bird-flu-mutations-outlook.

Center for Disease Control and Prevention. 2021. "Health Equity Considerations and Racial and Ethnic Groups." February 12, 2021. www.edu.gov-health-equity-race-ethnicity

Chen, Keith M., Judith A. Chevalier, and Elisa F. Long. 2021. "Nursing Home Staff Networks and COVID-19." *PNAS* (January 5, 2021). https://www.pnas.org/content/118/1/e2015455118. Accessed February 9, 2021.

CNBC.com staff. 2021. "COVID Updates: WHO Warns of Second Wave in Africa, U.S. Confirms Cases with New South African Strain." January 29, 2021. https://www.cnbc.com/2021/01/28/covid-live-updates-html.

Department of Health. 2011. "Severe Acute Respiratory Syndrome (SARS)." (October 2011). www.health.ny.gov/diseases/communicable/sars/.

Faryon, Joanne. 2020. "Nursing Homes Have Thousands of Ventilators that Hospitals Desperately Need." April 7, 2020. https://www.usnews.com/news/healthiest-communities/articles/2020-04-...nursing-homes-have-ventilators-posing-ethical-coronavirus-questions.

"Feds Unveil Plan to Get COVID-19 Shots to Nursing Homes." 2020. *Williamsport Sun-Gazette*, October 20, 2020. https://www.sungazette.com/news/2020/10/feds-unveil-plan-to-get-covid-19-shots-to-nursing-homes.

Goldfinger, Daina. 2020. "Looking Back: Toronto's 2003 SARS Outbreak." *Global News*, January 25, 2020.

Harrar, Sari, Joe Eaton, and Harris Meyer. 2021. "The Path Forward." *AARP Bulletin* 62, no. 1 (January/February 2021): 32–36.

Hoffman, Jacqueline B., Myla R. Reizer, and Adam S. Cooper. 2020, March 26. "COVID-19: Updated Nursing and Long-Term Care Facilities—Coronavirus (COVID-19) Considerations." *U.S. Health Care Alert*. https://www.klgates.com/COVID-19-Nursing-and-Long-Term-Care-Facilities-Coronavirus-COVID-19-Considerations-03-26-2020.

Kaplan, Karen. 2020. "As COVID-19 Vaccines Come Online, Fewer Americans Want to Take Them." *Los Angeles Times*, December 31, 2020.

Kennerly, Britt. "2020. COVID-19 Lockdowns Remind Those with Family at Care Facilities: We Miss That Human Touch." *Florida Today*, June 8, 2020.

Kestin, Sally. 2020. "COVID-19 Ravages Aston Park Nursing Home: Half of Patients Infected, 4 Deaths in 11 Days." *Citizen Times*, May 22, 2020.

Kim, E. Tammy. "Full Isolation." *The New York Times*, January 3, 2021: 4–5.

Kinder, Molly. 2020. "Essential But Undervalued: Millions of Health Care Workers Aren't Getting the Pay or Respect They Deserve in the COVID-19 Pandemic." *Brookings*. May 2020. www.brookings.edu-research-essential-but-underval...:

Kleindl, Jena. 2021. "Why Many Black Americans Are Fearful of the COVID-19 Vaccine." January 21, 2021. www.wrex.com-2021/01/21-why-many-black-americans...:

Lovelace, Beverly, and Noah Diggins. 2020. "CDC Says U.S. Should Have Enough Coronavirus Vaccine to Return to 'Regular Life' by Third Quarter of 2021." *CNBC*. September 18, 2020. www.cnbc.com-2020/09/16-coronavirus-cdc-v.

Lush, Tamara. 2020. "'Mom's Worth It': Why Americans are Traveling Despite Health Officials' Advice." *USA Today*, December 23, 2020. www.usatoday.com-story-travel-news-2020/12/23.

MacLellan, Lila. 2020. "Banning Family at Senior Care Homes Has Removed a Layer of Protection and Care." *Quartz*, April 29, 2020. https://qz.com/1845402/banning-family-at-senior-care-homes-has-removed-critical-care/.

McCausland, Phil. 2020. "Health Care Workers Have Sacrificed Their Lives Fighting COVID. It's Unclear How Many Have Died." *NBC News*, December 23, 2020. www.nbcnews.com-news-us-news-health-care-wor.

Meloa, Andrew. 2021. "The Aging US Population Is Creating Many Problems—Especially Regarding Elderly Healthcare Issues." *Insider*. (January 19, 2021).

Meyer, Harris. 2020, December. "A Failing Business Model." *AARP Bulletin* 61 (10): 26–28.

"North Carolina Coronavirus Map and Case Count." *The New York Times*, February 1, 2021. https://www.nytimes.com/interactive/2020/us/north-carolina-coronavirus-cases-html.

North Carolina Institute of Medicine. 2007. *Stockpiling Solutions: North Carolina's Ethical Guidelines for an Influenza Pandemic*, April 2007: 1–94.

Nunley, Christian. 2021. "State Legislatures Making Push to Limit Governors' Pandemic Response Ability." *CNBC*, January 28, 2021. https://www.cnbc.com/2021/28/covid-live-updates.html.

Ouslander, Joseph G. 2020. "COVID-19 in Nursing Homes: Calming the Perfect Storm." *Journal of the American Geriatrics Society*, July 31, 2020. https://onlinelibrary.wiley.com/doi/full/10.1111/jgs.16784.

Population Reference Bureau. 2019. "Fact Sheet: Aging in the United States." *Population Bulletin*, June 15, 2019. www.prb.org-aging-unitedstates-fact-sheet.

Rav, Jordan, Lauren Weber, and Rachans Pradham. 2020. "Nursing Homes Still See Dangerously Long Waits for COVID Test Results." November 12, 2020. https://hhn.org/news/article/nursing-homes-still-see-dangerously-long-waits-for-covid-test-results/.

Ravitz, Jessica. 2021, January/February. "A Tale of Two Nursing Homes." *AARP Bulletin* 62 (1): 27–32.

Riechmann, Deb. 2020. "As Virus Surges, Trump Rallies Keep Packing in Thousands." *AP News*, October 29, 2020. www.apnews.com-article-donald-trump-rallies-virus-surge.

Schiller, Meghan. "Firefighters and Nursing Homes Fighting to Get COVID-19 Vaccine First." *CBS Pittsburg*. https://pittsburg-chslocal.com/2020/11/30/fighting-for-priority-covid-19-vaccine/.

Schroeder, Kaitlin R. 2020. "Nursing Homes Battling Worker Turnover During Pandemic: What That Means." *Dayton Daily News*, September 15, 2020. www.daytondailynews.com-news-nursing-home-wo.

University of Toronto, Joint Center for Bioethics. "Standing Guard for Thee: Ethical Considerations for Pandemic Preparedness Planning." https://www.utoronto.ca.libroxy.lib.unc.edu/job/home/documents/pandemic.pdf.2005.

Wernau, Julie. 2021, February 1. "Some Health Workers Shun Vaccines." *The Wall Street Journal* A 7.

Zellman, Leah et al. 2019, June. "Care of America's Elderly and Disabled People Relies on Immigrant Labor." *Health Affairs* 38 (6): 919–26.

Zimmerman, Mike. "How to Beat COVID This Year." *AARP Bulletin* 62 (1) (January/February): 10–16.

Chapter 13
The UN System, COVID-19 Responses, and Building Back Better: Toward an Inclusive, Accessible and Sustainable World

Akiko Ito

Abstract At the time of the great disruption for the world due to the COVID-19 crisis, the situation of those with vulnerabilities, including women, persons with disabilities and other disadvantaged groups, is compounded by an unprecedented global health crisis with severe economic and social impacts. The international community, including Governments, the UN system, health communities and numerous networks of professional and experts across the disciplines and civil society worldwide, is addressing the situation of those with vulnerabilities to leave no one behind in their response to the COVID-19 crisis. In this context, the COVID-19 resource of the UN system has been developed for policy guidance, guidelines and tools for action by the Governments and other stakeholders to be inclusive and accessible for persons with disabilities and those who are marginalized with vulnerabilities, including women with disabilities.

Keywords Covid-19 crisis and disability · The SDGs and leaving no one behind · Women with disabilities · UN system and Covid-19

The COVID-19 pandemic has disrupted systems and societies globally. The unprecedented health crisis and its economic and social impacts have exacerbated the situation of those with vulnerabilities, including women, persons with disabilities, and other disadvantaged groups. This is particularly true for those who experience intersecting forms of discrimination, such as women and girls with disabilities, those with invisible or psychosocial disabilities, migrants, refugees, and racial and other minorities.[1]

The international community—Governments, the UN system, and health and expert networks across disciplines and civil society—has been tackling varying phases and situations of the impact of the pandemic on communities around the world, addressing "leaving no one behind" in its response to—and building back better from—the COVID-19 crisis. The topics of such initiatives range from conducting

A. Ito (✉)
New York, NY, USA
e-mail: ito@un.org
URL: https://www.un.org/en/coronavirus/UN-response

© The Author(s), under exclusive license to Springer Nature Switzerland AG 2022
M. Boylan (ed.), *Ethical Public Health Policy Within Pandemics*, The International Library of Bioethics 95, https://doi.org/10.1007/978-3-030-99692-5_12

socioeconomic impact assessments; combatting discrimination and its intersecting forms—including gender-based violence; improving access to and accessibility of health care and essential services and resources—including mental health and sexual and reproductive health care and accessible communication technologies; expanding social protection and income security; supporting those engaged in unpaid care and domestic work; and ensuring legal protection for all.[2]

To address the outsized impact of COVID-19 on persons with disabilities, the UN system mobilized through its various entities and their respective mandates. Its Inter-Agency Support Group on the Convention on the Rights of Persons with Disabilities (IASG-CRPD) and the UN Partnership on the Rights of Persons with Disabilities (UNPRPD)[3] undertook a series of consultations with Member States, expert communities, civil society, and other partners, in particular, with organizations of persons with disabilities. The results of this collaboration are summarized in the UN system's resource on COVID-19 and disability inclusion,[4] which includes policy guidance, guidelines, and tools for action by governments and other stakeholders to ensure that their crisis responses are inclusive of and accessible for persons with disabilities and other groups with vulnerabilities.

This resource is available and will be updated via the UN Enable gateway on COVID-19 and disability inclusion in coming months. A collaborative effort within the UN system and with its partners is underway to consolidate information and analyses on the subject from different sources and perspectives. The data, assessments, good practices, and reporting on steps taken to include persons with disabilities in the recovery and building back better processes are needed to support stakeholders to both comprehensively understand the situation of persons with disabilities and to develop effective policies, programmes, and plans of action. The gateway also includes a map of wheelchair-accessible COVID-19 testing sites worldwide, which is also available on Wheelmap.org.

Additionally, as a result of impact assessments of the COVID-19 crisis on persons with disabilities in humanitarian emergencies, recommendations have been developed for current and future disaster response initiatives to be inclusive of persons with disabilities.[5] These include a Guidance Note on the COVID-19 Crisis and the Rights of Persons with Disabilities,[6] a checklist for monitoring the rights of persons with disabilities in response and recovery,[7] with a view to collecting case studies on good practices for monitoring the human rights of persons with disabilities during the immediate response phase, recovery and building back better.

Further work by the UN system is underway to synthesize the most up-to-date information on the areas of life for persons with disabilities most impacted by COVID-19, such as education, employment, and health care. It will feature analyses informed by members of the international disability community, especially organizations of persons with disabilities, as well as a set of practical recommendations for stakeholders to better enhance, inform, and implement disability-inclusive recovery and building back better toward an inclusive, accessible and sustainable world, in line with the Convention on the Rights of Persons with Disabilities (CRPD) and the 2030 Agenda for Sustainable Development.

13.1 The Situation of Persons with Disabilities and Leaving no One Behind

The COVID-19 crisis has exposed the extent of the marginalization and inequalities faced by persons with disabilities. It heightened existing barriers to accessing necessities and raised new ones against the inclusion of persons with disabilities in responses to the COVID-19 crisis. Before the pandemic, persons with disabilities experienced poorer health outcomes, higher rates of poverty and un- and underemployment, and less access to education, the Internet, and information and communications technology (ICT) than those without disabilities. They were often prevented from living independently and faced exclusion from their communities, and they had difficulty accessing social services and important information due to inaccessibility or inadequate outreach from governments and other authorities. The COVID-19 crisis has worsened health outcomes for persons with disabilities due to higher risk of infection and discrimination in the provision of care; poverty and unemployment have worsened due to persons with disabilities' increased vulnerability to economic recession; furthermore, education has become less available and less accessible due to inaccessible distance learning platforms, a greater lack of Internet and ICT access among persons with disabilities to engage in distance learning, and the unavailability of key in-school support services, such as sign language translation. Moreover, lockdown and social distancing measures have deepened isolation and prevented many persons with disabilities from receiving community support, and COVID-19 response programmes and health information have often not been inclusive of or accessible for persons with disabilities.

The risk of infection from COVID-19 for persons with disabilities is often compounded by many other factors, which warrant targeted action. These include the disruption of essential services and support; a lack of accessible health information and exclusion from mainstream health provision; larger gaps in accessibility to essential resources and services; in some cases, pre-existing health conditions[8] that increase the severity of risk; and being more likely to live in institutional settings—psychiatric institutions, social institutions (orphanages, day care centres, rehabilitation centres), prisons, and institutions for older persons—in which transmission rates are higher and health outcomes are significantly less favourable.

For example, women and girls with disabilities are at further risk. Women with disabilities are three times more likely to have unmet needs for health care than women without disabilities. This is partly due to a lack of access to health information, as they are also three times more likely to be illiterate and two times less likely to use the Internet.[9] Moreover, women with disabilities are at heightened risk of suffering sexual violence,[10] which was exacerbated under COVID-19 lockdown measures.

In general, persons with disabilities tend to have more health care-related needs than persons without disabilities—both standard needs and needs linked to their impairments. Therefore, they are more vulnerable to disruptions in health care services than those without disabilities. Health emergencies and their recovery phases place pressure on national health services. When systems are stressed and resources are scarce, it is particularly important that national authorities establish non-discriminatory ethical medical guidelines. Health care authorities must put in place measures to reduce the risk of infection for persons with disabilities and their families and care-givers—while still upholding their dignity and autonomy—and to ensure that policies and practices on medical treatments—including triage decision-making and access to testing and vaccinations—do not discriminate based on age, gender, ethnicity, disability, or any other demographic factor. The World Health Organization (WHO) has issued disability-inclusive guidelines in line with international human rights conventions to address some urgent issues with regard to access and non-discrimination, which are directly applicable to ensuring the inclusion of persons with disabilities in the processes of immediate response and building back better in the COVID-19-impacted world.[11] Additionally, as part of the WHO's work with the UNPRPD, a number of initiatives have been taken through different tools and media, including through webinars on disability-inclusive strategic preparedness and response plants, disability-inclusive telehealth, and strengthening and expanding the availability of quality rehabilitation services during the recovery phase.[12]

Furthermore, health personnel, including in emergency response services, require further training to be able to meet the needs of persons with disabilities during any crisis and to include these needs from the planning stages of such services.[13] Other key recommendations include ensuring priority testing for symptomatic persons with disabilities; promoting research on the impact of COVID-19 on the health of persons with disabilities; identifying and removing barriers to treatment, including ensuring accessible environments (hospitals, testing, and containment centres) and the availability and dissemination of health information and communications in accessible means and formats; ensuring the provision of and continued access to medicines for persons with disabilities during the pandemic; and conducting training and awareness-raising activities for health-care workers to prevent discrimination based on prejudices and positions taken against persons with disabilities.

Accessible information is essential for persons with disabilities to protect themselves against infection and help them find care if they do become infected. Awareness-raising and risk communication strategies need to be specifically targeted to higher risk groups, including women and girls living in precarious conditions. Community-based and locally adaptive approaches to transfer information can be useful to reach persons with disabilities who have limited access to technology. Stakeholders engaged in prevention and recovery, including health care workers, education providers, disability service providers, and protection officers, among others, need to receive guidance and have access to resources that enable them to provide alternative formats and methods of communications, such as easy-to-read documents, braille, subtitling, and sign language. Further, information must be age-appropriate to facilitate the understanding of key information[14] by children.

To support disability-inclusive recovery, more data disaggregated by disability, gender, age, and other demographic factors are required. These are necessary for evidence-based impact assessments and to facilitate targeted and mainstreamed policies for persons with disabilities, including for women and girls with disabilities.

For accelerating evidence-based policy development, the UN system collaborated on an extensive series of policy briefs for disability-inclusive response and recovery. These focused on key issues around the inclusive realization of the Sustainable Development Goals (SDGs), such as disability-inclusive humanitarian emergency responses and social protection, aiming at building back better toward the implementation of the 2030 Agenda toward an inclusive, accessible, and sustainable world. The collaborative research of the UN system contributed to the policy brief of the Secretary-General of the United Nations, "A Disability-Inclusive Response to COVID-19".[15]

Poverty is a major barrier to accessing health care and other essential services. The proportion of persons with disabilities living in poverty is double the proportion of persons without disabilities in some countries, with the challenges compounded further for women and girls. However, countries that have built social protection systems and have age-, sex-, and disability-disaggregated census data and registry-based data are better able to provide universal allowance and support services for a fast and targeted relief. Social protection systems should also account for the fact that persons with disabilities are more likely to work in the informal sector—which often bars access to employment-based social security—and persons with disabilities who are employed or self-employed may not be able to work at home due to the lack of equipment and assistance normally available in the workplace. Further, persons with psychosocial disabilities and autism may require extra support due to the disproportionate stress they experience due to lockdown measures and disruptions in routine. To support these initiatives, UN system entities, individually and collectively, have created a series of webinars to adapt the good practices in disability-inclusive social protection responses to COVID-19 to different regional contexts.

Furthermore, persons with disabilities and their families require access to the same – or a greater – level of care and support during emergency situations to continue living independently. Governments and education providers must ensure that distance-learning platforms are accessible for children and other learners with disabilities, including those with developmental or intellectual disabilities or autism. The same applies to remote work, for which employer support should be disability-inclusive and gender-sensitive, such as reasonable accommodation at home and access to adapted and accessible materials. The International Labour Organization (ILO) Global Business and Disability Network, a consortium of business, non-profit, and disability organizations led by the ILO, has been developing accessibility guidelines, promoting reasonable accommodations for remote workers with disabilities and further Internet access for persons with disabilities to facilitate remote work and education.

Based on available information and resources, recommendations include ensuring legal protection of persons with disabilities and training of public officials and private agencies on the subject; prioritizing screening and promoting preventive measures in institutions to reduce the risk of infection, including by addressing overcrowding, implementing physical separation of residents, changing visiting hours, mandating the use of protective equipment, and improving hygiene conditions—all of which require that greater human and financial resources be dedicated to these institutions; ensuring that reporting mechanisms, hotlines, emergency shelters, and other forms of assistance are accessible to and inclusive of persons with disabilities; and monitoring the situation of persons with disabilities, especially those who are isolated, through upstream awareness raising, including through community and voluntary networks.

Overall, close and active involvement of persons with disabilities and their representative organizations in the development of a rights-based response to the pandemic—one that considers persons with disabilities in all their diversity – is crucial to building back better toward the realization of the SDGs. Organizations of persons with disabilities, women's organizations, and community-based groups of women and women with disabilities serve as indispensable agents and partners to local and national authorities, both in terms of consultation for policy and programme development and community outreach.

To elevate UN collaboration with persons with disabilities and their representative organizations, the UN system further advanced its research and good practices to promote the participation of persons with disabilities and their representative organizations in decision-making processes. An expert group meeting was recently organized by the UN Department of Economic and Social Affairs, from 3–6 August 2021, on "The participation and leadership of persons with disabilities in building a disability-inclusive, accessible, and sustainable post-COVID-19 world,"[16] which resulted in a set of recommendations to advance the meaningful participation of persons with disabilities in planning, implementing, and monitoring COVID-19 responses. Key networks were further strengthened and expanded through the 13th and 14th sessions of the Conference of States Parties to the Convention on the Rights of Disabilities,[17] whose respective themes were "A decade of action and delivery for inclusive sustainable development: implementing the CRPD and the 2030 Agenda for all persons with disabilities" and "Building back better: COVID-19 response and recovery; meeting the needs, realizing the rights, and addressing the socio-economic impacts on persons with disabilities," which brought together governments, UN entities, civil society, and expert communities around a shared goal. These multi-stakeholder coalitions took stock of issues, lessons learned, and good practices in achieving COVID-19 response and recovery that is both disability-inclusive and works toward achieving the SDGs by 2030—with persons with disabilities and their representative organizations at the forefront. Furthermore, the 2020 International Day of Persons with Disabilities, with the theme "Building Back Better: toward a disability-inclusive, accessible and sustainable post COVID-19 World", facilitated policy discourse, resource planning, and network-building between disability inclusion focal points from key UN entities and civil society.[18]

13.2 Building Back Better

The current recovery process is rife with opportunities to set new standards and norms, forge partnerships and strengthen institutions to build resilience against the devastating impact of the pandemic and other, future, crisis situations. The recovery and building back processes should inspire solidarity, flexibility, and motivation, thus, shaping the post-COVID-19 world in line with the CRPD and the 2030 Agenda for Sustainable Development.

One of the key cross-cutting principles of the SDGs is to leave no one behind. In the current phase of the COVID-19 recovery and building back better, the agency and leadership of persons with disabilities is not being secured. In fact, they are frequently "absent" in response and recovery measures and processes. But, to create a disability-inclusive, accessible and sustainable post-COVID-19 world – one in which no one is left behind – at least two shifts in approach are necessary: the rights, perspectives and well-being of persons with disabilities should be reflected in each step of the recovery process, and their capacity as leaders and agents of change should be strengthened. This should be the case especially for those who are furthest left behind, such as women and girls with disabilities.

Creating a more inclusive, accessible, and sustainable post-COVID-19 world requires more inclusive and resilient societies across borders, sectors, and generations. Current responses at every level are fundamental to the rights and well-being of women and girls and of persons with disabilities, and they will determine how soon the world can recover from this crisis and whether the SDGs can still be achieved by 2030. In applying the cross-cutting principle emanating from disability-inclusive disaster reduction: "building back better"[19] to COVID-19 recovery and building back better, it is a common aspiration of the international community, at this time in human history, that the world should emerge stronger and better equipped to build an inclusive and sustainable future for all—with persons with disabilities and others with vulnerabilities at the forefront, as agents and beneficiaries of building back for a better tomorrow.

Notes

1. UN Enable Resource on the COVID-19 crisis (https://www.un.org/development/desa/disabilities/covid-19.html).
2. Ibid.
3. UNPRPD, UN joint programme to support countries' design and implement disability inclusive response and recovery planning for COVID-19 (https://unprpd.org/our-programmes/160).
4. Ibid.
5. OHCHR, OHCHR and the rights of persons with disabilities (https://www.ohchr.org/en/issues/disability/pages/disabilityindex.aspx).
6. OHCHR, COVID-19 and the Rights of Persons with Disabilities: Guidance (https://www.ohchr.org/Documents/Issues/Disability/COVID-19_and_The_Rights_of_Persons_with_Disabilities.pdf).
7. Inter-Agency Working Group on Disability Inclusive COVID-19 Response and Recovery, Checklist for Planning a Disability Inclusive COVID-19 Socio-Economic Response and Recovery (https://www.un.org/sites/un2.un.org/files/disability-inclusion_checklist_socio-economic_response_july_2020.pdf).

8. UN Flagship Report on Disability and the Sustainable Development Goals (UNDESA 2018) (https://www.un.org/development/desa/disabilities/publication-disability-sdgs.html).
9. Ibid.
10. Ibid.
11. Disability considerations during the COVID-19 outbreak (https://www.who.int/who-documents-detail/disability-considerations-during-the-covid-19-outbreak).
12. https://unprpd.org/covid-19.
13. Voices of persons with disabilities during the COVID-19 outbreak (http://www.internationaldisabilityalliance.org/content/voices-persons-disabilities-during-covid19-outbreak).
14. https://www.un.org/development/desa/disabilities/covid-19.html.
15. Policy Brief: A Disability-Inclusive Response to COVID-19 (https://www.un.org/sites/un2.un.org/files/sg_policy_brief_on_persons_with_disabilities_final.pdf).
16. UN Enable, EGM on Building a Disability-Inclusive, Accessible and Sustainable post-COVID-19 World (https://www.un.org/development/desa/disabilities/egm-disability-inclusive-postcovid19.html).
17. UN Enable, Conference of States Parties to the Convention on the Rights of Persons with Disabilities (https://www.un.org/development/desa/disabilities/conference-of-states-parties-to-the-convention-on-the-rights-of-persons-with-disabilities-2.html).
18. UN Enable, International Day of Persons with Disabilities – 3 December (https://www.un.org/development/desa/disabilities/international-day-of-persons-with-disabilities-3-december.html).
19. The Sendai Framework for Disaster Risk Reduction 2015–2030 at the Third UN World Conference in Sendai, Japan, (March 2015).

Correction to: Ethical Public Health Policy Within Pandemics

Michael Boylan

Correction to:
M. Boylan (ed.), *Ethical Public Health Policy Within Pandemics*, The International Library of Bioethics 95, https://doi.org/10.1007/978-3-030-99692-5

In the original version of the book, the following corrections have been incorporated: In Chapter 8, comma has been removed after the word Fraud in the chapter title. The title has been corrected to "Principlist Pandemics: On Fraud Ethical Guidelines, and the Importance of Procedural Transparency". In Chapter 9, The author's name "Graf Keyserlingk Johannes" has been changed to "Johannes Graf Keyserlingk". The correction chapters have been updated with the changes.

The updated version of these chapters can be found at
https://doi.org/10.1007/978-3-030-99692-5_7
https://doi.org/10.1007/978-3-030-99692-5_8

© The Author(s), under exclusive license to Springer Nature Switzerland AG 2022
M. Boylan (ed.), *Ethical Public Health Policy Within Pandemics*, The International Library of Bioethics 95, https://doi.org/10.1007/978-3-030-99692-5_14

Index

A
American Medical Association (AMA), 6, 120, 123, 124, 127
Antonine Plague, 14
Axiology, 83, 84, 86, 87, 89

C
Common good, 45–56, 225, 231
Coronavirus, 45, 46, 53, 55, 63, 64, 82, 105, 121, 167, 168, 173, 186, 187, 199
COVID-19, 13–15, 21, 31, 33, 43, 44, 46, 47, 52–58, 63–69, 71, 73, 74, 78, 82, 84–86, 88, 90, 91, 95, 96, 105–110, 119, 121, 122, 125, 132, 133, 135, 136, 140, 141, 144, 150, 158, 164, 167–171, 173, 177, 178, 182, 185, 186, 188, 195, 196, 198–200, 203, 208–210, 220–231, 237–244
Covid-19 crisis and disability, 238, 239
COVID-19 pandemic, 13, 14, 32, 44, 46, 52, 64, 65, 70–74, 105, 106, 109, 132, 136, 138, 140, 144, 159, 164, 170, 178, 180, 185, 189, 195–202, 204, 205, 220, 221, 223–228, 231, 237
Crisis Standards of Care (CSC), 168, 170, 178–184, 186, 187, 205, 207, 208
Critical industry workers' responsibilities in a pandemic, 220, 225
Critical race theory, 102

D
Decision theory, 66, 68, 69, 71, 72
Distributive justice, 11, 29, 30

Duty, 25, 28, 32, 50, 51, 120–129, 152, 199
Duty to treat, 121–128, 222

E
Ebola pandemic, 20
Equal opportunity, 29, 179, 181, 202, 205, 207, 208, 211, 212
Essential goods, 28, 168–173, 175, 179, 182, 186–188
Ethical grounds for public health policy, 14, 23
Ethical guidelines, 132, 135–137, 140, 142–144, 220, 223
Ethics expert, 141–143
Ethics of care, 224, 231
Ethics of justice, 231
External perspective, 153, 156

F
Fair process, 212
Formal epistemology, 65, 68, 71, 77

G
Goods allocation, 29, 31, 32, 168

H
Habermas, 87, 88
Health care workers' responsibilities in a pandemic, 120
Health equity, 200, 201, 214
HIV/AIDS pandemic, 14, 18, 22, 99, 100, 104, 221

I
Internal perspective, 150, 151, 153, 154, 156
Iteration, 87, 91, 92, 104, 137

L
Long-Term Care Facilities (LTCFs), 220–224, 226–229

M
Moral obligations, 51, 122, 125–127, 139, 154, 176, 201
Multicriteria analysis (MCA), 65, 68, 73, 74, 76, 77

N
National responsibility, 154
Necropolitics, 109, 110

O
Oaths, 122, 123

P
Pandemic ethics, 133, 136, 140, 142, 143, 202
Pandemic(s), 13–22, 29–33, 43–48, 50–57, 63–69, 71, 72, 74, 77, 82–84, 87–91, 95, 96, 99–110, 120–125, 127–129, 132, 136–138, 140, 141, 144, 149–159, 163, 168–171, 173, 175, 177–179, 181, 183, 184, 186, 187, 195–207, 211, 212, 220–222, 225, 227, 229–231, 237, 239, 240, 242, 243
Peirce, 85–87
Performative contradiction, 83, 87–92
Principlism, 132–136, 140–142, 144, 175, 177, 178, 181, 182
Prioritizing limited health care resources in a pandemic, 230
Professional responsibility, 120
Public health ethics, 22
Public trust, 151, 164

R
Race, 96–107, 109, 110, 180–183, 196–198, 201–212, 230
Racial and ethnic health disparities, 197–201, 203, 204, 206, 208, 211, 212
Racialization, 96, 98, 99, 106
Racial projects, 102, 104, 105, 108, 110
Racism, 17, 98, 99, 103, 106, 107, 109, 185, 199
Rawls, John, 46, 125, 175, 179, 189
Rights, 10, 11, 23, 25, 27, 28, 45–47, 49–53, 55–57, 121, 123, 128, 136–138, 141, 149–165, 175, 176, 179, 180, 182, 220, 227, 231, 238, 240, 242, 243
Rule of the plan, 158–160

S
SARS and MERS pandemic, 14, 65, 119, 122, 125
SARS-CoV-19, 13, 21, 34, 64, 106, 167, 203
The SDGs and leaving no one behind, 237
Severe Acute Respiratory Syndrome (SARS), 20, 21, 64, 125–129, 137, 199, 220, 221
Spanish Flu pandemic, 14, 35
Sweden, 43–45, 53–55, 58, 68, 70, 77

T
2007 North Carolina Ethics Task Force on public health measures during a pandemic, 219

U
UN system and Covid-19, 238, 241
Utility, 45, 47, 48, 53–56, 73, 74, 78, 102, 103, 137, 138, 141, 143, 174, 178, 181

W
Women with disabilities, 239, 242
World Health Organization (WHO), 20, 21, 32, 64, 95, 108, 111, 137, 138, 140, 143, 173, 177, 221, 222, 240